Epigenetic Therapy of Cancer

Michael Lübbert • Peter A. Jones
Editors

Epigenetic Therapy of Cancer

Preclinical Models and Treatment Approaches

Springer

Editors
Michael Lübbert
Department of Hematology/Oncology
University Medical Center Freiburg
University of Freiburg
Freiburg
Germany

Peter A. Jones
Department of Biochemistry
and Molecular Biology
Norris Comprehensive Cancer Center
University of Southern California
Los Angeles, CA
USA

ISBN 978-3-642-38403-5 ISBN 978-3-642-38404-2 (eBook)
DOI 10.1007/978-3-642-38404-2
Springer Heidelberg New York Dordrecht London

Library of Congress Control Number: 2013956547

Printed on acid-free paper

Springer is part of Springer Science+Business Media (www.springer.com)

Preface

The view that cancer is primarily a genetic disease has been dramatically challenged by the recent discoveries demonstrating that malignancies are marked by multiple epigenetic abnormalities; the resultant gene silencing may be more ubiquitous than gene inactivation by genetic events. This paradigm change was accompanied by enormous advances in high-throughput sequencing of primary human tumors, leading to the discovery of "driver" mutations in a plethora of genes encoding chromatin-modifying enzymes. Finally, the last few years also saw a striking expansion in the clinical development of drugs inhibiting several of these enzymes. Whereas in the past, a crucial role for DNA hypermethylation in cancer and thus its pharmacologic reversal as a therapeutic principle were not at all generally accepted, finally two DNA hypomethylating agents are now in routine use in the treatment of several myeloid malignancies, and more in clinical development. Also several histone deacetylase (HDAC) inhibitors have found a place in the standard treatment of two types of T-cell lymphoma, providing robust proof of principle for *in vivo* inhibition of histone-modifying enzymes as a valid therapeutic approach. In order to systematically review these parallel and interlocking developments which drive fruitful cross-talk between basic epigenetic research, drug development and clinical application in hematology/oncology, we put together the present series of articles authored by leading experts in the field of cancer research and epigenetics.

The initial chapters review, from different perspectives, the central role of epigenetic regulation in coordinate normal cell growth, differentiation and the control of stemness, and delineate the consequences of its disturbances for cellular transformation. Thus in the first chapter, Manuel Rodríguez-Paredes and Manel Esteller provide a comprehensive view of different chromatin modifications, the enzymes setting the histone and DNA modification "marks" and their regulation during these processes. In Chap. 2, Irina Savelyeva and Frank Rosenbauer give in-depth descriptions of the murine models employed for *in vivo* studies of the effects of altered levels of DNA methylation or histone modifications, particularly as they relate to the induction and propagation of malignancies. In Chap. 3, Chaurasia, Berenzon and Hoffman take a similar view, but from the perspective of the normal hematopoietic cell differentiation model system. Specifically, they also provide their results of successful expansion of the hematopoietic progenitor cell pool through DNA methyltransferase (DNMT) and HDAC inhibitors. Focusing on one particular hematopoietic cell lineage – the erythropoietic system – Saunthararajah, Lavelle and

DeSimone in Chap. 4 review the concert of epigenetic regulatory mechanisms governing one of the "classical" cell differentiation models of tissue- and development-specific gene expression, i.e. globin gene regulation during the different stages of erythropoiesis. They elegantly demonstrate that (despite the non-malignant features of hemoglobinopathies) the study of dysregulated globin genes continues to deepen our understanding of epigenetic aberrations as therapeutic targets in the hematopoietic system, aside from the therapeutic implications of epigenetics for these very frequent genetic disorders.

Next, the focus is on the pathophysiological role of epigenetic abnormalities in hematopoietic cancers, as exemplified by myeloid neoplasias, with particular focus on acute myeloid leukemia (AML). Claus, Schmutz, Greve and Bullinger in Chap. 5 provide a timely look to the role of gene-specific and global DNA methylation abnormalities in these malignant disorders, expanding also on the new methodological possibilities provided by high-throughput technology. In Chap. 6, Duque-Afonso, Lübbert and Cleary describe several distinct AML syndromes, each bearing a striking genotype/phenotype relationship defined by chromosomal translocations generating fusion genes, which in turn act as epigenetic modifiers. These fusion genes, resulting in the AML1/ETO and MLL-rearranged oncofusion proteins, not only have a causal role in mediating the abnormal epigenotype of the resultant leukemias, but their pharmacologic antagonization has increasingly important therapeutic implications. Chapters 7 and 8 provide a comprehensive overview on clinical applications of DNA hypomethylating agents (primarily azanucleoside drugs) to treat hematologic malignancies, as well as on the – far from resolved – *in vivo* mechanism of action of these drugs. Specifically, Daskalakis, Joeckel, Lübbert and Kuendgen review published and ongoing clinical trials of hypomethylating agents being tested in myelodysplastic syndromes (MDS), AML and other hematopoietic malignancies. Their chapter is complemented by that of Griffiths, Momparler and Karpf on the pharmacodynamic responses to these drugs. Here the often debated similarities and differences of the two clinically approved DNA hypomethylating drugs are in focus.

Not only the introduction of DNMT inhibitors has significantly expanded our armamentarium to treat hematopoietic cancers, also cancer-associated histone modifications can be reversed by inhibition of the enzymes mediating them. Chapters 9 and 10 are devoted to drug development and clinical applications for inhibitor drugs of histone methyltransferases (as comprehensively reviewed by Richard Chesworth and colleagues), and of HDACs (with a timely update on clinical trials with HDAC inhibitors provided by Kristina Keller and Manfred Jung).

The final three chapters summarize our present knowledge of epigenetic disturbances in different solid tumor types, specifically in lung cancer, colorectal and ovarian cancer, and other frequent malignancies. Again, a firm link is provided between the description of these tissue-specific or ubiquitous abnormalities – conceptually as "druggable" as those found in hematopoietic cancers – to the present status of clinical trial development. In Chap. 11, David Schrump reviews the abnormal patterns of DNA methylation observed in primary lung cancer cells, with a particular focus on the cancer/testis antigens (CTAs); he then outlines the remarkable potential of epigenetic drug treatment to enhance lung cancer cell immunogenicity. In Chap. 12, Sarah Derks and Manon van Engeland detail the role of altered DNA methylation patterns in colorectal cancer, particularly as regards their predictive and prognostic impact. In the final chapter, Robert Brown and colleagues discuss the "priming" concept of combination treatment in ovarian cancer based on sequential exposure to DNMT inhibitors followed by platinum-based chemotherapy. They also provide a comprehensive and up-to-date overview on clinical trials with DNMT and HDAC inhibitors (alone and in combination with cytotoxic agents, differentiation-inducing or immunostimulating molecules etc.), in a broad array of solid tumors. The remarkable degree of activity in this area demonstrates how far the concept of epigenetic therapy has already entered the clinic, but the authors also discuss current challenges when comparing the results to those obtained in hematologic malignancies.

Being able to provide this broad overview over a field that has been active for decades but only entered center-stage over the last 5–10 years, we wish to thank all the authors for their dedicated and timely contributions, and gratefully acknowledge the editorial assistance provided by Juliane Steinmann, with support from Gregor Klaus, and the valuable input by Rainer Claus.

Freiburg, Germany Michael Lübbert
Los Angeles, CA, USA Peter A. Jones

Contents

1 The Fundamental Role of Epigenetic Regulation in Normal and Disturbed Cell Growth, Differentiation, and Stemness

Manuel Rodríguez-Paredes and Manel Esteller

1.1 Introduction

Originally coined by Conrad Waddington in the 1940s, the term *epigenetics* currently defines the mitotically and/or meiotically heritable changes in gene expression that take place without changes in the DNA sequence (Berger et al. 2009). More specifically, epigenetics includes a series of cellular mechanisms that, in response to external signals, are capable of modifying chromatin packaging, thus creating transient or permanent, global or local, condensed, and decondensed chromatin states that modulate access of the different enzymatic machineries involved in the main genetic processes (transcription, replication, recombination, and DNA repair). These patterns of more *closed* or *open* chromatin (also called heterochromatin and euchromatin, respectively) display special features during stemness. Subsequently, during differentiation, they undergo a series of changes, remain fixed, and become stably transmitted through multiple cycles of cell division. This gives rise to the different gene expression patterns that underlie cell-type identity and lineage specification, as well as adult cell renewal. Epigenetic layers also play a key role in processes like X-chromosome inactivation and genomic imprinting (Portela and Esteller 2010).

M. Rodríguez-Paredes (✉)
Cancer Epigenetics and Biology Program (PEBC),
Bellvitge Biomedical Research Institute (IDIBELL), L'Hospitalet, Barcelona, Spain
e-mail: mrodriguezp@idibell.cat

M. Esteller (✉)
Cancer Epigenetics and Biology Program (PEBC),
Bellvitge Biomedical Research Institute (IDIBELL), L'Hospitalet, Barcelona, Spain

Department of Physiological Sciences II, School of Medicine, University of Barcelona, Barcelona, Spain

Institució Catalana de Recerca i Estudis Avançats, Barcelona, Spain
e-mail: mesteller@iconcologia.net

M. Lübbert, P.A. Jones (eds.), *Epigenetic Therapy of Cancer*,
DOI 10.1007/978-3-642-38404-2_1, © Springer-Verlag Berlin Heidelberg 2014

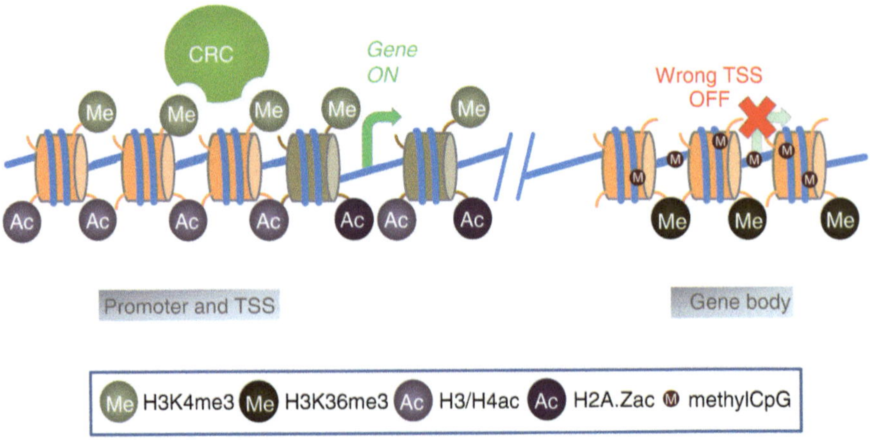

Fig. 1.1 Summary of the classical epigenetic mechanisms acting on a typical active gene in normal cells. This figure, depicting a typical transcriptionally active gene in a healthy cell, serves as an introduction to the various classic epigenetic mechanisms. Thus, the promoter and the region around the TSS present different activating covalent histone modifications which, recognized by ATP-dependent chromatin-remodeling complexes (CRCs), lead to a more *open* configuration of chromatin. Nucleosomes with histone variants like H2A.Z (in *brown*), upstream and downstream of the TSS, contribute to this transcriptionally permissive state. In the body of the gene, while other histone marks indicate active transcription, DNA methylation aborts spurious initiations

The classic epigenetic mechanisms are DNA methylation, a wide range of covalent histone modifications, and nucleosome positioning (through large ATP-dependent chromatin-remodeling complexes and the substitution of canonical histones with different variants) (Fig. 1.1). One should also highlight the role of noncoding RNAs (ncRNAs) such as microRNAs (miRNAs), which directly affect, or are affected by, all the former mechanisms. These are commonly included as part of the epigenetic setting phenomenon although, as with histone modifications, it is possible that not all of them may be self-perpetuating or inherited (Riddihough and Zahn 2010). Dysregulation of any of these mechanisms, which continuously work in close collaboration, is known to provoke misexpression of critical genes, problems in DNA repair, etc., leading to diseases like cancer (Portela and Esteller 2010; Rodriguez-Paredes and Esteller 2011).

Throughout this chapter, we will summarize the current knowledge about the operation of the main epigenetic mechanisms in normal cells, the way their disruption can promote tumorigenesis, and, finally, their importance in stemness. Along the way, we will also describe how all these mechanisms continuously coordinate in a given cell to yield what is currently called its *epigenome*, the epigenetic status that, starting from a single mammalian genome, gives rise to the diverse cell types and developmental stages of the organism.

1.2 Epigenetic Mechanisms in Normal and Cancer Cells

1.2.1 DNA Methylation

1.2.1.1 In Normal Cells

DNA methylation is historically the most extensively studied epigenetic mechanism, and its main effect is to silence genes and noncoding genomic regions. It normally consists of the covalent addition of a methyl group (-CH_3) at the 5′ position of the cytosine ring within CpG dinucleotides, but in embryonic stem (ES) cells, about 25 % of the total DNA methylation occurs in a non-CpG context (Lister et al. 2009). This unusual DNA methylation might be important for the origin and maintenance of pluripotency, as it disappears upon differentiation and is restored in induced pluripotent stem cells (Lister et al. 2009; Laurent et al. 2010).

The majority of the CpG dinucleotides are concentrated either in the so-called *CpG islands* or in regions of large repetitive sequences like centromeres and retrotransposon elements (Deaton and Bird 2011; Esteller 2008). CpG islands are CpG-rich DNA regions spanning, on average, 1,000 base pairs and are normally located near transcription start sites (TSSs) at approximately 70 % of annotated gene promoters (almost all those corresponding to housekeeping genes and some of the tissue-specific and developmental regulator gene promoters) (Larsen et al. 1992; Saxonov et al. 2006; Zhu et al. 2008). Although recent work has uncovered a large number of new CpG islands, called *orphan* CpG islands because they are located far away from the annotated TSSs, they may be canonical CpG islands associated with either alternative promoters of nearby annotated genes or with ncRNA promoters (Illingworth et al. 2010; Maunakea et al. 2010).

While the function of DNA methylation at repetitive sequences is to protect chromosomal integrity by preventing chromosome instability and transposition (parasitic sequence elements may represent more than 35 % of our genome), DNA methylation at CpG islands leads to the silencing of the corresponding genes (Esteller 2008). Intriguingly, while most CpG islands remain unmethylated during development and in differentiated tissues, only 6 % of the genes become methylated, and thus silenced, in this process. Among them are pluripotency and germ line-specific genes, different tissue-specific genes depending on each cell type, and, finally, genes involved in genomic imprinting and X-chromosome inactivation (Straussman et al. 2009; Suzuki and Bird 2008; Mohn et al. 2008). In this regard, it has been reported that extensive DNA methylation changes due to differentiation do occur at CpG island *shores*, regions of comparatively lower CpG density located near canonical CpG islands (Doi et al. 2009; Meissner et al. 2008). The fact that most tissue-specific DNA methylation takes place at these CpG island shores is supported by the observation that they account for 70 % of the differentially methylated regions when reprogramming somatic cells (Doi et al. 2009; Ji et al. 2010). The strong influence of DNA methylation upon cell identity is also underlined by the discovery that the efficiency of this reprogramming is greatly improved when methylation levels are artificially decreased (Huangfu et al. 2008).

On the other hand, it is important to point out that not only CpG dinucleotides within CpG islands may be methylated. Although they are not very abundant, there are also CpG dinucleotides located in the body of the genes, and in the case of those that are ubiquitously expressed, they commonly undergo methylation. Here, the function seems to be related to elongation efficiency and prevention of spurious initiations of transcription (Zilberman et al. 2007). Another interesting issue is the influence of DNA methylation on non-CpG island promoters, as it is known that methylation of the *POU5F1* and *SERPINB5* promoters, for instance, also has important negative effects on their expression levels (Futscher et al. 2002). In this regard, a recent study showed a clear nucleosome occupancy of these promoters after their methylation (Han et al. 2011).

The enzymes responsible for adding the methyl groups are called DNA methyltransferases (DNMTs). In mammals, there are five DNMTs—DNMT1, DNMT2, DNMT3a, DNMT3b, and DNMT3L—but only DNMT1, DNMT3a, and DNMT3b are able to transfer a methyl group from S-adenosylmethionine, the usual donor, to DNA. DNMT3a and DNMT3b, the so-called de novo DNMTs, are highly abundant in ES cells but very little expressed after differentiation (Portela and Esteller 2010). As a result, they are thought to be in charge of establishing the DNA methylation patterns during development. Despite being catalytically inactive, DNMT3L is expressed during gametogenesis, when it stimulates the de novo DNMTs and has an important role in genomic imprinting (Bourc'his et al. 2001; Holz-Schietinger and Reich 2010). The gene encoding DNMT1, the *maintenance* DNMT, is transcribed mostly during S phase and has a 30- to 40-fold preference for hemimethylated DNA. Hence, although it also possesses de novo activity, its role is far more important during semiconservative DNA replication, when it methylates the resulting hemimethylated sites. Its interaction with either the DNA polymerase processing factor, PCNA, mainly, or with the ubiquitin-like plant homeodomain and RING finger domain-containing protein 1 (UHRF1) promotes its localization at the replication fork (Chuang et al. 1997; Bostick et al. 2007). In a recent model proposed by Jones and Liang, DNMT3a and DNMT3b, which strongly anchor to nucleosomes containing methylated DNA, also help DNMT1 in this task (Jeong et al. 2009; Jones and Liang 2009). Finally, DNMT2, which does have all the catalytic signature motifs, is known to methylate $tRNA^{Asp}$ (Goll et al. 2006).

Two mechanisms could explain how DNA methylation leads to the inhibition of expression. First, for transcription factors such as CTCF, among others, DNA methylation represents a physical barrier to access to their binding sites (Rodriguez et al. 2010). Second, methylated DNA can recruit members of both the Kaiso-like or the methyl-CpG-binding domain (MBD) family of proteins (the latter being composed of MeCP2, MBD1, MBD2, MBD3, and MBD4) that, in turn, either interact with repressive histone-modifying enzymes, like histone deacetylases (HDACs) (as is the case of MeCP2), or directly belong to repressive chromatin-remodeling complexes like NuRD, which already includes these kinds of enzymes among its subunits (as is the case of MBD2) (Bogdanovic and Veenstra 2009; Lai and Wade 2011). All the latter actors eventually bring about the silencing.

Another example of the complex interplay between the different epigenetic mechanisms is provided by the way the DNA methylation machinery is probably targeted to particular genes throughout the genome. In this regard, numerous studies describe the recruitment of the DNMTs by histone-modifying enzymes and/or the marks they set on the chromatin (Esteve et al. 2009; Ooi et al. 2007; Tachibana et al. 2008; Wang et al. 2009; Zhao et al. 2009). X-linked CpG islands do not become methylated during X-chromosome inactivation until they acquire silencing marks like trimethylation of lysine (K) 27 on histone H3 (H3K27me3) (Okamoto and Heard 2009), and most CpG islands gaining methylation during differentiation are already silent in ES cells (Mohn et al. 2008), or the interaction between EZH2 (the enzyme that *writes* this mark) and DNMT3B (Viré et al. 2006). Considering these three points, it was proposed that, as a general rule, target genes were first marked by H3K27 methylation and the sequence was subsequently *locked* by the DNA methylation machinery (Ohm et al. 2007). Although it seems clear that there must be some connection between H3K27me3 and DNA methylation, the reality is that it has recently been reported in cancer cells that only up to 5 % of promoters containing CpGs are silenced by H3K27me3, independently of DNA methylation (Kondo et al. 2008). Another possibility for targeting the DNA methylation machinery comes from the plant world, where double-stranded small inhibitory RNAs (siRNAs) are known to initiate a stepwise process that targets DNMTs to specific regions—not only promoters but also repetitive sequences (Mosher and Melnyk 2010; Vrbsky et al. 2010). Although some of the components of this mechanism are conserved in mammals, the existence of an equivalent process in humans is still unclear.

Finally, the fact that 5-hydroxymethylcytosine could be an intermediary of DNA demethylation has recently focused considerable attention on either the mark itself, as has already been detected in ES cells and Purkinje neurons, or the enzymes capable of catalyzing it from the usual 5-methylcytosine, the three 2-oxoglutarate- and Fe(II)-dependent oxygenases TET1, TET2, and TET3 (Tahiliani et al. 2009). Further investigation is required to understand the role and nature of this modification, but it seems that while TET1 and, to a lesser extent, TET2 are essential players in maintaining pluripotency, TET3, which is not expressed in ES cells, may work with TET1 or TET2 to control hydroxylation in differentiated cells (Ito et al. 2010; Koh et al. 2011; Williams et al. 2011).

1.2.1.2 In Cancer Cells

Cancer cells show two major types of DNA methylation-related aberrancies that contribute to their malignant state: global hypomethylation of their genomes and CpG island promoter hypermethylation of different tumor suppressor genes.

Global hypomethylation at repetitive sequences, retrotransposons, CpG-poor promoters, introns, and gene deserts was the first epigenetic abnormality detected in cancer cells and is present in benign and malignant tumors (Esteller 2008). Its direct consequence is genomic instability, one of the most characteristic features of cancer cells, as a loss of methylation at repetitive sequences can favor mitotic recombination leading to deletions and translocations, as well as chromosome arrangements

(Eden et al. 2003; Esteller 2008). For example, cancer cells from ovarian and breast carcinomas, or Wilms tumors, which display severe hypomethylation of their pericentromeric satellite sequences, also present chromosomal translocations with breakpoints precisely in their pericentromeric DNA (Yeh et al. 2002). Moreover, hypomethylation of parasitic sequence elements can promote their transposition, once again generating chromosome rearrangements. One example is the hypomethylation of L1 retrotransposons in colorectal cancer (Howard et al. 2008). Finally, loss of methylation of latent viral sequences incorporated in the genome, and normally silent through DNA methylation, can activate them, again contributing to cancer. This is the case of genital human papillomaviruses in cervical tumors (Badal et al. 2003).

Global hypomethylation can contribute to tumorigenesis in two other ways. First of all, it can lead to the reactivation of some of the genes normally silenced in healthy cells by DNA methylation. Some examples are *SERPINB5*, whose aberrant reactivation promotes cell dedifferentiation in some cancers, *S100P* in pancreatic cancer, *SNCG* in breast and ovarian cancers, or *MAGE* and *DPP6* in melanomas (Portela and Esteller 2010). Of course, many genes encoding miRNAs are also affected by this abnormal process. A good example is the *let-7a-3* miRNA gene, which is reactivated in endometrial and colon cancer (Brueckner et al. 2007). Finally, DNA hypomethylation can promote loss of imprinting (LOI). For example, LOI of the insulin-like growth factor 2 (*IGF2*) gene has been reported in many different tumor types (Ito et al. 2008).

On the other hand, CpG island promoter hypermethylation leads to cancer by silencing tumor suppressor genes involved in the main cellular pathways related to tumorigenesis, such as cell cycle control, apoptosis, cell adhesion, and metastasis. Importantly, many silenced genes are also involved in DNA repair, which connects this kind of epigenetic dysregulation with all types of mutations, the classic genetic alterations linked to cancer. Some examples are listed in Table 1.1. Likewise, the expression of miRNA genes with tumor suppressor features is also known to be repressed by this epigenetic mechanism. Two examples of this are the silencing of *miR-124a*, leading to *CDK6* activation and Rb phosphorylation, and the silencing of *miR-148*, *miR-34b/c*, and *miR-9*, leading to metastatic phenotypes (Lujambio et al. 2007, 2008). This kind of epigenetic silencing of tumor suppressors has often been proposed as the second of the two essential events described by Knudson in his two-hit model of cancer initiation (Jones and Laird 1999). In this regard, this mechanism could silence the remaining active allele of a previously mutated tumor suppressor.

Recent findings suggest that most of the aberrant DNA methylation in cancer does not really occur at CpG islands, but at CpG island shores, although with equivalent consequences (Doi et al. 2009; Irizarry et al. 2009; Ji et al. 2010). In any case, this process is known to affect more genes than do mutations (Jones and Baylin 2002; Schuebel et al. 2007), and in fact, many genes, such as *RASSF1A*, owe their participation in tumorigenesis solely to this epigenetic alteration, as they are infrequently, if ever, mutated in cancer (Burbee et al. 2001; Dammann et al. 2000).

Hypermethylation patterns are not random. Each tumor type can be defined by its own *hypermethylome* (Esteller 2007), but what is not so clear is the way cancer

Table 1.1 Genes typically silenced by CpG island promoter hypermethylation in several frequent cancer types

Gene	Function	Cancer type/s
APC	Wnt signaling	Breast, colon, lung, prostate
ARNTL	Circadian clock	Hematological
BRCA1	DNA repair	Breast
CDH1	Cell adhesion	Multiple
CDH13	Cell adhesion	Breast, colon, hematological, lung
CDKN2A	Cell cycle control	Breast, colon, lung, lymphomas, prostate
CDKN2B	Cell cycle control	Breast, colon, leukemia, lung
CRBP1	Vitamin response	Colon, hematological
DAPK1	Apoptosis	Colon, hematological, lung
ESR1	Hormone response	Breast, hematological, lung, prostate
GATA4	Transcription factor	Colon
GATA5	Transcription factor	Colon
GSTP1	Detoxification	Lung, prostate
HIC1	p53 network	Breast, colon, hematological, lung
IGFBP3	Wnt signaling	Lung
MGMT	DNA repair	Colon, lymphomas and lung
MLH1	DNA repair	Colon
PTGS2	Prostaglandin biosynthesis	Colon
PYCARD	Apoptosis	Breast, lung
RARB2	Vitamin response	Colon, hematological, lung
RASSF1A	Ras signaling	Multiple
RASSF5	Ras signaling	Lung
SFRP1	Apoptosis	Breast, colon, leukemia, lung, prostate
TLE1	Transcription factor	Hematological
TP73	p53 network	Hematological
WIF1	Apoptosis	Breast, colon, lung
WRN	DNA repair	Colon

cells *decide* which genes must be aberrantly silenced. One obvious explanation is that silencing of particular genes can provide a growth advantage and, therefore, clonal selection (Esteller 2007). Another possibility comes from the interaction of DNMTs with oncogenic transcription factors, which, in turn, recruit them to their specific target genes. In acute promyelocytic leukemia (APL), for instance, the PML-RARA fusion protein interacts with DNMT1 and DNMT3a leading to the hypermethylation of the *RARB2* promoter (Di Croce et al. 2002). Moreover, the observation that large genomic regions become hypermethylated in cancer may mean that, just because of their location within those regions, many CpG islands could gain aberrant methylation (Frigola et al. 2006). Finally, as we saw for healthy cells in the last section, it is clear that histone marks and/or the enzymes that *write* them must also play a key role in the aberrant targeting of the DNA methylation machinery. In cancer cells, EZH2 also recruits DNMTs to the promoters of subsequently hypermethylated genes, like *TBX3* in breast cancer or *HOXD10*, *SIX3*, *KCNA1*, or *MYT1* in osteosarcoma (Vire et al. 2006).

Obviously, any kind of alteration in the normal levels of DNMTs can contribute to the abnormal methylation patterns present in cancer cells. In fact, increased expression of the genes encoding DNMT1, DNMT3a, and/or DNMT3b may be an early and important event in many tumor types (Daniel et al. 2011). Likewise, mutations in *DNMT1* and in *DNMT3A* in acute myeloid leukemia (AML) have also been described (Daniel et al. 2011; Ley et al. 2010). Upregulations and/or mutations of members of the MBD and Kaiso-like families of proteins have also been reported in many human cancers (Kanwal and Gupta 2010). Finally, as *MLL-TET1* fusions have been found in some cases of acute myeloid and lymphocytic leukemia, and homozygous null mutations and chromosomal deletions involving *TET2* have been observed in several myeloid malignancies, it seems that the disruption of the system in charge of placing 5-hydroxymethylcytosines throughout the genome is also connected to cancer (Mohr et al. 2011).

1.2.2 Covalent Histone Modifications

1.2.2.1 In Normal Cells

The various histones of the nucleosomes can undergo multiple posttranslational covalent modifications, mainly along their N-terminal *tails* but also in their core and C-terminal regions (Bannister and Kouzarides 2011). Hence, histones may be subject to acetylation, ubiquitination, sumoylation, or propionylation at their lysines; methylation at their lysines (one, two, or three groups) or arginines (one or two); phosphorylation mostly at their serines, threonines, or tyrosines; ADP ribosylation at their arginines or glutamates; β-*N*-acetylglucosamination of their serines and threonines; deimination of their arginines; and/or isomerization of their prolines (Bannister and Kouzarides 2011; Liu et al. 2009a; Sakabe et al. 2010). Intriguingly, their N-terminal tails can be even clipped (Duncan et al. 2008; Santos-Rosa et al. 2009).

All these modifications are established and removed by different enzymes. So far, histone acetyltransferases (HATs), deacetylases (HDACs), methyltransferases (HMTs), and demethylases (HDMs) have been the most extensively studied systems, although intensive research is currently being devoted to understanding the mode of action, specificity, and function of the other histone-modifying enzymes.

The acetyl groups are added by two types of HATs (Table 1.2). Type-B HATs, like HAT1, acetylate newly synthesized histones H3 and H4 in the cytoplasm to promote their deposition; the marks are subsequently removed (Parthun 2007). Type-A HATs can be classified into three families depending on their amino acid sequence homology and protein conformation: GNAT (HATs hGCN5, PCAF), MYST (TIP60, MYST1–4), and P300/CBP (P300, CBP) (Bannister and Kouzarides 2011). Type-A HATs are normally part of large multiprotein complexes that determine their recruitment and substrate specificity. Thus, while hGCN5 belongs to the SAGA complex (Rodriguez-Navarro 2009), TIP60 is the catalytic subunit of the NuA4 complex (Lu et al. 2009).

Table 1.2 Histone modifications in mammals: related enzymes and functions

Modification	Histone	Residue	Enzyme/s	Function/s
Acetylation	H2A	K5	HAT1, TIP60, P300/CBP	A
	H2B	K5	ATF2	A, Rep
		K12	ATF2, P300/CBP	A
		K15	ATF2, P300/CBP	A
		K20	P300	A
	H3	K9	hGCN5, PCAF, SRC-1, TFIIIC90	A, Rep
		K14	hGCN5, PCAF, TIP60, SRC-1, TFIIIC90, TAF1, MYST3-4	A, Rep, Repl
		K18	P300, CBP/hGCN5, PCAF, TFIIIC90	A, Rep
		K23	P300, CBP/hGCN5	A, Rep
		K27	hGCN5	A, Rep
	H4	K5	HAT1, TIP60, ATF2, MYST2	A, Rep, Repl
		K8	hGCN5, PCAF, TIP60, MYST2, ATF2	A, Rep, Repl
		K12	HAT1, TIP60/HAT1, MYST2	A, Rep, Repl
		K16	MYST1, MYST3, hGCN5, TIP60, ATF2/hGCN5	A, Rep
Methylation	H1	K26	EZH2	R
	H3	R2	CARM1, **JMJD6**	A
		$K4^{me1/2/3}$	MLL1-5, hSET1A-B, SET7/9, SMYD2-3, **LSD1-2**, **JHDM1B**, **JARID1A-D**, **NO66**	A
		R8	PMRT5	R
		$K9^{me1/2/3}$	SUV39H1-2, SETDB1, EHMT1-2, EZH2, PRDM2, **LSD1**, **JHDM1D**, **PHF8**, **JHDM2A**, **JHDM3A-D**	R>A, HF/S
		R17	CARM1	A
		R26	CARM1	A
		$K27^{me1/2/3}$	EZH2, EHMT2, **JHDM1D**, **UTX**, **JMJD3**	R>A, PS
		$K36^{me2/3}$	NSD1, SETD2, SMYD2, **JHDM1A-B**, **JHDM3A-C**, **NO66**	A
		$K79^{me1/2/3}$	DOT1L	A>R, Rep
	H4	R3	PRMT1, PRMT5, **JMJD6**	A
		$K20^{me1/2/3}$	SUV420H1, PR-SET7, PRDM6	R>A, Rep
Phosphorylation	H2B	S14	MST-1	Apoptosis
	H3	T3	Haspin	Mitosis
		S10	S6K-alpha-4, S6K-alpha-5, Aurora B	A, mitosis
		S28	S6K-alpha-4, S6K-alpha-5	A
	H2AX	S139	ATM, ATR, DNA-PK	Rep
Ubiquitination	H2A	K119	RING1b	R, Rep
	H2B	K120	BRE1-A/BRE1-B	A, Rep

K lysine, *R* arginine, *S* serine, *A* transcription activation, *R* transcription repression, *Rep* repair, *Repl* replication, *HF/S* heterochromatin formation/silencing, *PS* polycomb silencing
In bold font are enzymes which remove the mark

On the other hand, 18 different HDACs, classified into four classes according to their sequence homology to certain yeast proteins, are capable of removing this mark in mammals (Table 1.2) (Yang and Seto 2007). Class I contains the nuclear enzymes HDAC1–3 and 8; class II is formed by HDAC4–7, 9, and 10, which shuttle between nucleus and cytoplasm; and class IV only has one member, HDAC11; all of them are Zn-dependent HDACs (Yang and Seto 2007). Finally, class III, with seven members, called sirtuins due to their homology with yeast Sir2 (SIRT1–7), is the only one that requires NAD^+ as a cofactor (Vaquero 2009; Bannister and Kouzarides 2011). As many HDACs normally belong to different complexes, often together with other HDACs, their recruitment and substrate specificity is not as clear. For instance, HDAC1 has been found together with HDAC2 within the NuRD, Sin3A, and Co-REST complexes (Yang and Seto 2008).

There are two main classes of HMTs (Table 1.2): lysine and arginine methyltransferases (HKMTs and PRMTs, respectively). HKMTs, which catalyze the addition of methyl groups from S-adenosylmethionine (SAM) to the ε-amino group of lysines, can be further subdivided into the SET domain-containing and DOT1L families (Allis et al. 2007). Intriguingly, all the HKMTs methylate histones within their N-terminal tails except DOT1L, which is the only member of the family with the same name. It lacks the SET domain and methylates histones H3 at lysine 79 (H3K79), within their globular cores (Feng et al. 2002). HKMTs are relatively specific enzymes, and in general, it seems that the presence of a particular amino acid (a tyrosine or a phenylalanine) in their catalytic domain may determine their capability of proceeding past the monomethyl-lysine to the di- or trimethylated residues (Cheng et al. 2005; Collins et al. 2005b). On the other hand, PRMTs add methyl groups from SAM to the ω-guanidino group of arginines and can be subclassified into type-I and type-II enzymes; both produce monomethyl-arginines, but while type-I PRMTs also yield asymmetric dimethyl-arginines, type II generates symmetric ones (Bedford and Clarke 2009). The most relevant histone PRMTs are PRMT1, PRMT4, and PRMT6 (type I), as well as PRMT5 (type II) (Bedford and Clarke 2009). Intensive research is also focused on the PR-domain-containing family of proteins (PRDMs), as its members are structurally related to the SET domain-containing HKMTs and possess N-terminal PR domains which are 20–30 % similar to the SET domain (Davis et al. 2006). PRDM2 is already known to methylate histones H3 at lysine 9 (H3K9) (Kim et al. 2003), whereas PRDM6 has been reported to methylate histones H4 at lysine 20 (H4K20) (Funabiki et al. 1994).

Considered for many years to be a stable modification, we currently know a considerable number of HDMs (Table 1.2). LSD1 was the first to be discovered and uses FAD as a cofactor (Shi et al. 2004). Depending on the complex within which it works, LSD1 can be a transcription activator or a repressor. Thus, when associated with the Co-REST repressor complex, it demethylates mono- and dimethyl residues at H3K4 (H3K4me1/2) and acts as a repressor; when associated with the androgen receptor, it demethylates H3K9me1/2 and acts as an activator (Klose and Zhang 2007). Apart from LSD1 and the closely related LSD2, many other HDMs have been described, although their mode of action is completely different because their activity takes places within the shared JmjC jumonji domain; capable of demethylating some trimethyl-lysines, they use Fe(II) and α-ketoglutarate as cofactors and have a high level of substrate specificity (Pedersen and Helin 2010).

Genome-wide studies have confirmed that, like a sort of *histone code*, diverse combinations of histone modifications result in the different levels of chromatin packaging that, globally or locally, are necessary for (and thus define) the various nuclear functions: transcription, alternative splicing, replication, chromosome condensation, DNA repair, etc. (Kouzarides 2007; Luco et al. 2010; Li et al. 2007a). For instance, trimethylation of lysines 4, 36, or 79 on histone H3 (H3K4me3, H3K36me3, and H3K79me3, respectively), acetylation of its lysines 9 and 14 (H3K9ac and H3K14ac), and monomethylation of lysines 20 and 5 on histones H4 and H2B (H4K20me and H2BK5me), respectively, generally lead to a relaxed, *open* chromatin state (euchromatin) and gene activation, whereas di- or trimethylation of lysine 9 on histone H3 (H3K9me2 and H3K9me3) as well as trimethylation of its lysine 27 (H3K27me3) lead to a compact, *closed* chromatin state (heterochromatin) and gene repression (Barski et al. 2007; Li et al. 2007a; Rosenfeld et al. 2009). However, on a small scale, it is well known that histone modifications define the necessary chromatin states for the proper function of all the different sequences involved in transcription. Thus, boundary elements, regions separating heterochromatin and euchromatin that restrict the activity of enhancers, are enriched not only in histone variants like H2A.Z but also in modifications such as H3K9me1 (Barski et al. 2007). Active enhancers contain relatively high levels of H3K4me1 (Hon et al. 2009), transcription start sites (TSSs) are very enriched in H3K4me3, and the entire transcribed regions present a great deal of H3K36me3, among other examples (Barski et al. 2007; Hon et al. 2009; Li et al. 2007a). Together with histone variants and ATP-dependent chromatin-remodeling complexes, the histone code plays a key role in DNA replication and repair, processes that also need special relaxed chromatin conditions.

Replication requires not only access of its enzymatic machinery to DNA but also the removal of parental nucleosomes ahead of the replication fork and the assembly of new ones on the newly synthesized material. In this regard, the HAT MYST2 has been reported to associate with the replication factor MCM2 and the origin recognition complex 1 subunit of the human initiator protein (Burke et al. 2001). Furthermore, a complex containing MYST2 and ING5 (see later in this section) also interacts with the MCM2-7 helicase and seems to be essential for replication in humans (Doyon et al. 2006). On the other hand, one of the first events in DNA double-strand breaks (DBSs) is the phosphorylation of H2A.X in its serine 139 (H2AXS139ph) (Luijsterburg and van Attikum 2011). H2A.X is a histone variant that replaces H2A several megabases upstream and downstream of the break and that, upon phosphorylation, not only leads to massive targeting of repair proteins to the damaged sites (see later in this section) but also recruits HAT complexes such as NuA4, which, through histone acetylation, further enhance access of the DNA repair machinery to damaged chromatin (Luijsterburg and van Attikum 2011).

Although there are many possible combinations of histone modifications, it is important to highlight some peculiarities of their *cross talk*. Interplay among marks can take place at a single site, within the same histone tail (in *cis*) or between different tails (in *trans*). Some modifications cannot coexist at the same residue for steric reasons (Wang et al. 2008b). Some marks promote or block other modifications in *cis* or *trans*, such as the ubiquitylation of lysine 120 on histone H2B (H2BK120ub), which promotes trimethylation of H3K4 for eventual gene activation (Kim et al. 2009); the phosphorylation of the serine 10 on H3 (H3S10ph), which results in the acetylation of H3K14 for gene activation (Lo et al. 2000) and, also, in the inhibition of mono- and dimethylation of H3K9 during mitosis (Duan et al. 2008); or the phosphorylation of H3T6 (H3T6ph), which prevents LSD1 from demethylating H3K4 during androgen receptor-dependent gene activation (Metzger et al. 2010).

Histone modifications bring about chromatin remodeling by two main mechanisms.

First of all, marks such as acetylation or phosphorylation neutralize the positive charge of lysines, weakening interactions among nucleosomes and/or between DNA and histones and, thereby, relaxing chromatin (Luger and Richmond 1998; Steger and Workman 1996). For acetylation, this seems to be true, as the large number of possible acetylation sites within histone tails could enable the positive charge of lysines to be neutralized in hyperacetylated regions. Moreover, while hyperacetylation of histones is usually considered a hallmark of *open* chromatin, deacetylation is a hallmark of *closed* chromatin, and many acetylation marks are enriched at enhancers and promoters (Wang et al. 2008b). However, for phosphorylation, with fewer available sites within histone *tails*, this effect is not likely to be of great importance.

Histone modifications can serve as docking sites for recruiting many specific chromatin factors and/or complexes which, eventually, execute the remodeling (Kouzarides 2007). Likewise, regulators of any process related to chromatin, such as transcription factors, can also bind to their target regions through the same mechanism (Sims and Reinberg 2006). Several domains are capable of interacting with the different marks. For instance, PHD fingers and the domains of the Tudor *royal* family (chromodomains, Tudor, PWWP, and MBT domains) can bind to different methyl-lysines (Champagne and Kutateladze 2009; Kim et al. 2006), bromodomains and, again, PHD fingers interact with acetylated lysines (Mujtaba et al. 2007; Zeng et al. 2010), and, finally, 14-3-3 and BRCT domains can mediate targeting to phosphorylated serines (Macdonald et al. 2005; Stucki et al. 2005). A good example of this type of recruitment is the HP1 recognition of H3K9me2/3 through its single chromodomain; this binding targets the H3K9 HMTs SUV39H1/2 to chromatin (HP1 interacts with it), leading to the methylation of adjacent histones and, eventually, to heterochromatin silencing of sequences like telomeres and centromeres (Bannister et al. 2001; Lachner et al. 2001).

It is important to point out, however, that the same mark can be *read* by different domains, depending on the cellular context (de la Cruz et al. 2005). For example, H3K4me3 can be recognized not only by the PHD finger of the ING1-5 proteins that, in turn, recruit HATs or HDACs to chromatin (Champagne and Kutateladze 2009) but also by the tandem chromodomains of the ATP-dependent chromatin-remodeling enzyme CHD1 (see next section) (Sims et al. 2005) or by the Tudor domains of the HDM JMJD2A (Huang et al. 2006). To return to the subject of the *cross talk* between modifications, the binding of an effector to a particular mark can be blocked by other modifications or, even, DNA methylation, as occurs with HP1 binding to H3K9me2/3 during mitosis, due to H3S10ph (Fischle et al. 2005), or with JHDM1A binding to H3K9me3 due to methylcytosines (Bartke et al. 2010). Finally, different marks and, again, DNA methylation can also cooperate to recruit a factor more efficiently. This is the case with H3K4me3 and PHF8, whose interaction is enhanced when H3K9 and H3K14 are also acetylated (Vermeulen et al. 2010), or H3K9me3 and UHRF1, which, in a nucleosomal context, interact much better when CpG dinucleotides are also methylated (Bartke et al. 2010).

1.2.2.2 In Cancer Cells

Cancer cells present aberrant covalent histone modification profiles. It is well established that the disruption of particular histone marks can dysregulate normal expression patterns of oncogenes and tumor suppressor genes, as well as affect genome integrity and/or chromosome segregation, eventually leading to cancer. Typically, cancer cells show a global reduction of H4K16ac and H4K20me3 (Fraga et al. 2005) and also display different alterations in the enzymes in charge of *writing*, *erasing*, and *reading* the histone code (Ellis et al. 2009; Hatziapostolou and Iliopoulos 2011).

Disruption of histone acetylation has been reported in hematological and solid tumors. Chromosomal translocations, leading to aberrant fusion proteins involving HATs like CBP, P300, MYST3, or MYST4 and that eventually dysregulate the expression of multiple genes, have been described in different types of leukemia (Ayton and Cleary 2001; Champagne et al. 1999; Chan et al. 2007; Ida et al. 1997; Liang et al. 1998; Panagopoulos et al. 2001). Moreover, it is known that binding of adenoviral oncoproteins E1A and SV40 T to CBP and P300 leads to transformation due to a decrease in the global levels of H3K18ac, and the subsequent targeting of these HATs to genes promoting cell growth and division (Ferrari et al. 2008; Horwitz et al. 2008). Finally, missense mutations and monoallelic loss of *EP300* and *KAT5*, the genes encoding P300 and TIP60, respectively, have also been found in a range of solid and hematological tumors (Gayther et al. 2000; Gorrini et al. 2007).

In considering the role of histone deacetylation in cancer, it is worth mentioning that some malignant chromosomal translocations give rise to fusion proteins that, although they do not harbor their own deacetylation activity, can associate with HDACs (and other chromatin remodelers) with high affinity and target them to particular subsets of genes that end up repressed. This is the case of the PML-RARA and PLZF-RARA fusion proteins in APL (Minucci and Pelicci 2006), and AML1-ETO and CBFβ-MYH11 in AML (Bhalla 2005; Wang et al. 2007a). In B-cell-derived non-Hodgkin lymphomas, the transcriptional repressor BCL6 is upregulated and, similarly, provokes the silencing of its target genes by recruiting an exaggerated amount of HDACs (Bhalla 2005; Wang et al. 2007a). On the other hand, *HDAC1* and *HDAC2* are overexpressed in multiple tumor types; *HDAC3*, *HDAC7*, and *HDAC8* in colon cancer; *HDAC4* in prostate and breast cancer; and *HDAC6* in

AML and breast cancer (Ellis et al. 2009). However, the role of HDAC2 in colon cancer is not as clear because its gene was also found to be mutated in a subset of microsatellite unstable colorectal cell lines and primary tumors (Ropero et al. 2006). Reduced levels of HDACs have also been observed in the disease: HDAC1 and HDAC4 in colon cancer; HDAC5 in AML, lung, and, again, colon cancer; and HDAC10 in lung cancer (Ellis et al. 2009; Osada et al. 2004). With respect to sirtuins, overexpression of *SIRT1*, *SIRT3*, and *SIRT7* occurs in a wide range of tumors (Saunders and Verdin 2007). Interestingly, when inhibition of SIRT1 was seen to partially reactivate tumor suppressors like *CDH1*, *SFRP1*, *SFRP2*, and *MLH1*, their promoters remained heavily methylated, thus indicating a prevailing role for deacetylation, against DNA methylation, in gene silencing (Pruitt et al. 2006). Finally, SIRT1 and SIRT4 are downregulated in colon cancer and AML, respectively (Saunders and Verdin 2007).

Abnormal activity of the histone methylation enzymatic systems is also common in tumorigenesis. In the case of the methylation of H3K4, partial tandem duplication and more than 50 different fusions of the *MLL* gene are the cause of most infant leukemias, as well as of 5–10 % of AML and lymphoid leukemias (Krivtsov and Armstrong 2007). In some cases, the malignancy occurs due to an increase in activating marks like H3K4me2 and bulk histone acetylation at leukemia-promoting genes, but in other cases, these critical genes become activated by the anomalous recruitment of DOT1L, the H3K79 HMT (Chi et al. 2010; Dorrance et al. 2008). Another H3K4 HMT, SMYD3, is typically upregulated in colorectal and hepatocellular carcinoma cell lines (Hamamoto et al. 2004). Meanwhile, upregulation of the H3K27 HMT EZH2 provokes the silencing of key tumor suppressor genes in prostate, breast, colon, skin, and lung cancer (Bracken and Helin 2009). The increase of endothelial EZH2 promotes angiogenesis, at least in ovarian cancer, by silencing the *VASH1* gene (Lu et al. 2010). However, the mutation of *EZH2* can also yield malignant phenotypes, as was observed in some B-cell lymphomas (Lu et al. 2010; Morin et al. 2010). On the other hand, while high levels of the H3K9 HMTs EHMT2 and SETDB1 have been described in liver cancer and melanoma, respectively (Kondo et al. 2007; Ceol et al. 2011), NSD1, an HMT for H3K36 and H4K20, is involved in leukemogenic translocation and lost in gliomas and neuroblastomas by CpG island promoter hypermethylation (Wang et al. 2007c). The heterozygous mutation/loss of heterozygosity of the corresponding gene causes Sotos syndrome, a combination of symptoms that includes a higher risk of tumorigenesis (Berdasco et al. 2009). Highly similar to NSD1, the HMT NSD2 is involved in aggressive t(4;14)-associated multiple myelomas (MMs) (Marango et al. 2008). Finally, inactivation of PRDM2, an H3K9 HMT originally identified as a pRB-binding protein, either by mutations or promoter hypermethylation, is also found in many tumors (Gibbons 2005). The alteration of PRDM5, PRDM16, and the arginine methyltransferase PRMT4 is linked to cancer, too (Lahortiga et al. 2004; Majumder et al. 2006).

The role of HDMs in tumorigenesis is no less important. LSD1 is upregulated in many tumors (Kahl et al. 2006; Lim et al. 2010), and the disruption of many different JmjC domain-containing HDM genes has also been observed: while *KDM5A* (encoding JARID1A) is translocated in myeloid leukemia, overexpression of

KDM5B (encoding JARID1B) was found in advanced stages of breast and prostate cancers, where it facilitates the G1/S transition in the cell cycle, attenuates its mitotic checkpoint, or inactivates tumor suppressors like *BRCA1* and *CAV1* (Scibetta et al. 2007). In a recent study, inactivation of *KDM5C* (encoding JARID1C) by truncating mutations appeared in ≈3 % of renal cell carcinoma (RCC) samples (Dalgliesh et al. 2010). Moreover, JHDM1B, another HDM capable of repressing the tumor suppressor locus *CDKN2A-CDKN2B* by erasing both H3K36me1/2 and H3K4me3 marks, is known to be upregulated in T-cell lymphomas (Tzatsos et al. 2009). Mutations of the gene encoding the H3K27me2/3 HDM UTX become inactivated in a subset of MMs, esophageal squamous cell carcinomas, and RCC, and the expression of the related JMJD3, H3K27me2/3 HDM, is downregulated in many cancers (Agger et al. 2009; van Haaften et al. 2009). Finally, *KDM4C*, which encodes the H3K9me2/3 HDM JHDM3C/GASC1, is frequently overexpressed by gene amplification in esophageal squamous cell carcinoma, lung sarcomatoid carcinoma, desmoplastic medulloblastoma, and breast cancer (Italiano et al. 2006; Liu et al. 2009b).

Further research is needed to determine the importance of histone phosphorylation in cancer. For instance, it is known that JAK2, the tyrosine kinase for H3Y41, is frequently activated by chromosomal translocations or point mutations in different hematological malignancies (Dawson et al. 2009). Also, the upregulation of aurora kinase B, responsible for the H3S10ph mark, has been reported in several solid tumors (Dar et al. 2010; Hirota et al. 2005), and its collaboration with aurora kinase A is essential for the progression of Myc-driven B-cell lymphomas (den Hollander et al. 2010).

Malfunction of histone modification *readers* is also a significant event in tumorigenesis. Thus, the members of the ING family of H3K4me3 *readers* are components of different transcriptional regulation complexes controlling many cellular cancer-related processes: while ING1 and ING2 recruit HDAC-Sin3A repressive complexes, ING3, ING4, and ING5 recruit HATs to induce gene activation (Chi et al. 2010). Dysregulation of their expression or mutations affecting their binding capacity to the H3K4me3 mark has been described in many tumors (Chi et al. 2010).

1.2.3 Nucleosome Positioning

1.2.3.1 In Normal Cells

As previously stated, DNA methylation and covalent histone modifications determine, globally and locally, the levels of chromatin packaging, thereby controlling access to DNA of the enzymatic machineries in charge of the different genetic functions. However, in close collaboration with these, histone variants and ATP-dependent chromatin-remodeling factors/complexes are the cellular mechanisms that, ultimately, are capable of generating the different chromatin compaction patterns by physically executing the appropriate nucleosome displacement and/or removal. For example, it is well established that, in transcriptionally active genes, nucleosomes are positioned at fixed locations around promoters while they are more randomly distributed in the interior of the genes (Mavrich et al. 2008). Moreover, the 5′ and 3′ ends of these genes must also adopt nucleosome-free regions (NFRs) in order to expose binding sites for the different necessary transcription factors (Jiang and Pugh 2009; Schones et al. 2008). The loss of the nucleosome located directly upstream of the TSSs is strongly correlated with gene activation, whereas its presence is normally associated with gene repression (Portela and Esteller 2010).

The best studied histone variants are expressed outside S phase and incorporated into chromatin in a replication-independent manner (Santenard and Torres-Padilla 2009). They differ from canonical histones in their amino acid sequence and structure (Li et al. 2007a). Histone H2A may have three main variants: H2A.Z, H2A.X, and macroH2A. Preferentially enriched at promoters of active genes or genes poised for activation, H2A.Z contributes to their transcription by destabilizing the nucleosomes (Jin and Felsenfeld 2007). It is also known to protect those genes against possible repression by DNA methylation (Zilberman et al. 2008). As explained previously, the phosphorylation of H2A.X at its serine 139 (H2AXS139ph) occurs soon after a DNA double-strand break and promotes the recruitment of DNA repair complexes (Luijsterburg and van Attikum 2011). Finally, macroH2A is specifically placed throughout the inactive X chromosome in female mammals (Chadwick and Willard 2002). Histone H3 has two possible variants: CENP-A, which is essential for the highly condensed chromatin of centromeres and so for chromosome segregation, and H3.3, which is enriched at promoters of active genes like H2A.Z (Sarma and Reinberg 2005).

It is important to point out that not only H2A.X can undergo covalent modifications, as the acetylation of H2A.Z is commonly observed in active genes, whereas its ubiquitylation is associated with facultative heterochromatin (Svotelis et al. 2009); furthermore, H3.3 normally presents di- and trimethylation of lysine 4, as well as acetylation of lysines 9, 14, 18, and 23, marks which reflect transcriptional competence (Sarma and Reinberg 2005).

Several large multiprotein complexes have been found to move, destabilize, eject, or restructure nucleosomes using the energy of ATP hydrolysis (Clapier and Cairns 2009; Hargreaves and Crabtree 2011). They all have in common the presence of a DNA-dependent ATPase of the Snf2 family as their catalytic subunit. More precisely, these ATP-dependent chromatin-remodeling complexes always include an ATPase coming from up to seven different subfamilies of the Snf2 family: Snf2, ISWI, INO80, SWR1, CHD1, Mi-2, and CHD7 (Flaus et al. 2006). The ATPases of all these subfamilies are characterized by their particular combination of domains. Thus, apart from the SNF2_N and HELICc domains, which together form the catalytic center of all them, the ATPases of the Snf2 subfamily also have a bromodomain (Wilson and Roberts 2011), the ATPases of the ISWI subfamily present both a SANT and a SLIDE domain (Corona and Tamkun 2004), and the ones belonging to the CHD1 subfamily have two N-terminal chromodomains and a C-terminal DNA-binding domain (Hall and Georgel 2007; Marfella and Imbalzano 2007); the ATPases of the Mi-2 and CHD7 subfamilies also possess a couple of N-terminal chromodomains, but while the first ones also have two PHD domains, the others display a SANT domain and one or two BRK domains (Hall and Georgel 2007; Marfella and Imbalzano 2007). Finally, the very similar ATPases of the INO80 and SWR1 subfamilies do not have extra domains, but they are characterized by a typical spacer fragment within the amino acid sequence of their catalytic centers (Morrison and Shen 2009). The role of all these domains consists not only of stabilizing the binding of the entire complexes to the covalently modified histones and/or nucleosomal DNA typical of their target regions throughout the genome but also of mediating the necessary interactions between the different subunits of the complexes themselves, which include histone modification enzymes (such as TIP60 in the TRRAP/TIP60 complex or HDAC1 and HDAC2 in the NuRD complex) and, logically, histone modification *readers* (like ING3 or MBD3, in the same complexes, respectively), among other proteins with a wide variety of functions (Clapier and Cairns 2009; Bao and Shen 2007; Hargreaves and Crabtree 2011).

Thus, in humans, BAF and PBAF are the ATP-dependent chromatin-remodeling complexes with ATPases of the Snf2 subfamily. The ATPase of the BAF complex can be either hBRM or BRG1, whereas the ATPase of the PBAF complex can only be BRG1 (Bao and Shen 2007). These complexes are key regulators of gene expression and alternative splicing, controlling important processes such as cell cycle progression, organ development, and immune responses, among others (Wilson and Roberts 2011). NURF, hCHRAC, hACF/WCRF, or WICH, some of the complexes with ATPases of the ISWI subfamily, have been reported to repress transcription (rather than activate it), promote chromatin assembly during mitosis, and participate in DNA replication (Bao and Shen 2007; Corona and Tamkun 2004; Hargreaves and Crabtree 2011). Complexes with ATPases of the Mi-2 subfamily are mainly involved in transcription repression and DNA repair (Hargreaves and Crabtree 2011), and much less well-known, putative complexes harboring ATPases of the CHD7 subfamily may contribute to transcription, both its activation and repression, depending on the exact context (Lutz et al. 2006; Nishiyama et al. 2009; Rodriguez-Paredes et al. 2009; Schnetz et al. 2009; Shur et al. 2006; Takada et al. 2007). However, CHD1, ATPase of the subfamily with the same name, seems to work alone, without any complex, and its functions may be the promotion of transcription and splicing, as well as the deposition of the histone variant H3.3, as it does in *Drosophila* (Konev et al. 2007; Sims et al. 2007). Finally, complexes with ATPases of the INO80 subfamily have important roles in transcription, DNA replication and repair, chromosome segregation, and telomere regulation (Morrison and Shen 2009). Most importantly, the SRCAP complex, with the ATPase of the SWR1 subfamily of the same name, is essential for the deposition of the histone variant H2A.Z (Wong et al. 2007).

1.2.3.2 In Cancer Cells

In comparison with DNA methylation and covalent histone modifications, very little is known about the influence of aberrations in histone variants and/or ATP-dependent chromatin-remodeling factors on cancer.

First of all, although the histone variant H2A.Z is overexpressed in several cancer types where it seems to favor cell cycle progression, its loss has also been associated with the spread of repressive chromatin domains and de novo promoter hypermethylation of tumor suppressors (Svotelis et al. 2009); moreover, the H3 variant CENP-A becomes upregulated in colorectal cancer and may be responsible for aneuploidy (Tomonaga et al. 2003). On the other hand, bi-allelic loss of *SNF5*, encoding one of the core subunits of the BAF and PBAF complexes, is common in most human malignant rhabdoid tumors (MRTs) and leads to cancer through inactivation of the p21 and p16INK4A pathways (Chai et al. 2005). Nonetheless, it remains unclear whether its tumor suppressor function requires BAF-/PBAF-mediated chromatin remodeling. Loss of BRG1 and hBRM, the two mutually exclusive ATPases of these complexes, has been reported in up to 15–20 % of primary non-small-cell lung cancers, and bi-allelic loss of *SMARCA4* (encoding BRG1) takes place in prostate, lung, breast, and pancreatic cancer cell lines (Reisman et al. 2003; Medina and Sanchez-Cespedes 2008). Intriguingly, a recent study reveals that BRG1 also has an oncogenic role based on the destabilization of the p53 protein (Naidu et al. 2009). The NuRD complex was first connected to cancer through its metastasis-associated subunits MTA1, MTA2, and MTA3, but it has recently been found that, in leukemia, it also favors the targeting of the Polycomb repressive complex 2 (PRC2) and DNMT3A to the oncogenic transcription factor PML-RARA target promoters, leading to their permanent silencing (Morey et al. 2008; Wang et al. 2007b). It is well known that, in general terms, aberrant gene silencing through CpG island promoter hypermethylation normally involves the presence of a nucleosome that blocks the TSS (Lin et al. 2007). Finally, it is important to highlight the role in cancer of *CHD5*, which is required for the normal expression of *CDKN2A* (encoding p16INK4A and p19ARF) and is usually deleted in epithelial, neural, and hematopoietic malignancies (Bagchi et al. 2007).

1.3 The Epigenetic Role of miRNAs and Its Disruption in Cancer

miRNAs are the best studied type of ncRNAs. Generally speaking, these molecules, with an approximate length of 22 nucleotides, finely downregulate the expression of probably more than 60 % of protein-coding genes (Friedman et al. 2009b). However, in particular cases, miRNAs have also been found to increase the expression of their target genes (Vasudevan et al. 2007). Thus, miRNAs are involved in the majority of cellular functions, including proliferation, differentiation, and apoptosis (Davalos and Esteller 2010).

With respect to their biogenesis and mode of action, miRNAs are initially transcribed by RNA polymerase II as a pri-miRNA, a long, capped, polyadenylated transcript, which is further processed into a hairpin RNA precursor, the pre-miRNA, by the double-stranded RNA-specific ribonuclease Drosha, in collaboration with the microprocessor protein DGCR8 (Cai et al. 2004; Lee et al. 2004; Han et al. 2006). This pre-miRNA, a 70–100-nucleotide-long molecule, is then transported to the cytoplasm by Exportin-5 (XPO5) and, once there, cleaved by a large complex composed of Dicer, a ribonuclease III, and TRBP, a double-stranded RNA-binding protein (Hutvagner et al. 2001; Yi et al. 2003). The result is a duplex, 18–24 nucleotides long, which is then loaded into the RNA-induced silencing complex (RISC). In this complex, which includes proteins of the Argonaute family, one strand of the duplex remains stably associated, becoming the mature miRNA, and promotes RISC targeting normally (but not always) to the 3′ untranslated region (UTR) of the corresponding complementary mRNA (Davalos and Esteller 2010). If the miRNA and its target mRNA sequence match perfectly, the consequence is the cleavage and, hence, destruction of the latter. If they do not match perfectly, then mRNA translation is blocked (Davalos and Esteller 2010).

It is known that while each mRNA can be targeted by more than one miRNA (Vatolin et al. 2006), a single miRNA can regulate many different transcripts. In this regard, *miR-15a* and *miR-16* have been shown to regulate expression of ≈14 % of the human genome in a leukemic cell line (Calin et al. 2008).

It is widely accepted that an aberrant *miRNome*, with mainly downregulated but also upregulated miRNAs, is a hallmark of cancer (Croce 2009). In principle, these ncRNAs can regulate any gene and so in each tissue some of them act like *real* proto-oncogenes and some like *real* tumor suppressors. Therefore, it is not surprising that different chromosomal abnormalities, mutations, and/or polymorphisms (SNPs) affecting miRNA sequences have been described in many tumors, especially as miRNA genes are usually located in cancer-associated regions or fragile sites (Calin et al. 2004). Some examples include the deletion of the cluster *miR-15a/miR-16-1* (miRNAs are often found in clusters) in chronic B-cell lymphocytic leukemia (Calin et al. 2002), the amplification of *miR-26a* in glioblastoma (Huse et al. 2009), and the translocation of the *miR-17-92* cluster in T-cell acute lymphoblastic leukemia (Mavrakis et al. 2010). Moreover, the dysregulation of transcription factors like p53 or Myc, which are well established in cancer, promotes the misexpression of different miRNAs (in this case, the *miR-34* family and the *miR-17-92* cluster, respectively), thereby contributing to tumorigenesis (Davalos and Esteller 2010). Intriguingly, apart from particular examples, the pathological activation of Myc seems to globally repress miRNA expression and should be further investigated (Chang et al. 2008). Finally, defects in the miRNA processing machinery (see above) can also account for the altered miRNA levels related to cancer. For instance, frameshift mutations in the *TARBP2* gene, which encodes TARBP, lead to a decrease in normal miRNA levels, favoring tumorigenesis in sporadic and hereditary carcinomas with microsatellite instability (Melo et al. 2009). Likewise, mutations in *DICER1*, or the downregulation of the corresponding protein, have been shown to produce the same effect in some tumors (Bahubeshi et al. 2010; Merritt et al. 2008; Rio Frio et al. 2011).

However, most importantly, tumorigenic miRNA levels can also arise from the disruption of epigenetic mechanisms. Considering that approximately half of all miRNA genes are associated with CpG islands, it is not surprising that many of them have already been found to be silenced in cancer through CpG island promoter hypermethylation (Weber et al. 2007a). A good example is *miR-127*, which regulates the proto-oncogene *BCL6* and is silenced in several tumors (Saito et al. 2006). Others include *miR-9-1* in breast cancer, and *miR-34b* and *miR-34c* in colon cancer (Lehmann et al. 2008; Toyota et al. 2008). Additionally, this kind of aberrant silencing of *miR-9*, *miR-34b*, *miR-34c*, and *miR-148a*, which modulate *MYC*, *E2F3*, *CDK6*, and *TGIF2* expression, is known to give rise to metastatic capacities (Lujambio et al. 2008). Conversely, miRNAs controlling *real* tumor suppressors are activated in cancer by DNA hypomethylation, like *miR-21* in epithelial ovarian cancer (Iorio et al. 2007). As an example of the tissue specificity of epigenetic regulation, while *let-7a-3* is transcribed in lung adenocarcinoma due to DNA hypomethylation, it has also been found

Table 1.3 Epigenetically regulated miRNAs altered in human cancer

miRNA	Known target gene/s	Cancer type/s
let-7a-3	*IGF2*	Breast, lung, ovarian
miR-1	*FOXP1, MET, HDAC4*	HCC
miR-9-1	FGF and Claudin family genes	Multiple
miR-9-3	*CDH1*	Colorectal, head and neck, melanoma
miR-21	–	Ovarian
miR-29	–	Rabdomyosarcoma
miR-34a	*CD44, NOTCH1*	Multiple
miR-34b/c	*BCL2, CDK6, E2F3, MYC, NOTCH1, SIRT1*	Multiple
miR-107	*CDK6*	Pancreatic
miR-124	–	HCC
miR-124a	*CDK6, SMYD3, VIM*	Multiple
miR-126	–	Bladder, prostate
miR-127	*BCL6*	Bladder, prostate
miR-129-2	*SOX4*	Endometrial, gastric, colorectal
miR-137	*CDK6, E2F6, LSD1*	Oral, colorectal, glioblastoma
miR-141	*ZEB1, ZEB2*	Breast, colorectal, lung
miR145	*KLF4, OCT4, SOX2*	Prostate
miR-148a	*TGIF2*	Multiple
miR-181c	*KRAS, NOTCH4*	Gastric
miR-193b	–	Prostate
miR-196b	–	Gastric
miR-199a	*IKBKB, PODXL*	Ovarian, testicular
miR-200a/b	*ZEB2, ZFHX1B*	Breast, pancreatic
miR-200c	*ZEB1, ZEB2*	Breast, colorectal, lung
miR-203	*ABL1, ABCE1, CDK6*	ALL, HCC
miR-205	*ZEB1, ZEB2*	Bladder
miR-223	*MEF2C, NFIA*	AML
miR-335	*SOX4, TNC*	Breast
miR-342	*PDGFRA, RASA1*	Colorectal
miR-370	*MAP3K8*	Cholangiocarcinoma
miR-429	*ZEB1, ZEB2*	Breast, colorectal, lung
miR-449a/b	*CDC25A, CDK6, HDAC1*	Osteosarcoma, prostate
miR-512-5p	*MCL1*	Gastric

ALL acute lymphoblastic leukemia, *AML* acute myeloid leukemia, *HCC* hepatocellular carcinoma

to be silenced by promoter hypermethylation in ovarian cancer (Brueckner et al. 2007; Lu et al. 2007). However, DNA methylation cannot be the only epigenetic mechanism capable of leading to miRNA misexpression in cancer, given its strong relationship with covalent histone modifications and ATP-dependent chromatin-remodeling complexes. Thus, it is known that, upon inhibition of histone deacetylation, miRNA levels are profoundly altered in SKBR3 breast carcinoma cells (Scott et al. 2006). Moreover, it has been demonstrated in AML that the AML1/ETO fusion oncoprotein silences transcription of *miR-223* by recruiting HDAC activities (Fazi et al. 2007). For further examples, see Table 1.3.

Table 1.4 Epi-miRNAs altered in human cancer

miRNA	Known target gene/s	Cancer type/s
miR-1	*HDAC4*	Skeletal muscle tissue
miR-29a/b/c	*DNMT3a, DNMT3b*	AML, lung
miR-34b/c	*SIRT1*	Multiple
miR-101	*EZH2*	Bladder, prostate
miR-124a	*SMYD3*	Colorectal
miR-137	*LSD1*	Colorectal
miR-148a/b	*DNMT1, DNMT3b*	Cholangiocarcinoma, cervical
miR-152	*DNMT1*	Cholangiocarcinoma
miR-301	*DNMT1*	Cholangiocarcinoma
miR-449a	*HDAC1*	Prostate

AML acute myeloid leukemia

Finally, it is worth noting that epi-miRNAs, miRNAs which regulate the expression of members of the epigenetic machineries, can also be dysregulated in cancer. Good examples are *miR-29a*, *miR-29b*, and *miR-29c*, regulating *DNMT3a* and *DNMT3b*, in AML and lung cancer (Fabbri et al. 2007; Garzon et al. 2009) and *miR-101*, which regulates *EZH2*, in prostate and bladder cancer (Friedman et al. 2009; Varambally et al. 2008). Other examples are listed in Table 1.4.

1.4 Epigenetic Control of Stem Cell Behavior

1.4.1 Epigenetic Status in ES Cells

The definition of stemness includes two main capacities: indefinite self-renewal and pluripotency. The best experimental model for studying stemness is probably that of ES cells; derived from the inner cell mass of blastocyst-stage embryos, these cells are able to differentiate into any possible cell type, either fetal or adult, both in vivo and in vitro (Jaenisch and Young 2008). In general, and in contrast to what happens in differentiated cells, the chromatin of ES cells is in an *open* state; in fact, its constitutive heterochromatin (centromeres, telomeres, etc.) appears rather dispersed and there is a highly dynamic exchange of both histones and nonhistone proteins (including HP1) (Orkin and Hochedlinger 2011). These special chromatin features reflect the unusual nature of these cells; they are devoted not only to preserving their identity but also to maintaining their genomes in a flexible state capable of giving rise to any cell type. Although it is well established that stemness mainly requires a key set of transcription factors (Oct4, Nanog, Sox2, c-Myc, among others), it is also obvious that epigenetic mechanisms contribute decisively to providing the special chromatin characteristics of ES cells.

In the human genome, promoters can be divided into two main categories according to their CpG content: those with high CpG density (the vast majority), normally corresponding to housekeeping and tightly regulated developmental genes, and those with low CpG density, which are mainly associated with tissue-specific genes. The first group displays low DNA methylation levels and, in principle, should be transcriptionally active (Meissner et al. 2008; Mikkelsen et al. 2007), while the

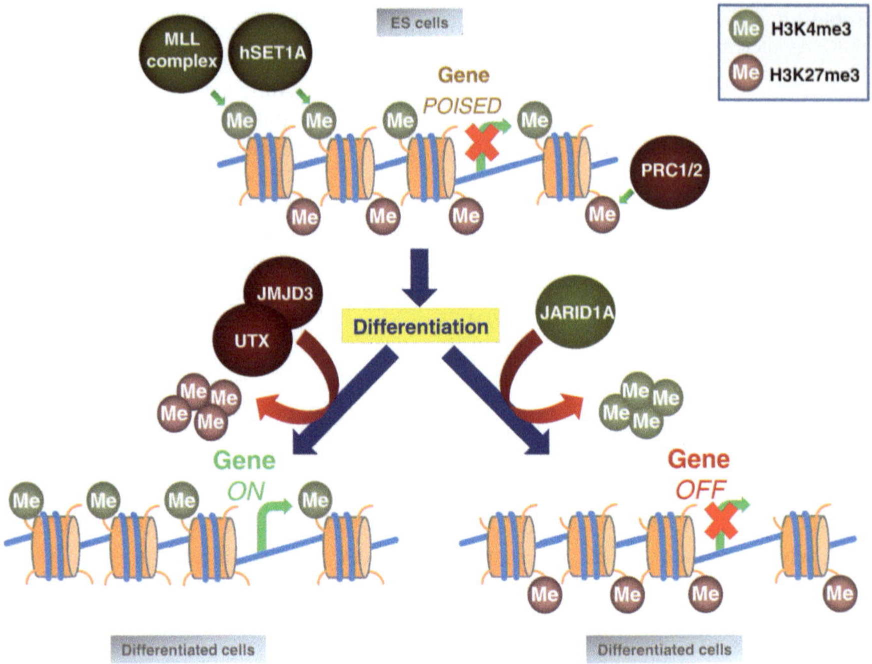

Fig. 1.2 Basic features of bivalent domains in ES and differentiated cells for a typical developmental gene. In ES cells, developmental genes are repressed but poised for full activation or repression upon differentiation. These genes present both activating (H3K4me3) and repressive (H3K27me3) covalent histone modifications around their TSSs. If differentiation involves a definitive activation of the gene, the HDMs UTX and JMJD3 *erase* the H3K27me3 mark; if it involves permanent repression, the HDM JARID1A removes the H3K4me3 mark. The figure also shows the enzymes and complexes in charge of placing H3K4me3 (hSET1A and different complexes with MLL proteins) and H3K27me3 (PRC1 and, mainly, PRC2 complexes)

other tends to be hypermethylated and, therefore, silenced (Meissner et al. 2008; Weber et al. 2007b). Nevertheless, to maintain stemness, the subgroup of developmental genes (the ones able to trigger the different differentiation programs) cannot be active. This problem is solved by additional covalent histone modifications. Thus, while housekeeping and tissue-specific genes present typical *active* and *inactive* histone marks, respectively, developmental genes present both (Bernstein et al. 2006; Mikkelsen et al. 2007). The so-called bivalent domains are characterized by the simultaneous presence of H3K4me3 and H3K27me3 marks, are frequently located on the binding sites of the transcription factors in charge of the decision stemness/differentiation (including Oct4, Nanog, and Sox2), and keep these genes repressed but poised to become fully active or silenced, depending on the triggering of particular differentiation programs (Bernstein et al. 2006; Mikkelsen et al. 2007). While the H3K4me3 mark is mediated through the hSET1A and/or diverse MLL complexes (Christophersen and Helin 2010), the H3K27me3 mark is placed by EZH1 or, mainly, EZH2, core members of the Polycomb repressive complexes 1 and 2 (PRC1 and PRC2), respectively (Fig. 1.2) (Margueron et al. 2008; Margueron and Reinberg 2011). These latter complexes are recruited to their target genes either by proteins like MTF2 and JARID2, a catalytically inactive HDM, or through short ncRNAs previously transcribed from them (Kanhere et al. 2010; Landeira et al. 2010; Walker et al. 2010). Their action sets not only the H3K27me3 mark but also the H2AK119ub (via PRC1), which blocks RNA polymerase II activity and is essential for maintaining ES cell identity (Endoh et al. 2008; Stock et al. 2007). The H2A variant H2A.Z has also been found enriched at some of these target genes (Creyghton et al. 2008).

As described in the DNA methylation section, upon differentiation, only a few genes become silenced by CpG island promoter hypermethylation, including germ line-specific and pluripotency genes (such as *POU5F1* and *NANOG*, which encode Oct4 and Nanog, respectively), different tissue-specific genes depending on each cell type, and genes involved in genomic imprinting and X-chromosome inactivation (Mohn et al. 2008; Straussman et al. 2009; Suzuki and Bird 2008). In fact, it also explained that most of the changes in DNA methylation were found, on the one hand, at CpG island shores and, on the other hand, in a non-CpG context (Doi et al. 2009; Laurent et al. 2010; Lister et al. 2009; Meissner et al. 2008). Genes with bivalent domains become less frequent as differentiation progresses (Fisher and Fisher 2011), usually ending up fully activated or repressed (Hawkins et al. 2010). In the former situation, the H3K27me3 mark is removed by the action of the HDMs UTX and JMJD3 (Christophersen and Helin 2010); in the latter, the H3K4me3 mark disappears by means of JARID1A (Fig. 1.2) (Pasini et al. 2008).

At this point, it is worth mentioning that other enzymes in charge of different covalent histone modifications have also been linked to stemness, for instance, the HMTs CARM1, EHMT1, EHMT2, and SETDB1 and the HDMs LSD1, JARID1B, JHDM2A, and JHDM3C (Lessard and Crabtree 2010; Orkin and Hochedlinger 2011).

Some ATP-dependent chromatin-remodeling complexes, on the other hand, play an important role in ES cells. Containing the ATPase BRG1 and subunits such as BAF155 and BAF60a, but never hBRM, BAF170, or BAF60c (like in differentiated cells), the ES cell-specific BAF complex, esBAF, is essential for self-renewal and pluripotency (Fisher and Fisher 2011; Ho et al. 2009). It is present in about the 25 % of promoters in ES cells, where it interacts with key transcription factors like Oct4, Sox2, Nanog, STAT3, and SMAD1 (Ho et al. 2009; Kidder et al. 2009); although it promotes the activation of many genes, its main functions related to stemness seem to be the repression of genes involved in differentiation, as well as the prevention of the overexpression of pluripotency-specific genes (Saladi and de la Serna 2010). Also essential for stemness, the TIP60-p400 complex is recruited to more than half of the promoters in ES cells by either the H3K4me3 mark (directly) or Nanog (indirectly); despite its normally activating HAT activity on histone H4, it mainly represses developmental genes in the context of other repressive marks (Fazzio et al. 2008). On the other hand, the ATPase CHD1 is key to maintaining the typical *open* chromatin of ES cells. Without it, an abnormal accumulation of heterochromatic foci makes correct differentiation impossible (Gaspar-Maia et al. 2009). It is tempting to speculate that CHD1 may accomplish its mission through the deposition of the histone variant H3.3, which is already found enriched at bivalent domains, as it does in *Drosophila* (Goldberg et al. 2010). Other ATP-dependent chromatin-remodeling factors involved in stemness are BPTF and MBD3, which are subunits of the NURF and NuRD complexes, respectively, and are mainly linked to the maintenance of pluripotency (Landry et al. 2008; Zhu et al. 2009). Finally, it has also been reported that CHD7 modulates ES cell-specific gene expression by targeting enhancers of active genes (Schnetz et al. 2010).

In mouse ES cells, the disruption of any enzyme involved in their biogenesis impairs stemness (Pauli et al. 2011). The ES cell-specific miRNAs, *miR-290-295*, were found to be able to complement the proliferative defects that appeared in *Dgcr8* knockout cells (Wang et al. 2008a). It has also been discovered that Oct4, Nanog, Sox2, or Tcf3 bind to the promoters of these and many other miRNAs, such as *let-7* and *miR-145* (Marson et al. 2008). However, the latter two remain normally repressed in ES cells by means of the PRC2 complex, and upon differentiation, both are transcribed and downregulate genes encoding key pluripotency factors like lin-28 and SALL4 (*let-7*) or Oct4, Sox2, and Klf4 (*miR-145*) (Melton et al. 2010; Xu et al. 2009). Consistently, repression of *let-7* in somatic cells contributes to their reprogramming (Melton et al. 2010). Related to the latter, it seems that the overexpression of the *miR-302-367* cluster alone could be enough as to induce pluripotency in fibroblasts (Anokye-Danso et al. 2011; Lin et al. 2011).

1.4.2 The Cancer Stem Cell Theory

Tumorigenesis is considered to be a complex multistep process whereby cells, after accumulating epigenetic and/or genetic alterations, display uncontrolled proliferation and aberrant patterns of differentiation due to the activation of oncogenes and/or silencing of tumor suppressors. However, the issue of cancer initiation remains under intense discussion. In the previous century, the clonal genetic model, which was based merely on subsequent genetic mutations in differentiated cells, was widely supported, but currently, the possibility that epigenetic dysregulation may precede genetic alterations and that stem cells may be the origin of some (if not all) tumors is an increasingly popular idea.

The cancer stem cell model postulates that epigenetic changes occurring in normal stem or progenitor cells may be the earliest events in tumorigenesis (Feinberg et al. 2006). Such an idea is consistent with several observations. First, it is known that certain epigenetic alterations indeed occur very early in various types of cancer and that, additionally, normal tissues have altered progenitor cells in cancer patients (Cui et al. 2003; Matsubayashi et al. 2003; Peters et al. 2007). Second, tumors normally include different cell populations with diverse tumorigenic and metastatic capacities (Al-Hajj et al. 2003). Third, it is well established, as we have already seen, that epigenetic mechanisms are essential for maintaining stemness (Surani et al. 2007; Wang et al. 2008b). Finally, human ES cells with cancer cell characteristics have already been found (Werbowetski-Ogilvie et al. 2009). Therefore, epigenetic disruption in a stem/progenitor cell of a particular tissue may create a different population with enhanced stemness, a high-risk cell population capable of undergoing transformation more easily after gaining subsequent genetic and epigenetic changes (Jones and Baylin 2007). Once generated, this resulting small cancer stem cell population would be able not only to self-renew but also to produce the phenotypically diverse cancer cells responsible for the usual massive tumor proliferation. Although this model remains a hypothesis, in the last decade, numerous studies have already described cancer-initiating cells in diverse solid tumors (Al-Hajj et al. 2003; Collins et al. 2005a; Dalerba et al. 2007; Li et al. 2007b; O'Brien et al. 2007; Prince et al. 2007; Ricci-Vitiani et al. 2007; Singh et al. 2004; Suetsugu et al. 2006). Most interestingly from a clinical point of view, others have reported that, unlike their derivatives, cancer stem cells are resistant to conventional chemo- and radiotherapy and could be responsible for eventual tumor repopulation and treatment failure (Bao et al. 2006; Matsui et al. 2008).

1.5 Concluding Remarks

Epigenetics is going through its golden age. Modern high-throughput technologies based on the combination of either bisulfite treatment of methylated DNA or chromatin immunoprecipitation with next-generation sequencing (methylC-seq and ChIP-seq, respectively) allow us to determine complete individual DNA methylomes and the exact position along the genome of any covalent histone modification or member of the epigenetic machineries. The information obtained by these kinds of epigenomic approach is now making the difference not only in basic epigenetic research but also to our understanding of stemness and tumorigenesis. The objective is to fully establish the role of epigenetic mechanisms in the origin and progression of the disease in order to be able to offer a more personalized treatment. However, there is still much work to do in many very exciting areas. For instance, we also need to expand our knowledge about DNA demethylation and the degree of participation of ncRNAs in the positioning of covalent histone modifications. In fact, there are still many marks of the histone code to identify and many combinations to understand in the different cellular contexts. The composition and function of some ATP-dependent chromatin-remodeling complexes also remain unknown, and moreover, connections between the epigenetic machineries and miRNAs still need to be much better understood. Finally, further research is needed to shed light on the epigenetic processes underlying stemness.

References

Agger K, Cloos PA, Rudkjaer L, Williams K, Andersen G, Christensen J, Helin K (2009) The H3K27me3 demethylase JMJD3 contributes to the activation of the INK4A-ARF locus in response to oncogene- and stress-induced senescence. Genes Dev 23(10):1171–1176. doi:10.1101/gad.510809, 23/10/1171 [pii]

Al-Hajj M, Wicha MS, Benito-Hernandez A, Morrison SJ, Clarke MF (2003) Prospective identification of tumorigenic breast cancer cells. Proc Natl Acad Sci U S A 100(7):3983–3988. doi:10.1073/pnas.0530291100, 0530291100 [pii]

Allis CD, Berger SL, Cote J, Dent S, Jenuwien T, Kouzarides T, Pillus L et al (2007) New nomenclature for chromatin-modifying enzymes. Cell 131(4):633–636. doi:10.1016/j.cell.2007.10.039, S0092-8674(07)01359-1 [pii]

Anokye-Danso F, Trivedi CM, Juhr D, Gupta M, Cui Z, Tian Y, Zhang Y et al (2011) Highly efficient miRNA-mediated reprogramming of mouse and human somatic cells to pluripotency. Cell Stem Cell 8(4):376–388. doi:10.1016/j.stem.2011.03.001, S1934-5909(11)00111-1 [pii]

Ayton PM, Cleary ML (2001) Molecular mechanisms of leukemogenesis mediated by MLL fusion proteins. Oncogene 20(40):5695–5707. doi:10.1038/sj.onc.1204639

Badal V, Chuang LS, Tan EH, Badal S, Villa LL, Wheeler CM, Li BF, Bernard HU (2003) CpG methylation of human papillomavirus type 16 DNA in cervical cancer cell lines and in clinical specimens: genomic hypomethylation correlates with carcinogenic progression. J Virol 77(11):6227–6234

Bagchi A, Papazoglu C, Wu Y, Capurso D, Brodt M, Francis D, Bredel M, Vogel H, Mills AA (2007) CHD5 is a tumor suppressor at human 1p36. Cell 128(3):459–475. doi:10.1016/j.cell.2006.11.052, S0092-8674(07)00053-0 [pii]

Bahubeshi A, Bal N, Frio TR, Hamel N, Pouchet C, Yilmaz A, Bouron-Dal Soglio D et al (2010) Germline DICER1 mutations and familial cystic nephroma. J Med Genet 47(12):863–866. doi:10.1136/jmg.2010.081216, jmg.2010.081216 [pii]

Bannister AJ, Kouzarides T (2011) Regulation of chromatin by histone modifications. Cell Res 21(3):381–395. doi:10.1038/cr.2011.22, cr201122 [pii]

Bannister AJ, Zegerman P, Partridge JF, Miska EA, Thomas JO, Allshire RC, Kouzarides T (2001) Selective recognition of methylated lysine 9 on histone H3 by the HP1 chromo domain. Nature 410(6824):120–124. doi:10.1038/35065138, 35065138 [pii]

Bao Y, Shen X (2007) SnapShot: chromatin remodeling complexes. Cell 129(3):632. doi:10.1016/j.cell.2007.04.018, S0092-8674(07)00524-7 [pii]

Bao S, Wu Q, McLendon RE, Hao Y, Shi Q, Hjelmeland AB, Dewhirst MW, Bigner DD, Rich JN (2006) Glioma stem cells promote radioresistance by preferential activation of the DNA damage response. Nature 444(7120):756–760. doi:10.1038/nature05236, nature05236 [pii]

Barski A, Cuddapah S, Cui K, Roh TY, Schones DE, Wang Z, Wei G, Chepelev I, Zhao K (2007) High-resolution profiling of histone methylations in the human genome. Cell 129(4):823–837. doi:10.1016/j.cell.2007.05.009, S0092-8674(07)00600-9 [pii]

Bartke T, Vermeulen M, Xhemalce B, Robson SC, Mann M, Kouzarides T (2010) Nucleosome-interacting proteins regulated by DNA and histone methylation. Cell 143(3):470–484. doi:10.1016/j.cell.2010.10.012, S0092-8674(10)01182-7 [pii]

Bedford MT, Clarke SG (2009) Protein arginine methylation in mammals: who, what, and why. Mol Cell 33(1):1–13. doi:10.1016/j.molcel.2008.12.013, S1097-2765(08)00856-3 [pii]

Berdasco M, Ropero S, Setien F, Fraga MF, Lapunzina P, Losson R, Alaminos M, Cheung NK, Rahman N, Esteller M (2009) Epigenetic inactivation of the Sotos overgrowth syndrome gene histone methyltransferase NSD1 in human neuroblastoma and glioma. Proc Natl Acad Sci U S A 106(51):21830–21835. doi:10.1073/pnas.0906831106, 0906831106 [pii]

Berger SL, Kouzarides T, Shiekhattar R, Shilatifard A (2009) An operational definition of epigenetics. Genes Dev 23(7):781–783. doi:10.1101/gad.1787609, 23/7/781 [pii]

Bernstein BE, Mikkelsen TS, Xie X, Kamal M, Huebert DJ, Cuff J, Fry B et al (2006) A bivalent chromatin structure marks key developmental genes in embryonic stem cells. Cell 125(2):315–326. doi:10.1016/j.cell.2006.02.041, S0092-8674(06)00380-1 [pii]

Bhalla KN (2005) Epigenetic and chromatin modifiers as targeted therapy of hematologic malignancies. J Clin Oncol 23(17):3971–3993. doi:10.1200/JCO.2005.16.600, JCO.2005.16.600 [pii]

Bogdanovic O, Veenstra GJ (2009) DNA methylation and methyl-CpG binding proteins: developmental requirements and function. Chromosoma 118(5):549–565. doi:10.1007/s00412-009 0221-9

Bostick M, Kim JK, Esteve PO, Clark A, Pradhan S, Jacobsen SE (2007) UHRF1 plays a role in maintaining DNA methylation in mammalian cells. Science 317(5845):1760–1764. doi:10.1126/science.1147939, 1147939 [pii]

Bourc'his D, Xu GL, Lin CS, Bollman B, Bestor TH (2001) Dnmt3L and the establishment of maternal genomic imprints. Science 294(5551):2536–2539

Bracken AP, Helin K (2009) Polycomb group proteins: navigators of lineage pathways led astray in cancer. Nat Rev Cancer 9(11):773–784. doi:10.1038/nrc2736, nrc2736 [pii]

Brueckner B, Stresemann C, Kuner R, Mund C, Musch T, Meister M, Sultmann H, Lyko F (2007) The human let-7a-3 locus contains an epigenetically regulated microRNA gene with oncogenic function. Cancer Res 67(4):1419–1423. doi:10.1158/0008-5472.CAN-06-4074, 67/4/1419 [pii]

Burbee DG, Forgacs E, Zochbauer-Muller S, Shivakumar L, Fong K, Gao B, Randle D et al (2001) Epigenetic inactivation of RASSF1A in lung and breast cancers and malignant phenotype suppression. J Natl Cancer Inst 93(9):691–699

Burke TW, Cook JG, Asano M, Nevins JR (2001) Replication factors MCM2 and ORC1 interact with the histone acetyltransferase HBO1. J Biol Chem 276(18):15397–15408. doi:10.1074/jbc.M011556200, M011556200 [pii]

Cai X, Hagedorn CH, Cullen BR (2004) Human microRNAs are processed from capped, polyadenylated transcripts that can also function as mRNAs. RNA 10(12):1957–1966. doi:10.1261/rna.7135204, rna.7135204 [pii]

Calin GA, Dumitru CD, Shimizu M, Bichi R, Zupo S, Noch E, Aldler H et al (2002) Frequent deletions and down-regulation of micro-RNA genes miR15 and miR16 at 13q14 in chronic lymphocytic leukemia. Proc Natl Acad Sci U S A 99(24):15524–15529. doi:10.1073/pnas.242606799, 242606799 [pii]

Calin GA, Sevignani C, Dumitru CD, Hyslop T, Noch E, Yendamuri S, Shimizu M et al (2004) Human microRNA genes are frequently located at fragile sites and genomic regions involved in cancers. Proc Natl Acad Sci U S A 101(9):2999–3004. doi:10.1073/pnas.0307323101, 0307323101 [pii]

Calin GA, Cimmino A, Fabbr M, Ferracin M, Wojcik SE, Shimizu M, Taccioli C et al (2008) MiR-15a and miR-16-1 cluster functions in human leukemia. Proc Natl Acad Sci U S A 105(13):5166–5171. doi:10.1073/pnas.0800121105, 0800121105 [pii]

Ceol CJ, Houvras Y, Jane-Valbuena J, Bilodeau S, Orlando DA, Battisti V, Fritsch L et al (2011) The histone methyltransferase SETDB1 is recurrently amplified in melanoma and accelerates its onset. Nature 471(7339):513–517. doi:10.1038/nature09806, nature09806 [pii]

Chadwick BP, Willard HF (2002) Cell cycle-dependent localization of macroH2A in chromatin of the inactive X chromosome. J Cell Biol 157(7):1113–1123. doi:10.1083/jcb.200112074, jcb.200112074 [pii]

Chai J, Charboneau AL, Betz BL, Weissman BE (2005) Loss of the hSNF5 gene concomitantly inactivates p21CIP/WAF1 and p16INK4a activity associated with replicative senescence in A204 rhabdoid tumor cells. Cancer Res 65(22):10192–10198. doi:10.1158/0008-5472.CAN-05-1896, 65/22/10192 [pii]

Champagne KS, Kutateladze TG (2009) Structural insight into histone recognition by the ING PHD fingers. Curr Drug Targets 10(5):432–441

Champagne N, Bertos NR, Pelletier N, Wang AH, Vezmar M, Yang Y, Heng HH, Yang XJ (1999) Identification of a human histone acetyltransferase related to monocytic leukemia zinc finger protein. J Biol Chem 274(40):28528–28536

Chan EM, Chan RJ, Comer EM, Goulet RJ 3rd, Crean CD, Brown ZD, Fruehwald AM et al (2007) MOZ and MOZ-CBP cooperate with NF-kappaB to activate transcription from NF-kappaB-dependent promoters. Exp Hematol 35(12):1782–1792. doi:10.1016/j.exphem.2007.07.015, S0301-472X(07)00437-7 [pii]

Chang TC, Yu D, Lee YS, Wentzel EA, Arking DE, West KM, Dang CV, Thomas-Tikhonenko A, Mendell JT (2008) Widespread microRNA repression by Myc contributes to tumorigenesis. Nat Genet 40(1):43–50. doi:10.1038/ng.2007.30, ng.2007.30 [pii]

Cheng X, Collins RE, Zhang X (2005) Structural and sequence motifs of protein (histone) methylation enzymes. Annu Rev Biophys Biomol Struct 34:267–294. doi:10.1146/annurev.biophys.34.040204.144452

Chi P, Allis CD, Wang GG (2010) Covalent histone modifications – miswritten, misinterpreted and mis-erased in human cancers. Nat Rev Cancer 10(7):457–469. doi:10.1038/nrc2876, nrc2876 [pii]

Christophersen NS, Helin K (2010) Epigenetic control of embryonic stem cell fate. J Exp Med 207(11):2287–2295. doi:10.1084/jem.20101438, em.20101438 [pii]

Chuang LS, Ian HI, Koh TW, Ng HH, Xu G, Li BF (1997) Human DNA-(cytosine-5) methyltransferase-PCNA complex as a target for p21WAF1. Science 277(5334):1996–2000

Clapier CR, Cairns BR (2009) The biology of chromatin remodeling complexes. Annu Rev Biochem 78:273–304. doi:10.1146/annurev.biochem.77.062706.153223

Collins AT, Berry PA, Hyde C, Stower MJ, Maitland NJ (2005a) Prospective identification of tumorigenic prostate cancer stem cells. Cancer Res 65(23):10946–10951. doi:10.1158/0008-5472.CAN-05-2018, 65/23/10946 [pii]

Collins RE, Tachibana M, Tamaru H, Smith KM, Jia D, Zhang X, Selker EU, Shinkai Y, Cheng X (2005b) In vitro and in vivo analyses of a Phe/Tyr switch controlling product specificity of histone lysine methyltransferases. J Biol Chem 280(7):5563–5570. doi:10.1074/jbc.M410483200, M410483200 [pii]

Corona DF, Tamkun JW (2004) Multiple roles for ISWI in transcription, chromosome organization and DNA replication. Biochim Biophys Acta 1677(1–3):113–119. doi:10.1016/j.bbaexp.2003.09.018, S0167478103002835 [pii]

Creyghton MP, Markoulaki S, Levine SS, Hanna J, Lodato MA, Sha K, Young RA, Jaenisch R, Boyer LA (2008) H2AZ is enriched at polycomb complex target genes in ES cells and is necessary for lineage commitment. Cell 135(4):649–661. doi:10.1016/j.cell.2008.09.056, S0092-8674(08)01252-X [pii]

Croce CM (2009) Causes and consequences of microRNA dysregulation in cancer. Nat Rev Genet 10(10):704–714. doi:10.1038/nrg2634, nrg2634 [pii]

Cui H, Cruz-Correa M, Giardiello FM, Hutcheon DF, Kafonek DR, Brandenburg S, Wu Y, He X, Powe NR, Feinberg AP (2003) Loss of IGF2 imprinting: a potential marker of colorectal cancer risk. Science 299(5613):1753–1755. doi:10.1126/science.1080902 299/5613/1753 [pii]

Dalerba P, Dylla SJ, Park IK, Liu R, Wang X, Cho RW, Hoey T et al (2007) Phenotypic characterization of human colorectal cancer stem cells. Proc Natl Acad Sci U S A 104(24):10158–10163. doi:10.1073/pnas.0703478104, 0703478104 [pii]

Dalgliesh GL, Furge K, Greenman C, Chen L, Bignell G, Butler A, Davies H et al (2010) Systematic sequencing of renal carcinoma reveals inactivation of histone modifying genes. Nature 463(7279):360–363. doi:10.1038/nature08672, nature08672 [pii]

Dammann R, Li C, Yoon JH, Chin PL, Bates S, Pfeifer GP (2000) Epigenetic inactivation of a RAS association domain family protein from the lung tumour suppressor locus 3p21.3. Nat Genet 25(3):315–319. doi:10.1038/77083

Daniel FI, Cherubini K, Yurgel LS, de Figueiredo MA, Salum FG (2011) The role of epigenetic transcription repression and DNA methyltransferases in cancer. Cancer 117(4):677–687. doi:10.1002/cncr.25482

Dar AA, Goff LW, Majid S, Berlin J, El-Rifai W (2010) Aurora kinase inhibitors – rising stars in cancer therapeutics? Mol Cancer Ther 9(2):268–278. doi:10.1158/1535-7163.MCT-09-0765, 1535-7163.MCT-09-0765 [pii]

Davalos V, Esteller M (2010) MicroRNAs and cancer epigenetics: a macrorevolution. Curr Opin Oncol 22(1):35–45. doi:10.1097/CCO.0b013e328333dcbb

Davis CA, Haberland M, Arnold MA, Sutherland LB, McDonald OG, Richardson JA, Childs G, Harris S, Owens GK, Olson EN (2006) PRISM/PRDM6, a transcriptional repressor that promotes the proliferative gene program in smooth muscle cells. Mol Cell Biol 26(7):2626–2636. doi:10.1128/MCB.26.7.2626-2636.2006, 26/7/2626 [pii]

Dawson MA, Bannister AJ, Gottgens B, Foster SD, Bartke T, Green AR, Kouzarides T (2009) JAK2 phosphorylates histone H3Y41 and excludes HP1alpha from chromatin. Nature 461(7265):819–822. doi:10.1038/nature08448, nature08448 [pii]

de la Cruz X, Lois S, Sanchez-Molina S, Martinez-Balbas MA (2005) Do protein motifs read the histone code? Bioessays 27(2):164–175. doi:10.1002/bies.20176

Deaton AM, Bird A (2011) CpG islands and the regulation of transcription. Genes Dev 25(10):1010–1022. doi:10.1101/gad.2037511, 25/10/1010 [pii]

den Hollander J, Rimpi S, Doherty JR, Rudelius M, Buck A, Hoellein A, Kremer M et al (2010) Aurora kinases A and B are up-regulated by Myc and are essential for maintenance of the malignant state. Blood 116(9):1498–1505. doi:10.1182/blood-2009-11-251074, blood-2009-11-251074 [pii]

Di Croce L, Raker VA, Corsaro M, Fazi F, Fanelli M, Faretta M, Fuks F et al (2002) Methyltransferase recruitment and DNA hypermethylation of target promoters by an oncogenic transcription factor. Science 295(5557):1079–1082. doi:10.1126/science.1065173, 295/5557/1079 [pii]

Doi A, Park IH, Wen B, Murakami P, Aryee MJ, Irizarry R, Herb B et al (2009) Differential methylation of tissue- and cancer-specific CpG island shores distinguishes human induced pluripotent stem cells, embryonic stem cells and fibroblasts. Nat Genet 41(12):1350–1353. doi:10.1038/ng.471, ng.471 [pii]

Dorrance AM, Liu S, Chong A, Pulley B, Nemer D, Guimond M, Yuan W et al (2008) The Mll partial tandem duplication: differential, tissue-specific activity in the presence or absence of the wild-type allele. Blood 112(6):2508–2511. doi:10.1182/blood-2008-01-134338, blood-2008-01-134338 [pii]

Doyon Y, Cayrou C, Ullah M, Landry AJ, Cote V, Selleck W, Lane WS, Tan S, Yang XJ, Cote J (2006) ING tumor suppressor proteins are critical regulators of chromatin acetylation required for genome expression and perpetuation. Mol Cell 21(1):51–64. doi:10.1016/j.molcel.2005.12.007, S1097-2765(05)01849-6 [pii]

Duan Q, Chen H, Costa M, Dai W (2008) Phosphorylation of H3S10 blocks the access of H3K9 by specific antibodies and histone methyltransferase. Implication in regulating chromatin dynamics and epigenetic inheritance during mitosis. J Biol Chem 283(48):33585–33590. doi:10.1074/jbc.M803312200, M803312200 [pii]

Duncan EM, Muratore-Schroeder TL, Cook RG, Garcia BA, Shabanowitz J, Hunt DF, Allis CD (2008) Cathepsin L proteolytically processes histone H3 during mouse embryonic stem cell differentiation. Cell 135(2):284–294. doi:10.1016/j.cell.2008.09.055, S0092-8674(08)01248-8 [pii]

Eden A, Gaudet F, Waghmare A, Jaenisch R (2003) Chromosomal instability and tumors promoted by DNA hypomethylation. Science 300(5618):455. doi:10.1126/science.1083557, 300/5618/455 [pii]

Ellis L, Atadja PW, Johnstone RW (2009) Epigenetics in cancer: targeting chromatin modifications. Mol Cancer Ther 8(6):1409–1420

Endoh M, Endo TA, Endoh T, Fujimura Y, Ohara O, Toyoda T, Otte AP et al (2008) Polycomb group proteins Ring1A/B are functionally linked to the core transcriptional regulatory circuitry to maintain ES cell identity. Development 135(8):1513–1524. doi:10.1242/dev.014340, dev.014340 [pii]

Esteller M (2007) Cancer epigenomics: DNA methylomes and histone-modification maps. Nat Rev Genet 8(4):286–298. doi:10.1038/nrg2005, nrg2005 [pii]

Esteller M (2008) Epigenetics in cancer. N Engl J Med 358(11):1148–1159. doi:10.1056/NEJMra072067, 358/11/1148 [pii]

Esteve PO, Chin HG, Benner J, Feehery GR, Samaranayake M, Horwitz GA, Jacobsen SE, Pradhan S (2009) Regulation of DNMT1 stability through SET7-mediated lysine methylation in mammalian cells. Proc Natl Acad Sci U S A 106(13):5076–5081. doi:10.1073/pnas.0810362106, 0810362106 [pii]

Fabbri M, Garzon R, Cimmino A, Liu Z, Zanesi N, Callegari E, Liu S et al (2007) MicroRNA-29 family reverts aberrant methylation in lung cancer by targeting DNA methyltransferases 3A and 3B. Proc Natl Acad Sci U S A 104(40):15805–15810. doi:10.1073/pnas.0707628104, 0707628104 [pii]

Fazi F, Racanicchi S, Zardo G, Starnes LM, Mancini M, Travaglini L, Diverio D et al (2007) Epigenetic silencing of the myelopoiesis regulator microRNA-223 by the AML1/ETO oncoprotein. Cancer Cell 12(5):457–466. doi:10.1016/j.ccr.2007.09.020, S1535-6108(07)00268-1 [pii]

Fazzio TG, Huff JT, Panning B (2008) Tip60-p400 as a regulator of embryonic stem cell identity. Cell 1 134(1):162–174. doi:10.1016/j.cell.2008.05.031, S0092-8674(08)00692-2 [pii]

Feinberg AP, Ohlsson R, Henikoff S (2006) The epigenetic progenitor origin of human cancer. Nat Rev Genet 7(1):21–33. doi:10.1038/nrg1748, nrg1748 [pii]

Feng Q, Wang H, Ng HH, Erdjument-Bromage H, Tempst P, Struhl K, Zhang Y (2002) Methylation of H3-lysine 79 is mediated by a new family of HMTases without a SET domain. Curr Biol 12(12):1052–1058, S0960982202009016 [pii]

Ferrari R, Pellegrini M, Horwitz GA, Xie W, Berk AJ, Kurdistani SK (2008) Epigenetic reprogramming by adenovirus e1a. Science 321(5892):1086–1088. doi:10.1126/science.1155546, 321/5892/1086 [pii]

Fischle W, Tseng BS, Dormann HL, Ueberheide BM, Garcia BA, Shabanowitz J, Hunt DF, Funabiki H, Allis CD (2005) Regulation of HP1-chromatin binding by histone H3 methylation and phosphorylation. Nature 438(7071):1116–1122

Fisher CL, Fisher AG (2011) Chromatin states in pluripotent, differentiated, and reprogrammed cells. Curr Opin Genet Dev 21(2):140–146. doi:10.1016/j.gde.2011.01.015, S0959-437X(11)00019-0 [pii]

Flaus A, Martin DM, Barton GJ, Owen-Hughes T (2006) Identification of multiple distinct Snf2 subfamilies with conserved structural motifs. Nucleic Acids Res 34(10):2887–2905. doi:10.1093/nar/gkl295, 34/10/2887 [pii]

Fraga MF, Ballestar E, Villar-Garea A, Boix-Chornet M, Espada J, Schotta G, Bonaldi T et al (2005) Loss of acetylation at Lys16 and trimethylation at Lys20 of histone H4 is a common hallmark of human cancer. Nat Genet 37(4):391–400. doi:10.1038/ng1531, ng1531 [pii]

Friedman JM, Liang G, Liu CC, Wolff EM, Tsai YC, Ye W, Zhou X, Jones PA (2009a) The putative tumor suppressor microRNA-101 modulates the cancer epigenome by repressing the polycomb group protein EZH2. Cancer Res 69(6):2623–2629. doi:10.1158/0008-5472.CAN-08-3114, 0008-5472.CAN-08-3114 [pii]

Friedman RC, Farh KK, Burge CB, Bartel DP (2009b) Most mammalian mRNAs are conserved targets of microRNAs. Genome Res 19(1):92–105. doi:10.1101/gr.082701.108, gr.082701.108 [pii]

Frigola J, Song J, Stirzaker C, Hinshelwood RA, Peinado MA, Clark SJ (2006) Epigenetic remodeling in colorectal cancer results in coordinate gene suppression across an entire chromosome band. Nat Genet 38(5):540–549. doi:10.1038/ng1781, ng1781 [pii]

Funabiki T, Kreider BL, Ihle JN (1994) The carboxyl domain of zinc fingers of the Evi-1 myeloid transforming gene binds a consensus sequence of GAAGATGAG. Oncogene 9(6):1575–1581

Futscher BW, Oshiro MM, Wozniak RJ, Holtan N, Hanigan CL, Duan H, Domann FE (2002) Role for DNA methylation in the control of cell type specific maspin expression. Nat Genet 31(2):175–179. doi:10.1038/ng886, ng886 [pii]

Garzon R, Liu S, Fabbri M, Liu Z, Heaphy CE, Callegari E, Schwind S et al (2009) MicroRNA-29b induces global DNA hypomethylation and tumor suppressor gene reexpression in acute myeloid leukemia by targeting directly DNMT3A and 3B and indirectly DNMT1. Blood 113(25):6411–6418. doi:10.1182/blood-2008-07-170589, blood-2008-07-170589 [pii]

Gaspar-Maia A, Alajem A, Polesso F, Sridharan R, Mason MJ, Heidersbach A, Ramalho-Santos J et al (2009) Chd1 regulates open chromatin and pluripotency of embryonic stem cells. Nature 460(7257):863–868. doi:10.1038/nature08212, nature08212 [pii]

Gayther SA, Batley SJ, Linger L, Bannister A, Thorpe K, Chin SF, Daigo Y et al (2000) Mutations truncating the EP300 acetylase in human cancers. Nat Genet 24(3):300–303. doi:10.1038/73536

Gibbons RJ (2005) Histone modifying and chromatin remodelling enzymes in cancer and dysplastic syndromes. Hum Mol Genet 14(Spec No 1):R85–R92. doi:10.1093/hmg/ddi106, 14/suppl_1/R85 [pii]

Goldberg AD, Banaszynski LA, Noh KM, Lewis PW, Elsaesser SJ, Stadler S, Dewell S et al (2010) Distinct factors control histone variant H3.3 localization at specific genomic regions. Cell 140(5):678–691. doi:10.1016/j.cell.2010.01.003, S0092-8674(10)00004-8 [pii]

Goll MG, Kirpekar F, Maggert KA, Yoder JA, Hsieh CL, Zhang X, Golic KG, Jacobsen SE, Bestor TH (2006) Methylation of tRNAAsp by the DNA methyltransferase homolog Dnmt2. Science 311(5759):395–398. doi:10.1126/science.1120976, 311/5759/395 [pii]

Gorrini C, Squatrito M, Luise C, Syed N, Perna D, Wark L, Martinato F et al (2007) Tip60 is a haplo-insufficient tumour suppressor required for an oncogene-induced DNA damage response. Nature 448(7157):1063–1067. doi:10.1038/nature06055, nature06055 [pii]

Hall JA, Georgel PT (2007) CHD proteins: a diverse family with strong ties. Biochem Cell Biol 85(4):463–476. doi:10.1139/O07-063, o07-063 [pii]

Hamamoto R, Furukawa Y, Morita M, Iimura Y, Silva FP, Li M, Yagyu R, Nakamura Y (2004) SMYD3 encodes a histone methyltransferase involved in the proliferation of cancer cells. Nat Cell Biol 6(8):731–740. doi:10.1038/ncb1151, ncb1151 [pii]

Han J, Lee Y, Yeom KH, Nam JW, Heo I, Rhee JK, Sohn SY, Cho Y, Zhang BT, Kim VN (2006) Molecular basis for the recognition of primary microRNAs by the Drosha-DGCR8 complex. Cell 125(5):887–901. doi:10.1016/j.cell.2006.03.043, S0092-8674(06)00516-2 [pii]

Han H, Cortez CC, Yang X, Nichols PW, Jones PA, Liang G (2011) DNA methylation directly silences genes with non-CpG island promoters and establishes a nucleosome occupied promoter. Hum Mol Genet. doi:10.1093/hmg/ddr356, ddr356 [pii]

Hargreaves DC, Crabtree GR (2011) ATP-dependent chromatin remodeling: genetics, genomics and mechanisms. Cell Res 21(3):396–420. doi:10.1038/cr.2011.32, cr201132 [pii]

Hatziapostolou M, Iliopoulos D (2011) Epigenetic aberrations during oncogenesis. Cell Mol Life Sci 68(10):1681–1702. doi:10.1007/s00018-010-0624-z

Hawkins RD, Hon GC, Lee LK, Ngo Q, Lister R, Pelizzola M, Edsall LE et al (2010) Distinct epigenomic landscapes of pluripotent and lineage-committed human cells. Cell Stem Cell 6(5):479–491. doi:10.1016/j.stem.2010.03.018, S1934-5909(10)00147-5 [pii]

Hirota T, Lipp JJ, Toh BH, Peters JM (2005) Histone H3 serine 10 phosphorylation by Aurora B causes HP1 dissociation from heterochromatin. Nature 438(7071):1176–1180. doi:10.1038/nature04254, nature04254 [pii]

Ho L, Ronan JL, Wu J, Staahl BT, Chen L, Kuo A, Lessard J, Nesvizhskii AI, Ranish J, Crabtree GR (2009) An embryonic stem cell chromatin remodeling complex, esBAF, is essential for embryonic stem cell self-renewal and pluripotency. Proc Natl Acad Sci U S A 106(13):5181–5186. doi:10.1073/pnas.0812889106, 0812889106 [pii]

Holz-Schietinger C, Reich NO (2010) The inherent processivity of the human de novo methyltransferase 3A (DNMT3A) is enhanced by DNMT3L. J Biol Chem 285(38):29091–29100. doi:10.1074/jbc.M110.142513, M110.142513 [pii]

Hon GC, Hawkins RD, Ren B (2009) Predictive chromatin signatures in the mammalian genome. Hum Mol Genet 18(R2):R195–R201. doi:10.1093/hmg/ddp409, ddp409 [pii]

Horwitz GA, Zhang K, McBrian MA, Grunstein M, Kurdistani SK, Berk AJ (2008) Adenovirus small e1a alters global patterns of histone modification. Science 321(5892):1084–1085. doi:10.1126/science.1155544, 321/5892/1084 [pii]

Howard G, Eiges R, Gaudet F, Jaenisch R, Eden A (2008) Activation and transposition of endogenous retroviral elements in hypomethylation induced tumors in mice. Oncogene 27(3):404–408. doi:10.1038/sj.onc.1210631, 1210631 [pii]

Huang Y, Fang J, Bedford MT, Zhang Y, Xu RM (2006) Recognition of histone H3 lysine-4 methylation by the double tudor domain of JMJD2A. Science 312(5774):748–751. doi:10.1126/science.1125162, 1125162 [pii]

Huangfu D, Osafune K, Maehr R, Guo W, Eijkelenboom A, Chen S, Muhlestein W, Melton DA (2008) Induction of pluripotent stem cells from primary human fibroblasts with only Oct4 and Sox2. Nat Biotechnol 26(11):1269–1275. doi:10.1038/nbt.1502, nbt.1502 [pii]

Huse JT, Brennan C, Hambardzumyan D, Wee B, Pena J, Rouhanifard SH, Sohn-Lee C et al (2009) The PTEN-regulating microRNA miR-26a is amplified in high-grade glioma and facilitates gliomagenesis in vivo. Genes Dev 23(11):1327–1337. doi:10.1101/gad.1777409, 23/11/1327 [pii]

Hutvagner G, McLachlan J, Pasquinelli AE, Balint E, Tuschl T, Zamore PD (2001) A cellular function for the RNA-interference enzyme Dicer in the maturation of the let-7 small temporal RNA. Science 293(5531):834–838. doi:10.1126/science.1062961, 1062961 [pii]

Ida K, Kitabayashi I, Taki T, Taniwaki M, Noro K, Yamamoto M, Ohki M, Hayashi Y (1997) Adenoviral E1A-associated protein p300 is involved in acute myeloid leukemia with t(11;22)(q23;q13). Blood 90(12):4699–4704

Illingworth RS, Gruenewald-Schneider U, Webb S, Kerr AR, James KD, Turner DJ, Smith C, Harrison DJ, Andrews R, Bird AP (2010) Orphan CpG islands identify numerous conserved promoters in the mammalian genome. PLoS Genet 6(9):e1001134. doi:10.1371/journal.pgen.1001134

Iorio MV, Visone R, Di Leva G, Donati V, Petrocca F, Casalini P, Taccioli C et al (2007) MicroRNA signatures in human ovarian cancer. Cancer Res 67(18):8699–8707. doi:10.1158/0008-5472.CAN-07-1936, 67/18/8699 [pii]

Irizarry RA, Ladd-Acosta C, Wen B, Wu Z, Montano C, Onyango P, Cui H et al (2009) The human colon cancer methylome shows similar hypo- and hypermethylation at conserved tissue-specific CpG island shores. Nat Genet 41(2):178–186. doi:10.1038/ng.298, ng.298 [pii]

Italiano A, Attias R, Aurias A, Perot G, Burel-Vandenbos F, Otto J, Venissac N, Pedeutour F (2006) Molecular cytogenetic characterization of a metastatic lung sarcomatoid carcinoma: 9p23 neocentromere and 9p23-p24 amplification including JAK2 and JMJD2C. Cancer Genet Cytogenet 167(2):122–130. doi:10.1016/j.cancergencyto.2006.01.004, S0165-4608(06)00049-5 [pii]

Ito Y, Koessler T, Ibrahim AE, Rai S, Vowler SL, Abu-Amero S, Silva AL et al (2008) Somatically acquired hypomethylation of IGF2 in breast and colorectal cancer. Hum Mol Genet 17(17):2633–2643. doi:10.1093/hmg/ddn163, ddn163 [pii]

Ito S, D'Alessio AC, Taranova OV, Hong K, Sowers LC, Zhang Y (2010) Role of Tet proteins in 5mC to 5hmC conversion, ES-cell self-renewal and inner cell mass specification. Nature 466(7310):1129–1133. doi:10.1038/nature09303, nature09303 [pii]

Jaenisch R, Young R (2008) Stem cells, the molecular circuitry of pluripotency and nuclear reprogramming. Cell 132(4):567–582. doi:10.1016/j.cell.2008.01.015, S0092-8674(08)00115-3 [pii]

Jeong S, Liang G, Sharma S, Lin JC, Choi SH, Han H, Yoo CB, Egger G, Yang AS, Jones PA (2009) Selective anchoring of DNA methyltransferases 3A and 3B to nucleosomes containing methylated DNA. Mol Cell Biol 29(19):5366–5376. doi:10.1128/MCB.00484-09, MCB.00484-09 [pii]

Ji H, Ehrlich LI, Seita J, Murakami P, Doi A, Lindau P, Lee H et al (2010) Comprehensive methylome map of lineage commitment from haematopoietic progenitors. Nature 467(7313):338–342. doi:10.1038/nature09367, nature09367 [pii]

Jiang C, Pugh BF (2009) Nucleosome positioning and gene regulation: advances through genomics. Nat Rev Genet 10(3):161–172. doi:10.1038/nrg2522, nrg2522 [pii]

Jin C, Felsenfeld G (2007) Nucleosome stability mediated by histone variants H3.3 and H2A.Z. Genes Dev 21(12):1519–1529. doi:10.1101/gad.1547707, 21/12/1519 [pii]

Jones PA, Baylin SB (2002) The fundamental role of epigenetic events in cancer. Nat Rev Genet 3(6):415–428. doi:10.1038/nrg816, nrg816 [pii]

Jones PA, Baylin SB (2007) The epigenomics of cancer. Cell 128(4):683–692. doi:10.1016/j.cell.2007.01.029, S0092-8674(07)00127-4 [pii]

Jones PA, Laird PW (1999) Cancer epigenetics comes of age. Nat Genet 21(2):163–167. doi:10.1038/5947

Jones PA, Liang G (2009) Rethinking how DNA methylation patterns are maintained. Nat Rev Genet 10(11):805–811. doi:10.1038/nrg2651, nrg2651 [pii]

Kahl P, Gullotti L, Heukamp LC, Wolf S, Friedrichs N, Vorreuther R, Solleder G et al (2006) Androgen receptor coactivators lysine-specific histone demethylase 1 and four and a half LIM domain protein 2 predict risk of prostate cancer recurrence. Cancer Res 66(23):11341–11347. doi:10.1158/0008-5472.CAN-06-1570, 66/23/11341 [pii]

Kanhere A, Viiri K, Araujo CC, Rasaiyaah J, Bouwman RD, Whyte WA, Pereira CF et al (2010) Short RNAs are transcribed from repressed polycomb target genes and interact with polycomb repressive complex-2. *Mol.* Cell 38(5):675–688. doi:10.1016/j.molcel.2010.03.019, S1097-2765(10)00327-8 [pii]

Kanwal R, Gupta S (2010) Epigenetics and cancer. J Appl Physiol 109(2):598–605. doi:10.1152/japplphysiol.00066.2010, 00066.2010 [pii]

Kidder BL, Palmer S, Knott JG (2009) SWI/SNF-Brg1 regulates self-renewal and occupies core pluripotency-related genes in embryonic stem cells. Stem Cells 27(2):317–328. doi:10.1634/stemcells.2008-0710, stemcells.2008-0710 [pii]

Kim KC, Geng L, Huang S (2003) Inactivation of a histone methyltransferase by mutations in human cancers. Cancer Res 63(22):7619–7623

Kim J, Daniel J, Espejo A, Lake A, Krishna M, Xia L, Zhang Y, Bedford MT (2006) Tudor, MBT and chromo domains gauge the degree of lysine methylation. EMBO Rep 7(4):397–403. doi:10.1038/sj.embor.7400625, 7400625 [pii]

Kim J, Guermah M, McGinty RK, Lee JS, Tang Z, Milne TA, Shilatifard A, Muir TW, Roeder RG (2009) RAD6-mediated transcription-coupled H2B ubiquitylation directly stimulates H3K4 methylation in human cells. Cell 137(3):459–471. doi:10.1016/j.cell.2009.02.027, S0092-8674(09)00203-7 [pii]

Klose RJ, Zhang Y (2007) Regulation of histone methylation by demethylimination and demethylation. Nat Rev Mol Cell Biol 8(4):307–318. doi:10.1038/nrm2143, nrm2143 [pii]

Koh KP, Yabuuchi A, Rao S, Huang Y, Cunniff K, Nardone J, Laiho A et al (2011) Tet1 and Tet2 regulate 5-hydroxymethylcytosine production and cell lineage specification in mouse embryonic stem cells. Cell Stem Cell 8(2):200–213. doi:10.1016/j.stem.2011.01.008, S1934-5909(11)00009-9 [pii]

Kondo Y, Shen L, Suzuki S, Kurokawa T, Masuko K, Tanaka Y, Kato H et al (2007) Alterations of DNA methylation and histone modifications contribute to gene silencing in hepatocellular carcinomas. Hepatol Res 37(11):974–983. doi:10.1111/j.1872-034X.2007.00141.x, HEP141 [pii]

Kondo Y, Shen L, Cheng AS, Ahmed S, Boumber Y, Charo C, Yamochi T et al (2008) Gene silencing in cancer by histone H3 lysine 27 trimethylation independent of promoter DNA methylation. Nat Genet 40(6):741–750. doi:10.1038/ng.159, ng.159 [pii]

Konev AY, Tribus M, Park SY, Podhraski V, Lim CY, Emelyanov AV, Vershilova E et al (2007) CHD1 motor protein is required for deposition of histone variant H3.3 into chromatin in vivo. Science 317(5841):1087–1090. doi:10.1126/science.1145339, 317/5841/1087 [pii]

Kouzarides T (2007) Chromatin modifications and their function. Cell 128(4):693–705. doi:10.1016/j.cell.2007.02.005, S0092-8674(07)00184-5 [pii]

Krivtsov AV, Armstrong SA (2007) MLL translocations, histone modifications and leukaemia stem-cell development. Nat Rev Cancer 7(11):823–833. doi:10.1038/nrc2253, nrc2253 [pii]

Lachner M, O'Carroll D, Rea S, Mechtler K, Jenuwein T (2001) Methylation of histone H3 lysine 9 creates a binding site for HP1 proteins. Nature 410(6824):116–120. doi:10.1038/35065132, 35065132 [pii]

Lahortiga I, Agirre X, Belloni E, Vazquez I, Larrayoz MJ, Gasparini P, Lo Coco F, Pelicci PG, Calasanz MJ, Odero MD (2004) Molecular characterization of a t(1;3)(p36;q21) in a patient with MDS. MEL1 is widely expressed in normal tissues, including bone marrow, and it is not overexpressed in the t(1;3) cells. Oncogene 23(1):311–316. doi:10.1038/sj.onc.1206923, 1206923 [pii]

Lai AY, Wade PA (2011) Cancer biology and NuRD: a multifaceted chromatin remodelling complex. Nat Rev Cancer 11(8):588–596. doi:10.1038/nrc3091, nrc3091 [pii]

Landeira D, Sauer S, Poot R, Dvorkina M, Mazzarella L, Jorgensen HF, Pereira CF et al (2010) Jarid2 is a PRC2 component in embryonic stem cells required for multi-lineage differentiation and recruitment of PRC1 and RNA Polymerase II to developmental regulators. Nat Cell Biol 12(6):618–624. doi:10.1038/ncb2065, ncb2065 [pii]

Landry J, Sharov AA, Piao Y, Sharova LV, Xiao H, Southon E, Matta J et al (2008) Essential role of chromatin remodeling protein Bptf in early mouse embryos and embryonic stem cells. PLoS Genet 4(10):e1000241. doi:10.1371/journal.pgen.1000241

Larsen F, Gundersen G, Lopez R, Prydz H (1992) CpG islands as gene markers in the human genome. Genomics 13(4):1095–1107

Laurent L, Wong E, Li G, Huynh T, Tsirigos A, Ong CT, Low HM et al (2010) Dynamic changes in the human methylome during differentiation. Genome Res 20(3):320–331. doi:10.1101/gr.101907.109, gr.101907.109 [pii]

Lee Y, Kim M, Han J, Yeom KH, Lee S, Baek SH, Kim VN (2004) MicroRNA genes are transcribed by RNA polymerase II. EMBO J 23(20):4051–4060. doi:10.1038/sj.emboj.7600385, 7600385 [pii]

Lehmann U, Hasemeier B, Christgen M, Muller M, Romermann D, Langer F, Kreipe H (2008) Epigenetic inactivation of microRNA gene hsa-mir-9-1 in human breast cancer. J Pathol 214(1):17–24. doi:10.1002/path.2251

Lessard JA, Crabtree GR (2010) Chromatin regulatory mechanisms in pluripotency. Annu Rev Cell Dev Biol 26:503–532. doi:10.1146/annurev-cellbio-051809-102012

Ley TJ, Ding L, Walter MJ, McLellan MD, Lamprecht T, Larson DE, Kandoth C et al (2010) DNMT3A mutations in acute myeloid leukemia. N Engl J Med 363(25):2424–2433. doi:10.1056/NEJMoa1005143

Li B, Carey M, Workman JL (2007a) The role of chromatin during transcription. Cell 128(4):707–719. doi:10.1016/j.cell.2007.01.015, S0092-8674(07)00109-2 [pii]

Li C, Heidt DG, Dalerba P, Burant CF, Zhang L, Adsay V, Wicha M, Clarke MF, Simeone DM (2007b) Identification of pancreatic cancer stem cells. Cancer Res 67(3):1030–1037. doi:10.1158/0008-5472.CAN-06-2030, 67/3/1030 [pii]

Liang J, Prouty L, Williams BJ, Dayton MA, Blanchard KL (1998) Acute mixed lineage leukemia with an inv(8)(p11q13) resulting in fusion of the genes for MOZ and TIF2. Blood 92(6):2118–2122

Lim S, Janzer A, Becker A, Zimmer A, Schule R, Buettner R, Kirfel J (2010) Lysine-specific demethylase 1 (LSD1) is highly expressed in ER-negative breast cancers and a biomarker predicting aggressive biology. Carcinogenesis 31(3):512–520. doi:10.1093/carcin/bgp324, bgp324 [pii]

Lin JC, Jeong S, Liang G, Takai D, Fatemi M, Tsai YC, Egger G, Gal-Yam EN, Jones PA (2007) Role of nucleosomal occupancy in the epigenetic silencing of the MLH1 CpG island. Cancer Cell 12(5):432–444. doi:10.1016/j.ccr.2007.10.014, S1535-6108(07)00299-1 [pii]

Lin SL, Chang DC, Lin CH, Ying SY, Leu D, Wu DT (2011) Regulation of somatic cell reprogramming through inducible mir-302 expression. Nucleic Acids Res 39(3):1054–1065. doi:10.1093/nar/gkq850, gkq850 [pii]

Lister R, Pelizzola M, Dowen RH, Hawkins RD, Hon G, Tonti-Filippini J, Nery JR et al (2009) Human DNA methylomes at base resolution show widespread epigenomic differences. Nature 462(7271):315–322. doi:10.1038/nature08514, nature08514 [pii]

Liu B, Lin Y, Darwanto A, Song X, Xu G, Zhang K (2009a) Identification and characterization of propionylation at histone H3 lysine 23 in mammalian cells. J Biol Chem 284(47):32288–32295. doi:10.1074/jbc.M109.045856, M109.045856 [pii]

Liu G, Bollig-Fischer A, Kreike B, van de Vijver MJ, Abrams J, Ethier SP, Yang ZQ (2009b) Genomic amplification and oncogenic properties of the GASC1 histone demethylase gene in breast cancer. Oncogene 28(50):4491–4500. doi:10.1038/onc.2009.297, onc2009297 [pii]

Lo WS, Trievel RC, Rojas JR, Duggan L, Hsu JY, Allis CD, Marmorstein R, Berger SL (2000) Phosphorylation of serine 10 in histone H3 is functionally linked in vitro and in vivo to Gcn5-mediated acetylation at lysine 14. Mol Cell 5(6):917–926, S1097-2765(00)80257-9 [pii]

Lu L, Katsaros D, de la Longrais IA, Sochirca O, Yu H (2007) Hypermethylation of let-7a-3 in epithelial ovarian cancer is associated with low insulin-like growth factor-II expression and favorable prognosis. Cancer Res 67(21):10117–10122. doi:10.1158/0008-5472.CAN-07-2544, 67/21/10117 [pii]

Lu PY, Levesque N, Kobor MS (2009) NuA4 and SWR1-C: two chromatin-modifying complexes with overlapping functions and components. Biochem Cell Biol 87(5):799–815. doi:10.1139/O09-062, o09-062 [pii]

Lu C, Han HD, Mangala LS, Ali-Fehmi R, Newton CS, Ozbun L, Armaiz-Pena GN et al (2010) Regulation of tumor angiogenesis by EZH2. Cancer Cell 18(2):185–197. doi:10.1016/j.ccr.2010.06.016, S1535-6108(10)00250-3 [pii]

Luco RF, Pan Q, Tominaga K, Blencowe BJ, Pereira-Smith OM, Misteli T (2010) Regulation of alternative splicing by histone modifications. Science 327(5968):996–1000. doi:10.1126/science.1184208, science.1184208 [pii]

Luger K, Richmond TJ (1998) The histone tails of the nucleosome. Curr Opin Genet Dev 8(2):140–146, S0959-437X(98)80134-2 [pii]

Luijsterburg MS, van Attikum H (2011) Chromatin and the DNA damage response: the cancer connection. Mol Oncol 5(4):349–367. doi:10.1016/j.molonc.2011.06.001, S1574-7891(11)00069-X [pii]

Lujambio A, Ropero S, Ballestar E, Fraga MF, Cerrato C, Setien F, Casado S et al (2007) Genetic unmasking of an epigenetically silenced microRNA in human cancer cells. Cancer Res 67(4):1424–1429. doi:10.1158/0008-5472.CAN-06-4218, 67/4/1424 [pii]

Lujambio A, Calin GA, Villanueva A, Ropero S, Sanchez-Cespedes M, Blanco D, Montuenga LM et al (2008) A microRNA DNA methylation signature for human cancer metastasis. Proc Natl Acad Sci U S A 105(36):13556–13561. doi:10.1073/pnas.0803055105, 0803055105 [pii]

Lutz T, Stoger R, Nieto A (2006) CHD6 is a DNA-dependent ATPase and localizes at nuclear sites of mRNA synthesis. FEBS Lett 580(25):5851–5857. doi:10.1016/j.febslet.2006.09.049, S0014-5793(06)01156-2 [pii]

Macdonald N, Welburn JP, Noble ME, Nguyen A, Yaffe MB, Clynes D, Moggs JG et al (2005) Molecular basis for the recognition of phosphorylated and phosphoacetylated histone h3 by 14-3-3. Mol Cell 20(2):199–211. doi:10.1016/j.molcel.2005.08.032, S1097-2765(05)01596-0 [pii]

Majumder S, Liu Y, Ford OH 3rd, Mohler JL, Whang YE (2006) Involvement of arginine methyltransferase CARM1 in androgen receptor function and prostate cancer cell viability. Prostate 66(12):1292–1301. doi:10.1002/pros.20438

Marango J, Shimoyama M, Nishio H, Meyer JA, Min DJ, Sirulnik A, Martinez-Martinez Y et al (2008) The MMSET protein is a histone methyltransferase with characteristics of a transcriptional corepressor. Blood 111(6):3145–3154. doi:10.1182/blood-2007-06-092122, blood-2007-06-092122 [pii]

Marfella CG, Imbalzano AN (2007) The Chd family of chromatin remodelers. Mutat Res 618(1–2):30–40. doi:10.1016/j.mrfmmm.2006.07.012, S0027-5107(07)00030-9 [pii]

Margueron R, Reinberg D (2011) The Polycomb complex PRC2 and its mark in life. Nature 469(7330):343–349. doi:10.1038/nature09784, nature09784 [pii]

Margueron R, Li G, Sarma K, Blais A, Zavadil J, Woodcock CL, Dynlacht BD, Reinberg D (2008) Ezh1 and Ezh2 maintain repressive chromatin through different mechanisms. Mol Cell 32(4):503–518. doi:10.1016/j.molcel.2008.11.004, S1097-2765(08)00770-3 [pii]

Marson A, Levine SS, Cole MF, Frampton GM, Brambrink T, Johnstone S, Guenther MG et al (2008) Connecting microRNA genes to the core transcriptional regulatory circuitry of embryonic stem cells. Cell 134(3):521–533. doi:10.1016/j.cell.2008.07.020, S0092-8674(08)00938-0 [pii]

Matsubayashi H, Sato N, Fukushima N, Yeo CJ, Walter KM, Brune K, Sahin F, Hruban RH, Goggins M (2003) Methylation of cyclin D2 is observed frequently in pancreatic cancer but is also an age-related phenomenon in gastrointestinal tissues. Clin Cancer Res 9(4): 1446–1452

Matsui W, Wang Q, Barber JP, Brennan S, Smith BD, Borrello I, McNiece I et al (2008) Clonogenic multiple myeloma progenitors, stem cell properties, and drug resistance. Cancer Res 68(1):190–197. doi:10.1158/0008-5472.CAN-07-3096, 68/1/190 [pii]

Maunakea AK, Nagarajan RP, Bilenky M, Ballinger TJ, D'Souza C, Fouse SD, Johnson BE et al (2010) Conserved role of intragenic DNA methylation in regulating alternative promoters. Nature 466(7303):253–257. doi:10.1038/nature09165, nature09165 [pii]

Mavrakis KJ, Wolfe AL, Oricchio E, Palomero T, de Keersmaecker K, McJunkin K, Zuber J et al (2010) Genome-wide RNA-mediated interference screen identifies miR-19 targets in Notch-induced T-cell acute lymphoblastic leukaemia. Nat Cell Biol 12(4):372–379. doi:10.1038/ncb2037, ncb2037 [pii]

Mavrich TN, Ioshikhes IP, Venters BJ, Jiang C, Tomsho LP, Qi J, Schuster SC, Albert I, Pugh BF (2008) A barrier nucleosome model for statistical positioning of nucleosomes throughout the yeast genome. Genome Res 18(7):1073–1083. doi:10.1101/gr.078261.108, gr.078261.108 [pii]

Medina PP, Sanchez-Cespedes M (2008) Involvement of the chromatin-remodeling factor BRG1/SMARCA4 in human cancer. Epigenetics 3(2):64–68, 6153 [pii]

Meissner A, Mikkelsen TS, Gu H, Wernig M, Hanna J, Sivachenko A, Zhang X et al (2008) Genome-scale DNA methylation maps of pluripotent and differentiated cells. Nature 454(7205):766–770. doi:10.1038/nature07107, nature07107 [pii]

Melo SA, Ropero S, Moutinho C, Aaltonen LA, Yamamoto H, Calin GA, Rossi S et al (2009) A TARBP2 mutation in human cancer impairs microRNA processing and DICER1 function. Nat Genet 41(3):365–370. doi:10.1038/ng.317, ng.317 [pii]

Melton C, Judson RL, Blelloch R (2010) Opposing microRNA families regulate self-renewal in mouse embryonic stem cells. Nature 463(7281):621–626. doi:10.1038/nature08725, nature08725 [pii]

Merritt WM, Lin YG, Han LY, Kamat AA, Spannuth WA, Schmandt R, Urbauer D et al (2008) Dicer, Drosha, and outcomes in patients with ovarian cancer. N Engl J Med 359(25):2641–2650. doi:10.1056/NEJMoa0803785, 359/25/2641 [pii]

Metzger E, Imhof A, Patel D, Kahl P, Hoffmeyer K, Friedrichs N, Muller JM et al (2010) Phosphorylation of histone H3T6 by PKCbeta(I) controls demethylation at histone H3K4. Nature 464(7289):792–796. doi:10.1038/nature08839, nature08839 [pii]

Mikkelsen TS, Ku M, Jaffe DB, Issac B, Lieberman E, Giannoukos G, Alvarez P et al (2007) Genome-wide maps of chromatin state in pluripotent and lineage-committed cells. Nature 448(7153):553–560. doi:10.1038/nature06008, nature06008 [pii]

Minucci S, Pelicci PG (2006) Histone deacetylase inhibitors and the promise of epigenetic (and more) treatments for cancer. Nat Rev Cancer 6(1):38–51. doi:10.1038/nrc1779, nrc1779 [pii]

Mohn F, Weber M, Rebhan M, Roloff TC, Richter J, Stadler MB, Bibel M, Schubeler D (2008) Lineage-specific polycomb targets and de novo DNA methylation define restriction and potential of neuronal progenitors. Mol Cell 30(6):755–766. doi:10.1016/j.molcel.2008.05.007, S1097-2765(08)00358-4 [pii]

Mohr F, Dohner K, Buske C, Rawat VP (2011) TET genes: new players in DNA demethylation and important determinants for stemness. Exp Hematol 39(3):272–281. doi:10.1016/j.exphem.2010.12.004, S0301-472X(10)00605-3 [pii]

Morey L, Brenner C, Fazi F, Villa R, Gutierrez A, Buschbeck M, Nervi C, Minucci S, Fuks F, Di Croce L (2008) MBD3, a component of the NuRD complex, facilitates chromatin alteration and deposition of epigenetic marks. Mol Cell Biol 28(19):5912–5923. doi:10.1128/MCB.00467-08, MCB.00467-08 [pii]

Morin RD, Johnson NA, Severson TM, Mungall AJ, An J, Goya R, Paul JE et al (2010) Somatic mutations altering EZH2 (Tyr641) in follicular and diffuse large B-cell lymphomas of germinal-center origin. Nat Genet 42(2):181–185. doi:10.1038/ng.518, ng.518 [pii]

Morrison AJ, Shen X (2009) Chromatin remodelling beyond transcription: the INO80 and SWR1 complexes. Nat Rev Mol Cell Biol 10(6):373–384. doi:10.1038/nrm2693, nrm2693 [pii]

Mosher RA, Melnyk CW (2010) siRNAs and DNA methylation: seedy epigenetics. Trends Plant Sci 15(4):204–210. doi:10.1016/j.tplants.2010.01.002, S1360-1385(10)00005-1 [pii]

Mujtaba S, Zeng L, Zhou MM (2007) Structure and acetyl-lysine recognition of the bromodomain. Oncogene 26(37):5521–5527. doi:10.1038/sj.onc.1210618, 1210618 [pii]

Naidu SR, Love IM, Imbalzano AN, Grossman SR, Androphy EJ (2009) The SWI/SNF chromatin remodeling subunit BRG1 is a critical regulator of p53 necessary for proliferation of malignant cells. Oncogene 28(27):2492–2501. doi:10.1038/onc.2009.121, onc2009121 [pii]

Nishiyama M, Oshikawa K, Tsukada Y, Nakagawa T, Iemura S, Natsume T, Fan Y, Kikuchi A, Skoultchi AI, Nakayama KI (2009) CHD8 suppresses p53-mediated apoptosis through histone H1 recruitment during early embryogenesis. Nat Cell Biol 11(2):172–182. doi:10.1038/ncb1831, ncb1831 [pii]

O'Brien CA, Pollett A, Gallinger S, Dick JE (2007) A human colon cancer cell capable of initiating tumour growth in immunodeficient mice. Nature 445(7123):106–110. doi:10.1038/nature05372, nature05372 [pii]

Ohm JE, McGarvey KM, Yu X, Cheng L, Schuebel KE, Cope L, Mohammad HP et al (2007) A stem cell-like chromatin pattern may predispose tumor suppressor genes to DNA hypermethylation and heritable silencing. Nat Genet 39(2):237–242. doi:10.1038/ng1972, ng1972 [pii]

Okamoto I, Heard E (2009) Lessons from comparative analysis of X-chromosome inactivation in mammals. Chromosome Res 17(5):659–669. doi:10.1007/s10577-009-9057-7

Ooi SK, Qiu C, Bernstein E, Li K, Jia D, Yang Z, Erdjument-Bromage H et al (2007) DNMT3L connects unmethylated lysine 4 of histone H3 to de novo methylation of DNA. Nature 448(7154):714–717. doi:10.1038/nature05987, nature05987 [pii]

Orkin SH, Hochedlinger K (2011) Chromatin connections to pluripotency and cellular reprogramming. Cell 145(6):835–850. doi:10.1016/j.cell.2011.05.019, S0092-8674(11)00576-9 [pii]

Osada H, Tatematsu Y, Saito H, Yatabe Y, Mitsudomi T, Takahashi T (2004) Reduced expression of class II histone deacetylase genes is associated with poor prognosis in lung cancer patients. Int J Cancer 112(1):26–32. doi:10.1002/ijc.20395

Panagopoulos I, Fioretos T, Isaksson M, Samuelsson U, Billstrom R, Strombeck B, Mitelman F, Johansson B (2001) Fusion of the MORF and CBP genes in acute myeloid leukemia with the t(10;16)(q22;p13). Hum Mol Genet 10(4):395–404

Parthun MR (2007) Hat1: the emerging cellular roles of a type B histone acetyltransferase. Oncogene 26(37):5319–5328. doi:10.1038/sj.onc.1210602, 1210602 [pii]
Pasini D, Hansen KH, Christensen J, Agger K, Cloos PA, Helin K (2008) Coordinated regulation of transcriptional repression by the RBP2 H3K4 demethylase and Polycomb-Repressive Complex 2. Genes Dev 22(10):1345–1355. doi:10.1101/gad.470008, 22/10/1345 [pii]
Pauli A, Rinn JL, Schier AF (2011) Non-coding RNAs as regulators of embryogenesis. Nat Rev Genet 12(2):136–149. doi:10.1038/nrg2904, nrg2904 [pii]
Pedersen MT, Helin K (2010) Histone demethylases in development and disease. Trends Cell Biol 20(11):662–671. doi:10.1016/j.tcb.2010.08.011, S0962-8924(10)00179-0 [pii]
Peters I, Vaske B, Albrecht K, Kuczyk MA, Jonas U, Serth J (2007) Adiposity and age are statistically related to enhanced RASSF1A tumor suppressor gene promoter methylation in normal autopsy kidney tissue. Cancer Epidemiol Biomarkers Prev 16(12):2526–2532. doi:10.1158/1055-9965.EPI-07-0203, 16/12/2526 [pii]
Portela A, Esteller M (2010) Epigenetic modifications and human disease. Nat Biotechnol 28(10):1057–1068. doi:10.1038/nbt.1685, nbt.1685 [pii]
Prince ME, Sivanandan R, Kaczorowski A, Wolf GT, Kaplan MJ, Dalerba P, Weissman IL, Clarke MF, Ailles LE (2007) Identification of a subpopulation of cells with cancer stem cell properties in head and neck squamous cell carcinoma. Proc Natl Acad Sci U S A 104(3):973–978. doi:10.1073/pnas.0610117104, 0610117104 [pii]
Pruitt K, Zinn RL, Ohm JE, McGarvey KM, Kang SH, Watkins DN, Herman JG, Baylin SB (2006) Inhibition of SIRT1 reactivates silenced cancer genes without loss of promoter DNA hypermethylation. PLoS Genet 2(3):e40. doi:10.1371/journal.pgen.0020040
Reisman DN, Sciarrotta J, Wang W, Funkhouser WK, Weissman BE (2003) Loss of BRG1/BRM in human lung cancer cell lines and primary lung cancers: correlation with poor prognosis. Cancer Res 63(3):560–566
Ricci-Vitiani L, Lombardi DG, Pilozzi E, Biffoni M, Todaro M, Peschle C, De Maria R (2007) Identification and expansion of human colon-cancer-initiating cells. Nature 445(7123):111–115. doi:10.1038/nature05384, nature05384 [pii]
Riddihough G, Zahn LM (2010) Epigenetics. What is epigenetics? Introduction. Science 330(6004):611. doi:10.1126/science.330.6004.611, 330/6004/611 [pii]
Rio Frio T, Bahubeshi A, Kanellopoulou C, Hamel N, Niedziela M, Sabbaghian N, Pouchet C et al (2011) DICER1 mutations in familial multinodular goiter with and without ovarian Sertoli-Leydig cell tumors. JAMA 305(1):68–77. doi:10.1001/jama.2010.1910, 305/1/68 [pii]
Rodriguez C, Borgel J, Court F, Cathala G, Forne T, Piette J (2010) CTCF is a DNA methylation-sensitive positive regulator of the INK/ARF locus. Biochem Biophys Res Commun 392(2):129–134. doi:10.1016/j.bbrc.2009.12.159, S0006-291X(09)02557-1 [pii]
Rodriguez-Navarro S (2009) Insights into SAGA function during gene expression. EMBO Rep 10(8):843–850. doi:10.1038/embor.2009.168, embor2009168 [pii]
Rodriguez-Paredes M, Esteller M (2011) Cancer epigenetics reaches mainstream oncology. Nat Med 17(3):330–339. doi:10.1038/nm.2305, nm.2305 [pii]
Rodriguez-Paredes M, Ceballos-Chavez M, Esteller M, Garcia-Dominguez M, Reyes JC (2009) The chromatin remodeling factor CHD8 interacts with elongating RNA polymerase II and controls expression of the cyclin E2 gene. Nucleic Acids Res 37(8):2449–2460. doi:10.1093/nar/gkp101, gkp101 [pii]
Ropero S, Fraga MF, Ballestar E, Hamelin R, Yamamoto H, Boix-Chornet M, Caballero R et al (2006) A truncating mutation of HDAC2 in human cancers confers resistance to histone deacetylase inhibition. Nat Genet 38(5):566–569. doi:10.1038/ng1773, ng1773 [pii]
Rosenfeld JA, Wang Z, Schones DE, Zhao K, DeSalle R, Zhang MQ (2009) Determination of enriched histone modifications in non-genic portions of the human genome. BMC Genomics 10:143. doi:10.1186/1471-2164-10-143, 1471-2164-10-143 [pii]
Saito Y, Liang G, Egger G, Friedman JM, Chuang JC, Coetzee GA, Jones PA (2006) Specific activation of microRNA-127 with downregulation of the proto-oncogene BCL6 by chromatin-modifying drugs in human cancer cells. Cancer Cell 9(6):435–443. doi:10.1016/j.ccr.2006.04.020, S1535-6108(06)00143-7 [pii]

Sakabe K, Wang Z, Hart GW (2010) Beta-N-acetylglucosamine (O-GlcNAc) is part of the histone code. Proc Natl Acad Sci U S A 107(46):19915–19920. doi:10.1073/pnas.1009023107, 1009023107 [pii]

Saladi SV, de la Serna IL (2010) ATP dependent chromatin remodeling enzymes in embryonic stem cells. Stem Cell Rev 6(1):62–73. doi:10.1007/s12015-010-9120-y

Santenard A, Torres-Padilla ME (2009) Epigenetic reprogramming in mammalian reproduction: contribution from histone variants. Epigenetics 4(2):80–84, 7838 [pii]

Santos-Rosa H, Kirmizis A, Nelson C, Bartke T, Saksouk N, Cote J, Kouzarides T (2009) Histone H3 tail clipping regulates gene expression. Nat Struct Mol Biol 16(1):17–22. doi:10.1038/nsmb.1534, nsmb.1534 [pii]

Sarma K, Reinberg D (2005) Histone variants meet their match. Nat Rev Mol Cell Biol 6(2):139–149. doi:10.1038/nrm1567, nrm1567 [pii]

Saunders LR, Verdin E (2007) Sirtuins: critical regulators at the crossroads between cancer and aging. Oncogene 26(37):5489–5504. doi:10.1038/sj.onc.1210616, 1210616 [pii]

Saxonov S, Berg P, Brutlag DL (2006) A genome-wide analysis of CpG dinucleotides in the human genome distinguishes two distinct classes of promoters. Proc Natl Acad Sci U S A 103(5):1412–1417. doi:10.1073/pnas.0510310103, 0510310103 [pii]

Schnetz MP, Bartels CF, Shastri K, Balasubramanian D, Zentner GE, Balaji R, Zhang X et al (2009) Genomic distribution of CHD7 on chromatin tracks H3K4 methylation patterns. Genome Res 19(4):590–601. doi:10.1101/gr.086983.108, gr.086983.108 [pii]

Schnetz MP, Handoko L, Akhtar-Zaidi B, Bartels CF, Pereira CF, Fisher AG, Adams DJ et al (2010) CHD7 targets active gene enhancer elements to modulate ES cell-specific gene expression. PLoS Genet 6(7):e1001023. doi:10.1371/journal.pgen.1001023

Schones DE, Cui K, Cuddapah S, Roh TY, Barski A, Wang Z, Wei G, Zhao K (2008) Dynamic regulation of nucleosome positioning in the human genome. Cell 132(5):887–898. doi:10.1016/j.cell.2008.02.022, S0092-8674(08)00270-5 [pii]

Schuebel KE, Chen W, Cope L, Glockner SC, Suzuki H, Yi JM, Chan TA et al (2007) Comparing the DNA hypermethylome with gene mutations in human colorectal cancer. PLoS Genet 3(9):1709–1723. doi:10.1371/journal.pgen.0030157, 07-PLGE-RA-0242 [pii]

Scibetta AG, Santangelo S, Coleman J, Hall D, Chaplin T, Copier J, Catchpole S, Burchell J, Taylor-Papadimitriou J (2007) Functional analysis of the transcription repressor PLU-1/JARID1B. Mol Cell Biol 27(20):7220–7235. doi:10.1128/MCB.00274-07, MCB.00274-07 [pii]

Scott GK, Mattie MD, Berger CE, Benz SC, Benz CC (2006) Rapid alteration of microRNA levels by histone deacetylase inhibition. Cancer Res 66(3):1277–1281. doi:10.1158/0008-5472.CAN-05-3632, 66/3/1277 [pii]

Shi Y, Lan F, Matson C, Mulligan P, Whetstine JR, Cole PA, Casero RA (2004) Histone demethylation mediated by the nuclear amine oxidase homolog LSD1. Cell 119(7):941–953. doi:10.1016/j.cell.2004.12.012, S0092867404011997 [pii]

Shur I, Socher R, Benayahu D (2006) In vivo association of CReMM/CHD9 with promoters in osteogenic cells. J Cell Physiol 207(2):374–378. doi:10.1002/jcp.20586

Sims RJ 3rd, Reinberg D (2006) Histone H3 Lys 4 methylation: caught in a bind? Genes Dev 20(20):2779–2786. doi:10.1101/gad.1468206, 20/20/2779 [pii]

Sims RJ 3rd, Chen CF, Santos-Rosa H, Kouzarides T, Patel SS, Reinberg D (2005) Human but not yeast CHD1 binds directly and selectively to histone H3 methylated at lysine 4 via its tandem chromodomains. J Biol Chem 280(51):41789–41792. doi:10.1074/jbc.C500395200, C500395200 [pii]

Sims RJ 3rd, Millhouse S, Chen CF, Lewis BA, Erdjument-Bromage H, Tempst P, Manley JL, Reinberg D (2007) Recognition of trimethylated histone H3 lysine 4 facilitates the recruitment of transcription postinitiation factors and pre-mRNA splicing. Mol Cell 28(4):665–676. doi:10.1016/j.molcel.2007.11.010, S1097-2765(07)00744-7 [pii]

Singh SK, Hawkins C, Clarke ID, Squire JA, Bayani J, Hide T, Henkelman RM, Cusimano MD, Dirks PB (2004) Identification of human brain tumour initiating cells. Nature 432(7015):396–401. doi:10.1038/nature03128, nature03128 [pii]

Steger DJ, Workman JL (1996) Remodeling chromatin structures for transcription: what happens to the histones? Bioessays 18(11):875–884. doi:10.1002/bies.950181106

Stock JK, Giadrossi S, Casanova M, Brookes E, Vidal M, Koseki H, Brockdorff N, Fisher AG, Pombo A (2007) Ring1-mediated ubiquitination of H2A restrains poised RNA polymerase II at bivalent genes in mouse ES cells. Nat Cell Biol 9(12):1428–1435. doi:10.1038/ncb1663, ncb1663 [pii]

Straussman R, Nejman D, Roberts D, Steinfeld I, Blum B, Benvenisty N, Simon I, Yakhini Z, Cedar H (2009) Developmental programming of CpG island methylation profiles in the human genome. Nat Struct Mol Biol 16(5):564–571. doi:10.1038/nsmb.1594, nsmb.1594 [pii]

Stucki M, Clapperton JA, Mohammad D, Yaffe MB, Smerdon SJ, Jackson SP (2005) MDC1 directly binds phosphorylated histone H2AX to regulate cellular responses to DNA double-strand breaks. Cell 123(7):1213–1226. doi:10.1016/j.cell.2005.09.038, S0092-8674(05)01165-7 [pii]

Suetsugu A, Nagaki M, Aoki H, Motohashi T, Kunisada T, Moriwaki H (2006) Characterization of CD133+ hepatocellular carcinoma cells as cancer stem/progenitor cells. Biochem Biophys Res Commun 351(4):820–824. doi:10.1016/j.bbrc.2006.10.128, S0006-291X(06)02324-2 [pii]

Surani MA, Hayashi K, Hajkova P (2007) Genetic and epigenetic regulators of pluripotency. Cell 128(4):747–762. doi:10.1016/j.cell.2007.02.010, S0092-8674(07)00191-2 [pii]

Suzuki MM, Bird A (2008) DNA methylation landscapes: provocative insights from epigenomics. Nat Rev Genet 9(6):465–476. doi:10.1038/nrg2341, nrg2341 [pii]

Svotelis A, Gevry N, Gaudreau L (2009) Regulation of gene expression and cellular proliferation by histone H2A.Z. Biochem Cell Biol 87(1):179–188. doi:10.1139/O08-138, o08-138 [pii]

Tachibana M, Matsumura Y, Fukuda M, Kimura H, Shinkai Y (2008) G9a/GLP complexes independently mediate H3K9 and DNA methylation to silence transcription. EMBO J 27(20):2681–2690. doi:10.1038/emboj.2008.192, emboj2008192 [pii]

Tahiliani M, Koh KP, Shen Y, Pastor WA, Bandukwala H, Brudno Y, Agarwal S et al (2009) Conversion of 5-methylcytosine to 5-hydroxymethylcytosine in mammalian DNA by MLL partner TET1. Science 324(5929):930–935. doi:10.1126/science.1170116, 1170116 [pii]

Takada I, Mihara M, Suzawa M, Ohtake F, Kobayashi S, Igarashi M, Youn MY et al (2007) A histone lysine methyltransferase activated by non-canonical Wnt signalling suppresses PPAR-gamma transactivation. Nat Cell Biol 9(11):1273–1285. doi:10.1038/ncb1647, ncb1647 [pii]

Tomonaga T, Matsushita K, Yamaguchi S, Oohashi T, Shimada H, Ochiai T, Yoda K, Nomura F (2003) Overexpression and mistargeting of centromere protein-A in human primary colorectal cancer. Cancer Res 63(13):3511–3516

Toyota M, Suzuki H, Sasaki Y, Maruyama R, Imai K, Shinomura Y, Tokino T (2008) Epigenetic silencing of microRNA-34b/c and B-cell translocation gene 4 is associated with CpG island methylation in colorectal cancer. Cancer Res 68(11):4123–4132. doi:10.1158/0008-5472.CAN-08-0325, 68/11/4123 [pii]

Tzatsos A, Pfau R, Kampranis SC, Tsichlis PN (2009) Ndy1/KDM2B immortalizes mouse embryonic fibroblasts by repressing the Ink4a/Arf locus. Proc Natl Acad Sci U S A 106(8):2641–2646. doi:10.1073/pnas.0813139106, 0813139106 [pii]

van Haaften G, Dalgliesh GL, Davies H, Chen L, Bignell G, Greenman C, Edkins S et al (2009) Somatic mutations of the histone H3K27 demethylase gene UTX in human cancer. Nat Genet 41(5):521–523. doi:10.1038/ng.349, ng.349 [pii]

Vaquero A (2009) The conserved role of sirtuins in chromatin regulation. Int J Dev Biol 53(2–3):303–322. doi:10.1387/ijdb.082675av, 082675av [pii]

Varambally S, Cao Q, Mani RS, Shankar S, Wang X, Ateeq B, Laxman B et al (2008) Genomic loss of microRNA-101 leads to overexpression of histone methyltransferase EZH2 in cancer. Science 322(5908):1695–1699. doi:10.1126/science.1165395, 1165395 [pii]

Vasudevan S, Tong Y, Steitz JA (2007) Switching from repression to activation: microRNAs can up-regulate translation. Science 318(5858):1931–1934. doi:10.1126/science.1149460, 1149460 [pii]

Vatolin S, Navaratne K, Weil RJ (2006) A novel method to detect functional microRNA targets. J Mol Biol 358(4):983–996. doi:10.1016/j.jmb.2006.02.063, S0022-2836(06)00279-8 [pii]

Vermeulen M, Eberl HC, Matarese F, Marks H, Denissov S, Butter F, Lee KK et al (2010) Quantitative interaction proteomics and genome-wide profiling of epigenetic histone marks and their readers. Cell 142(6):967–980. doi:10.1016/j.cell.2010.08.020, S0092-8674(10)00951-7 [pii]
Viré E, Brenner C, Deplus R, Blanchon L, Fraga M, Didelot C, Morey L et al (2006) The polycomb group protein EZH2 directly controls DNA methylation. Nature 439(7078):871–874. doi:10.1038/nature04431, nature04431 [pii]
Vrbsky J, Akimcheva S, Watson JM, Turner TL, Daxinger L, Vyskot B, Aufsatz W, Riha K (2010) siRNA-mediated methylation of Arabidopsis telomeres. PLoS Genet 6(6):e1000986. doi:10.1371/journal.pgen.1000986
Walker E, Chang WY, Hunkapiller J, Cagney G, Garcha K, Torchia J, Krogan NJ, Reiter JF, Stanford WL (2010) Polycomb-like 2 associates with PRC2 and regulates transcriptional networks during mouse embryonic stem cell self-renewal and differentiation. Cell Stem Cell 6(2):153–166. doi:10.1016/j.stem.2009.12.014, S1934-5909(09)00637-7 [pii]
Wang GG, Allis CD, Chi P (2007a) Chromatin remodeling and cancer, part I: covalent histone modifications. Trends Mol Med 13(9):363–372. doi:10.1016/j.molmed.2007.07.003, S1471-4914(07)00146-3 [pii]
Wang GG, Allis CD, Chi P (2007b) Chromatin remodeling and cancer, part II: ATP-dependent chromatin remodeling. Trends Mol Med 13(9):373–380. doi:10.1016/j.molmed.2007.07.004, S1471-4914(07)00147-5 [pii]
Wang GG, Cai L, Pasillas MP, Kamps MP (2007c) NUP98-NSD1 links H3K36 methylation to Hox-A gene activation and leukaemogenesis. Nat Cell Biol 9(7):804–812. doi:10.1038/ncb1608, ncb1608 [pii]
Wang Y, Baskerville S, Shenoy A, Babiarz JE, Baehner L, Blelloch R (2008a) Embryonic stem cell-specific microRNAs regulate the G1-S transition and promote rapid proliferation. Nat Genet 40(12):1478–1483. doi:10.1038/ng.250, ng.250 [pii]
Wang Z, Zang C, Rosenfeld JA, Schones DE, Barski A, Cuddapah S, Cui K et al (2008b) Combinatorial patterns of histone acetylations and methylations in the human genome. Nat Genet 40(7):897–903. doi:10.1038/ng.154, ng.154 [pii]
Wang J, Hevi S, Kurash JK, Lei H, Gay F, Bajko J, Su H et al (2009) The lysine demethylase LSD1 (KDM1) is required for maintenance of global DNA methylation. Nat Genet 41(1):125–129. doi:10.1038/ng.268, ng.268 [pii]
Weber B, Stresemann C, Brueckner B, Lyko F (2007a) Methylation of human microRNA genes in normal and neoplastic cells. Cell Cycle 6(9):1001–1005, 4209 [pii]
Weber M, Hellmann I, Stadler MB, Ramos L, Paabo S, Rebhan M, Schubeler D (2007b) Distribution, silencing potential and evolutionary impact of promoter DNA methylation in the human genome. Nat Genet 39(4):457–466. doi:10.1038/ng1990, ng1990 [pii]
Werbowetski-Ogilvie TE, Bosse M, Stewart M, Schnerch A, Ramos-Mejia V, Rouleau A, Wynder T et al (2009) Characterization of human embryonic stem cells with features of neoplastic progression. Nat Biotechnol 27(1):91–97. doi:10.1038/nbt.1516, nbt.1516 [pii]
Williams K, Christensen J, Pedersen MT, Johansen JV, Cloos PA, Rappsilber J, Helin K (2011) TET1 and hydroxymethylcytosine in transcription and DNA methylation fidelity. Nature 473(7347):343–348. doi:10.1038/nature10066, nature10066 [pii]
Wilson BG, Roberts CW (2011) SWI/SNF nucleosome remodellers and cancer. Nat Rev Cancer 11(7):481–492. doi:10.1038/nrc3068, nrc3068 [pii]
Wong MM, Cox LK, Chrivia JC (2007) The chromatin remodeling protein, SRCAP, is critical for deposition of the histone variant H2A.Z at promoters. J Biol Chem 282(36):26132–26139. doi:10.1074/jbc.M703418200, M703418200 [pii]
Xu N, Papagiannakopoulos T, Pan G, Thomson JA, Kosik KS (2009) MicroRNA-145 regulates OCT4, SOX2, and KLF4 and represses pluripotency in human embryonic stem cells. Cell 137(4):647–658. doi:10.1016/j.cell.2009.02.038, S0092-8674(09)00252-9 [pii]
Yang XJ, Seto E (2007) HATs and HDACs: from structure, function and regulation to novel strategies for therapy and prevention. Oncogene 26(37):5310–5318. doi:10.1038/sj.onc.1210599, 1210599 [pii]

Yang XJ, Seto E (2008) The Rpd3/Hda1 family of lysine deacetylases: from bacteria and yeast to mice and men. Nat Rev Mol Cell Biol 9(3):206–218. doi:10.1038/nrm2346, nrm2346 [pii]

Yeh A, Wei M, Golub SB, Yamashiro DJ, Murty VV, Tycko B (2002) Chromosome arm 16q in Wilms tumors: unbalanced chromosomal translocations, loss of heterozygosity, and assessment of the CTCF gene. Genes Chromosomes Cancer 35(2):156–163. doi:10.1002/gcc.10110

Yi R, Qin Y, Macara IG, Cullen BR (2003) Exportin-5 mediates the nuclear export of pre-microRNAs and short hairpin RNAs. Genes Dev 17(24):3011–3016. doi:10.1101/gad.1158803, 1158803 [pii]

Zeng L, Zhang Q, Li S, Plotnikov AN, Walsh MJ, Zhou MM (2010) Mechanism and regulation of acetylated histone binding by the tandem PHD finger of DPF3b. Nature 466(7303):258–262. doi:10.1038/nature09139, nature09139 [pii]

Zhao Q, Rank G, Tan YT, Li H, Moritz RL, Simpson RJ, Cerruti L et al (2009) PRMT5-mediated methylation of histone H4R3 recruits DNMT3A, coupling histone and DNA methylation in gene silencing. Nat Struct Mol Biol 16(3):304–311. doi:10.1038/nsmb.1568, nsmb.1568 [pii]

Zhu J, He F, Hu S, Yu J (2008) On the nature of human housekeeping genes. Trends Genet 24(10):481–484. doi:10.1016/j.tig.2008.08.004, S0168-9525(08)00223-0 [pii]

Zhu D, Fang J, Li Y, Zhang J (2009) Mbd3, a component of NuRD/Mi-2 complex, helps maintain pluripotency of mouse embryonic stem cells by repressing trophectoderm differentiation. PLoS One 4(11):e7684. doi:10.1371/journal.pone.0007684

Zilberman D, Gehring M, Tran RK, Ballinger T, Henikoff S (2007) Genome-wide analysis of Arabidopsis thaliana DNA methylation uncovers an interdependence between methylation and transcription. Nat Genet 39(1):61–69. doi:10.1038/ng1929, ng1929 [pii]

Zilberman D, Coleman-Derr D, Ballinger T, Henikoff S (2008) Histone H2A.Z and DNA methylation are mutually antagonistic chromatin marks. Nature 456(7218):125–129. doi:10.1038/nature07324, nature07324 [pii]

Mouse Models to Study DNA Methylation in Cancer Research

2

Irina Savelyeva and Frank Rosenbauer

2.1 Introduction

The epigenetic state of chromatin is a major factor by which expression of adequate gene programs is maintained during cell divisions. DNA methylation and histone tail modifications are the two main epigenetic chromatin control mechanisms in mammalian cells, both of which are closely connected (Cedar and Bergman 2009). Epigenetic modifications aroused a high level of interest in both basic and clinical research because of two reasons: they are altered in various diseases, in particular cancer and neurological disorders (Feinberg et al. 2006), and principally have a reversible nature – a very attractive quality from the therapeutical point of view.

A main function of DNA methylation and other epigenetic mechanisms as well is to regulate gene activities in a heritable fashion. However, besides gene regulation, DNA methylation is essential for many cellular processes such as silencing transposable and retroviral elements and maintaining genomic integrity, control of imprinting, and X-chromosome inactivation (Jaenisch 1997; Liang et al. 2002; Norris et al. 1994; Monk et al. 1987). All these biological functions require dynamic and flexible regulation, and the methylation pattern must therefore underlie a tight spatial-temporal control. Three groups of proteins are important for the dynamic methylation control of cells: those that catalyze the addition of the methyl groups to the DNA, those that bind to methylated DNA sequences and translate the methylation information into biological functions, and those that may remove the marks. Additionally, there is a group of factors that control DNA methylation indirectly, which includes mainly histone-modifying enzymes.

Much of what we know today on the function of DNA methylation in higher vertebrates, particularly with respect to its role in development and disease, has

I. Savelyeva • F. Rosenbauer (✉)
Laboratory of Molecular Stem Cell Biology,
Institute of Molecular Tumor Biology – IMTB, University of Münster,
Robert Koch Str. 43, Münster D-48149, Germany
e-mail: frank.rosenbauer@ukmuenster.de

M. Lübbert, P.A. Jones (eds.), *Epigenetic Therapy of Cancer*,
DOI 10.1007/978-3-642-38404-2_2, © Springer-Verlag Berlin Heidelberg 2014

been derived from genetic experiments in mice. Therefore, after briefly introducing the proteins that establish, maintain, translate, and potentially erase DNA methylation in mammals, this chapter focuses on the genetic mouse models which have been useful to decipher the functional role of DNA methylation in cancer.

2.2 The Mammalian DNA Methylation System: Writers, Readers, Erasers, and Cooperation Partners

2.2.1 Writing DNA Methylation: DNA Methyltransferases

DNA methylation was discovered in mammals soon after the genetic nature of DNA was understood (Hotchkiss 1948). It represents a covalent modification of DNA which is catalyzed by a conserved family of DNA methyltransferases (DNMTs) (Adams 1990). DNMTs transfer methyl group from S-adenosylmethionine (SAM) to the fifth carbon of the unmethylated cytosine, in mammals almost exclusively in the context of CG dinucleotide (CpG), forming the base 5-methylcytosine (5mC) (Bird 2002; Bestor 2000).

2.2.1.1 DNMT Proteins

In mammalian cells five members of the DNMT family have been identified – DNMT1, DNMT2, DNMT3A, DNMT3B, and DNMT3L. Structurally all proteins, with the exception of DNMT2 and DNMT3L, are divided into two domains – regulatory *N*-terminal and catalytic *C*-terminal domain. The largest protein of the DNMT family, DNMT1, is the first mammalian methyltransferase purified and cloned (Bestor 1988). The catalytic domain in the *C*-terminus of DNMT1 contains six conserved motifs, which are present in all DNMTs (except DNMT3L), and is highly related to bacterial restriction methyltransferases (Bestor 1988). DNMT1 possesses a long *N*-terminal domain that profoundly differs from the *N*-terminus of DNMT3 proteins. It contains a nuclear localization signal (NLS) motif, a replication-foci-targeting (TRF) sequence, a Zn-binding domain of the CXXC type, a poly-bromo-1 homology domain (PHD), and a proliferating cell nuclear antigen (PCNA)-binding motif (Leonhardt et al. 1992; Liu et al. 1998; Bestor 1992; Glickman et al. 1997; Chuang et al. 1997). The members of the DNMT3 family have shorter *N*-termini, bearing a PWWP domain (except DNMT3L), presumably required for nonspecific DNA binding (Qiu et al. 2002; Aapola et al. 2000; Aapola et al. 2001), and cystein-rich 3-Zn-binding domain (containing six CXXC motifs). The smallest member of the DNMT family, DNMT2, possesses the shortest *N*-terminus but retains all ten conserved motifs found in the *C*-termini of the other DNMTs. Nevertheless, DNMT2 lacks DNA methyltransferase activity.

2.2.1.2 Activities of DNMTs: De Novo and Maintenance Methylation

The de novo establishment of methylation is catalyzed by DNMT3A and DNMT3B, both of which are highly expressed in undifferentiated embryonic stem (ES) cells as compared to differentiated cells and adult tissues (Yokochi and

Robertson 2002). DNMT3s are thought to establish methylation patterns on un- and hemi-methylated DNA, but do not maintain them after cell division (Okano et al. 1999). The maintenance of DNA methylation after replication is a prerequisite for proper execution of differentiation programs in a cell. It is controlled by DNMT1, which has a 5- to 30-fold higher preference for hemi-methylated DNA strands as compared to unmethylated DNA, and therefore is considered to act as the major maintenance methyltransferase (Hermann et al. 2004). DNMT1 is highly expressed in S phase and is recruited to the replication foci by the proliferating cell nuclear antigen (PCNA) (Leonhardt et al. 1992). It was shown that DNMT1 requires chromatin-associated/remodeling factors, such as ubiquitin-like PHD and RING finger domain1 (UHRF1) protein, and lymphoid-specific helicase (LSH1) for methylation maintenance (Bostick et al. 2007; Sharif et al. 2007; Dennis et al. 2001; Huang et al. 2004).

DNMT1 and DNMT3A/3B are believed to be sufficient to catalyze all DNA methylation reactions in a cell, since DNMT3L and DNMT2 proteins do not possess DNA methyltransferase activity. However, DNMT3L co-localizes and physically interacts with both de novo methyltransferases (Jia et al. 2007; Hata et al. 2002) and represents an essential cofactor for the establishment of imprinting methylation in germ cells (Hata et al. 2002; Bourc'his et al. 2001). DNMT3L has been suggested to stabilize the active center of DNMT3A by forming a DNMT3L-DNMT3A tetramer (Hata et al. 2002; Jia et al. 2007). DNMT2, though not required for DNA methylation, has been recognized to catalyze $tRNA^{Asp}$ cytosine methylation (Yoder and Bestor 1998; Okano et al. 1998; Goll et al. 2006).

2.2.2 Reading and Executing DNA Methylation

DNA methylation bears instructions for execution of biological programs. Several mechanisms explaining how DNA methylation controls gene silencing have been proposed so far. First, methylation of DNA sequences may interfere with the binding of regulatory proteins to DNA. Binding of transcription factors c-MYC, AP-2, E2F, NFkB, and CTCF to their target sequences is prevented by methylation (Prendergast and Ziff 1991; Comb and Goodman 1990; Singal and Ginder 1999; Bell and Felsenfeld 2000). Second, DNA methylation provides target sites for methyl-CpG-binding domain (MBD) proteins (MDPs) – MeCP2, MBD1-4, and Kaiso (Hendrich and Bird 1998) – that were reported to repress transcription through recruitment of histone deacetylases (HDACs), affecting the chromatin structure (Jones et al. 1998; Nan et al. 1998). Of note, MDPs can also be linked to disease because mutations in the MeCP2 gene cause the neuronal disorder Rett syndrome (Amir et al. 1999). This syndrome can be recapitulated in the mouse by deletion of the MeCP2 gene, underscoring the impact of mouse models in the investigation of epigenetic causes of human disease (Guy et al. 2001). Third, DNMTs can cooperate with other members of epigenetic machinery such as histone (de)acetylases (HATs and HDACs) and histone methyltransferases (HMTs) to regulate gene expression.

2.2.3 Erasing and Editing DNA Methylation

DNA methylation is a stable epigenetic mark that is established and removed during different steps of development. The loss of methylation can either occur by a passive mechanism, when methylation is diluted out by DNA replication in the absence of DNMT activity, or by an active enzymatic removal of 5mC. In contrast to plants, in which 5mC is removed by the DNA repair enzymes glycosylases (Zhu 2009), no homologous enzyme has been found in mammals. Current models propose indirect mechanisms that include several conversion steps of 5mC into different oxidized intermediates which in the end are removed by the base excision repair (BER) machinery. The conversion is mediated by recently identified members of ten-eleven translocation (TET) family of proteins which first oxidize 5mC to 5 hydroxymethylcytosine (5hmC) and then to 5-formylcytosine (5fC) and 5-carboxylcytosine (5caC) (Tahiliani et al. 2009; Pfaffeneder et al. 2011; He et al. 2011; Ito et al. 2010). One of the models suggests that 5mC and 5hmC undergo deamination by the deaminases of AID (activation-induced cytidine deaminase)/APOBEC (apoprotein B mRNA-editing enzyme complex) family, creating mismatches recognized by the thymine DNA glycosylase (TDG) and subsequently repaired by the BER machinery (Zhu et al. 2010; Ito et al. 2010). Another possible scenario includes an excision of 5fC and 5caC by the TDG, again involving the BER pathway in the DNA demethylation process (Cortellino et al. 2011; Maiti and Drohat 2011).

2.2.4 Interplay Between DNA Methylation and Histone Modifications

DNA methylation is part of a well-orchestrated epigenetic network which also includes various histone modifications. Histone-modifying enzymes together with DNMTs dynamically mediate chromatin remodeling and transcriptional control. Histones are posttranslationally modified primarily in their *N*-terminal tails at lysines, arginines, and serines/threonines and more rarely in the globular domain by the addition of acetyl-, methyl-, phospho-, ubiquitin-, sumo-, or ADP-ribosyl groups. At least two modifications – acetylation and methylation – have been identified to cooperate with DNA methylation to control gene transcription. Histone acetylation is believed to control transcription independently of DNA methylation by neutralizing positive charges in *N*-terminal histone tails and thereby relaxing the condensed chromatin structure (Hong et al. 1993). Histone methylation, in turn, does not affect the overall charge of histones, but often closely cooperates with DNA methylation for gene expression control (Fuks 2005). Therefore here we will focus on histone methylation and its interaction with DNA methylation in regulation of gene expression.

2.2.4.1 Histone Methylation: Writing and Erasing

While histone acetylation at gene regulatory elements primarily correlates with active transcription, histone methylation can be associated with either transcriptional activation or silencing. All core histones are subject of modification by histone methyltransferases (HMTs) which transfer mono- (me1), di- (me2), or trimethyl (me3) groups to lysines (K) or arginines (R, only me1-2). However, the most extensively studied methylation events are those on histones H3 and H4. The establishment of histone methylation is mediated by two families of HMTs: protein arginine methyltransferases (PRMTs) and lysine HMTs which are subdivided into two groups, SET (suppressor of variegation, enhancer of zeste, trithorax) domain-containing HMTs (include 38 enzymes, targeting lysines in the histone tails) and non-SET domain-containing HMTs (represented by DOT 1-like (DOT1L) methyltransferase, targeting lysines in the globular core of the histones).

HMTs of the SET family form part of two important protein complexes identified in *Drosophila melanogaster* as trithorax (Trx) and polycomb (PcG), which are critical regulators of gene expression during development and differentiation. Mammalian homologues include mixed-lineage leukemia (MLL) and enhancer of zeste 2 (EZH2) proteins that catalyze H3K4me3 and H3K27me3, respectively. With the aid of high-throughput techniques, it became possible to show that distinct combinations of histone modifications correlate with specific patterns of gene expression genome wide. Thus, initiation of transcription is reported to be marked by the H3K4me3 as well as H3K9/K14 acetylation at gene promoters (Bernstein et al. 2002; Liang et al. 2004; Pokholok et al. 2005; Schneider et al. 2004; Schubeler et al. 2004), whereas H3K27me3 and H3K9me3 are found to be markers of more compact, silent chromatin (Cao et al. 2002; Lachner et al. 2001). Many lineage-specific genes in ES cells contain both activating H3K4me3 and repressive H3K27me3 marks, known as "bivalent histone modification." During development, these bivalent marks are resolved into either H3K4me3 or H3K27me3 only, leading to transcriptional activation or repression of corresponding genes, respectively. By this way, ES cells retain pluripotency and prime lineage-specific genes for rapid activation/inhibition in subsequent phases of differentiation (Bernstein et al. 2006). Removal of histone marks in mammals is mediated by two groups of proteins known so far – lysine-specific demethylase 1 (LSD1), responsible for the cleavage of mono- and dimethylation of H3K4 and H3K9 (Metzger et al. 2005; Shi et al. 2004), and Jumonji C (JmjC) domain-containing proteins (Kouzarides 2007; Metzger and Schüle 2007).

2.2.4.2 Crosstalk Between DNA and Histone Methylation

Gene expression in mammals is regulated by dynamic changes in chromatin configuration, switching between "open" euchromatic and compact heterochromatic states. Multiple studies have suggested that DNA methylation and histone methylation affect gene expression in an interdependent way. This relationship includes multiple feedback loops in which HMTs/histone methylation can influence DNA methylation and vice versa.

Initial studies showing that DNA methylation levels drop at specific genomic loci upon loss of H3K9 HMT activity were performed in fungi and plants (Tamaru et al. 2003; Jackson et al. 2002). Similar results were later obtained in mammalian ES cells lacking activity of the H3K9-specific HMTs G9A or SUV39H1/H2

(Dong et al. 2008; Epsztejn-Litman et al. 2008; Tachibana et al. 2008; Xin et al. 2003; Lehnertz et al. 2003). One genome-wide study suggested that G9A regulates DNA methylation in a locus-specific manner, because its knockdown in ES cells did not lead to global DNA demethylation but affected only 1.6 % of the analyzed genomic regions (Ikegami et al. 2007). Both G9A and SUV39H1/H2 control de novo DNA methylation by recruiting DNMT3A/B to their target sites, as was shown for postimplantation embryonic genes (Epsztejn-Litman et al. 2008; Feldman et al. 2006) and satellite repeats (Lehnertz et al. 2003; Fuks et al. 2003). It has also been suggested that all types of H3K4 methylation can protect CpG islands from de novo DNA methylation during early development (Ooi et al. 2007). This mechanism is mediated by DNMT3L which recruits DNMT3A only to those nucleosomes that are free of H3K4 methylation. In contrast, PcG proteins – in particular EZH2 which catalyzes the repressive H3K27me3 mark and interacts with DNMTs in vitro and in vivo (Vire et al. 2006) – are likely to mediate de novo DNA methylation in order to resolve bivalent domains into repressive during differentiation.

Many studies report the importance of DNA methylation in the establishment of histone modification patterns. Initially, this was shown in a mouse model in which DNA methylation of a transgenic construct prevented H3K4 methylation and promoted H3K9 methylation (Hashimshony et al. 2003). Another study, performed in *Arabidopsis* null mutants for the plant DNMT1-like methyltransferase MET1, showed profound loss of H3K9 methylation in heterochromatic areas (Tariq et al. 2003). Similarly, DNMT1 deficiency has been reported to influence H3K9me1,2,3 patterns in human cancer cell lines (Espada et al. 2004; Esteve et al. 2006). The possible mechanism of H3K9 methylation establishment by DNMT1 was proposed for replication foci where DNMT1 co-localizes and interacts with G9a (Esteve et al. 2006). However, in murine ES cells, H3K9 methylation does not change globally or locally upon knockout of de novo and maintenance DNMTs, raising the idea that the above-discussed phenomenon may be cell type specific (Tsumura et al. 2006).

Taken together, tight cooperation of DNA methylation and histone modifications in gene expression control often makes it difficult to reveal the unique role of an individual epigenetic modification in development and cancer when correlative studies are performed. Therefore, gene-targeting techniques in mice provide the most useful tools for investigating the functional roles of epigenetic modifications.

2.3 Experimental Manipulation of DNA Methylation in the Context of Cancer in Mice

Based on the recent revolution in genomic technologies, enormous efforts are currently being made to map DNA methylation marks in the genome of multiple cell types including cancer cells (Meissner et al. 2008; Weber et al. 2005; Schilling et al. 2009; Lister et al. 2009). This undertaking has already led to groundbreaking discoveries and will rapidly further our ideas on the role of DNA methylation in cellular processes such as development and cancer. However, it remains essential to continuously complement such descriptive approaches with experiments in vivo using animal models to fully elucidate the functional nature of DNA methylation within complex biological systems and to fully be able to exploit the potential of DNA methylation-targeting for therapeutic interventions.

For nearly 40 years, investigators have been addressing the role of DNA methylation in rodents by using either pharmacological inhibition of methyltransferase activity, dietary restriction of methyl sources, or targeted ablation of the methyltransferase genes.

2.3.1 Pharmacological and Dietary-Induced DNA Hypomethylation

In the era before targeted deletion of genes in mice was possible, the causal link between tumorigenesis and genomic methylation was initially addressed by the use of pharmacological inhibitors of methyltransferases and by dietary restrictions of methyl-group sources. The cytosine analogues 5-azacytidine and 5-aza-2′-deoxycytidine (=decitabine or DAC) have been the most widely used mechanism-based pharmacological inhibitors of methyltransferase activity (Jones 1985; Flotho et al. 2009). Both agents (in low dose!) have successfully been introduced into the clinical practice for treatment of myelodysplasia and selected patients with acute myeloid leukemia, following the idea that these substances would reactivate the expression of hypermethylated tumor-suppressor genes (Claus and Lübbert 2003). Methyl-group transfer during catalysis is inhibited by the N5 in these compounds and leads to covalent trapping of the methyltransferases by the base analogue incorporated into the DNA (Santi et al. 1984). In consequence, these compounds deplete the cell of DNMTs which indirectly leads to genomic hypomethylation. In experiments with rodents, several studies have suggested pro-oncogenic effects of pharmacological and dietary-induced DNA hypomethylation. Administration of 5-azacytidine to mice increased lung tumor incidences, led to lymphomas and granulocytic sarcomas, and produced a variety of different tumors in drug-treated rats (Stoner et al. 1973; Carr et al. 1984). However, these studies are difficult to interpret because 5-azacytidine (at least at a higher dose) can cause cytotoxicity (which may or may not be attributed to its demethylating effect) (Juttermann et al. 1994). It can also incorporate into RNA and is mutagenic, leaving some doubt whether its pro-oncogenic effect is indeed due to induction of DNA hypomethylation. It should be noted that an improved DNA cytosine methylation inhibitor, zebularine, which is preferentially incorporated into DNA, inhibits tumor cell growth in culture and prevents intestinal tumors in mice with minimal side effects, suggesting that this drug may be a promising candidate for anticancer therapy (Cheng et al. 2004; Yoo et al. 2008).

During the methyl-transfer reaction, the methyl-donor SAM is converted to S-adenosylhomocysteine (SAH). SAH is subsequently converted to homocysteine, which is then re-methylated to yield methionine in a folate- and cobalamin-dependent reaction before being converted back to SAM. This cycle can be blocked by dietary-based restriction of the methyl-group sources methionine, choline, folate, and/or vitamin B12. Dietary restriction of methyl sources increased the incidence of liver cancer in rodents, further supporting the notion that DNA hypomethylation is pro-oncogenic (Ghoshal and Farber 1984; Mikol et al. 1983; Sawada et al. 1990). However, this approach is also problematic because altering SAM levels by dietary methyl-deficiency would inhibit other cellular *trans*-methylation reactions as well, again providing no clear answer on whether DNA hypomethylation was indeed the (sole) cause of cancer in these studies.

2.3.2 Genetic Targeting of DNA Methyltransferases

The most straightforward approach to reduce DNA methylation levels in mice and cell culture systems is targeting of the *Dnmts* directly. In vitro, this can be achieved by small inhibiting (si) RNA and small hairpin (sh) RNA approaches. However, gene targeting in ES cells proved to be the most useful in vivo approach to manipulate expression of methyltransferases in the mouse genome. Here we summarize *Dnmt* mouse models used to study the role of DNA methylation in normal development and tumorigenesis (Table 2.1).

2.3.2.1 *Dnmt1* Knockout Mice

Dnmt1 is the first methyltransferase that was deleted by gene targeting in ES cells (Li et al. 1992). Several knockout alleles of *Dnmt1* have been described. The first mutant allele was generated by insertion of a neomycin selection cassette near the 5′ end of the gene and deletes *N*-terminal sequences (Li et al. 1992). This allele is usually called *Dnmt1*^{n} allele. *Dnmt1*$^{n/n}$ embryos show profound (but not complete) loss of genomic methylation and die during embryogenesis around 10 d.p.c. (Li et al. 1992). However, in the meantime, the *Dnmt1*^{n} allele turned out not to be a real null allele and expresses still low levels of functional DNMT1 activity. Therefore, two different true *Dnmt1* null-alleles have been generated: one allele carries a neomycin selection cassette insertion in the replication-foci-targeting region (termed *Dnmt1*^{s} allele for the *Sal*I site used for insertion into the locus); the other allele is a deletion of the conserved motifs in the *C*-terminal catalytic domain (termed *Dnmt1*^{c} allele) (Lei et al. 1996). The homozygous phenotypes of both null mutants resemble that of the *Dnmt1*$^{n/n}$ embryos, although they show even lower (but still not complete) methylation levels and die approximately 2 days earlier (Lei et al. 1996).

The embryonic lethality of the *Dnmt1* knockout mice precluded their use for studying the role of DNA methylation in tumorigenesis. Laird et al. partially solved this problem by combining *Dnmt1* heterozygosity with low-dose treatment of 5-azacytidine (Laird et al. 1995). When combining a *Dnmt1*^{s} allele with an *Apc*^{Min} allele, which predisposes mice to develop intestinal neoplasia, the authors observed that 5-azacydidine treatment substantially decreased the incidence of intestinal adenomas.

2.3.2.2 Conditional *Dnmt1* Knockout Mice

Jackson-Grusby et al. produced a conditional *Dnmt1* mutant allele in which exons 4 and 5 of the gene were flanked by *lox*P sites, leading to loss of catalytic activity (Jackson-Grusby et al. 2001). In the original study, embryonic fibroblasts from

Table 2.1 DNMT mouse models used in cancer research. *5-AZA* 5-azacytidine, *ESC* embryonic stem cell, *HSC* hematopoietic stem cell, *Cre* Cre recombinase, *MEF* mouse embryonic fibroblast, *CNS* central nervous system

Gene	Additional mutations/ treatment/ transgene	Mutant/cancer phenotype	References
Dnmt1$^{n/n}$		Global DNA demethylation, embryonic lethality	Li et al., (1992)
Dnmt1$^{s/s}$		DNA demethylation stronger than in *Dnmt1*$^{n/n}$, embryonic lethality	Lei et al., (1996)
Dnmt1$^{c/c}$		DNA demethylation stronger than in *Dnmt1*$^{n/n}$, embryonic lethality	Lei et al., (1996)
Dnmt1$^{s/+}$	*Apc*$^{Min/+}$ 5–AZA	Reduction in the number of intestinal adenomas after 5–AZA	Laird et al., (1995)
Dnmt1$^{flox/flox}$	Retroviral Cre	DNA demethylation in primary fibroblasts, activation of retro-elements, deregulation of gene expression, p53–mediated apoptosis	Jackson- Grusby et al., (2001)
	lckCre CD4Cre	Deregulation of T-cell development	Lee et al., (2001)
	Mx1-Cre	Hematopoietic cell depletion, rapid death of animals	Broske et al., (2009)
		Defects in HSC self-renewal, niche retention, enhanced cell cycling of myeloid progenitors	Trowbridge et al., (2009)
	nestin-Cre CamK-Cre	Rapid death of animals with high number of hypomethylated cells in CNS	Fan et al., (2001)
Dnmt1$^{n/chip}$		Runted hypomorphic mice, developing T cell lymphomas, gain of chromosome 15, genomic instability	Gaudet et al., (2003) Eden et al., (2003)
		Impairment of HSC self-renewal and lymphoid differentiation	Broske et al., (2009)
Dnmt1$^{c/chip}$	*Apc*$^{Min/+}$	Inhibition of intestinal tumorigenesis at the late stages, promotion of early colon and liver lesions	Yamada et al., (2005)
Dnmt3a$^{-/-}$		Normal at birth mice with subsequent death after 4 weeks, retention of de novo DNA methylation capacity by ESCs	Okano et al., (1999)
Dnmt3b$^{-/-}$		Embryonic lethality, retention of de novo DNA methylation capacity by ESCs	Okano et al., (1999)
Dnmt3a$^{-/-}$ *Dnmt3b*$^{-/-}$		Severe embryonic defects, loss of de novo DNA methylation capacity by ESCs	Okano et al., (1999)
Dnmt3a$^{flox/flox}$	Nes- Cre1	Neuromuscular defects and premature death of mice	Nguyen et al., (2007)
	TNAP- Cre	Defects in imprinting	Kaneda et al., (2004)
	Mx1- Cre	Enhanced self-renewal and disrupted differentiation of HSCs	Challen et al., (2012)
Dnmt3a$^{flox/flox}$	K-ras$^{LSL-G12D}$ Ad- Cre	Promotion of lung tumour growth and progression	Gao et al., (2011)
Dnmt3b$^{flox/flox}$	Ad- Cre	Global hypomethylation, aneuploidy, chromosomal breaks, spontaneous immortalization and senescence of MEFs	Dodge et al., (2005)
Dnmt3b$^{flox/flox}$	*Apc*$^{Min/+}$ Fabp- Cre	Inhibition of early stage macroscopic intestinal tumors	Lin et al., (2006)
Dnmt3a *Dnmt3b* inducible transgenes	*Apc*$^{Min/+}$	***Dnmt3a*** induction: increase in the number and size of colon tumors ***Dnmt3b*** induction: loss of imprinting, increased DNA methylation at the tumour suppressor loci	Linhart et al., (2007)

Dnmt1$^{loxP/loxP}$ mice were transduced with a CRE-bearing retrovirus to ablate *Dnmt1* in somatic cells. This approach led to severe demethylation, activation of endogenous retroviral elements, grossly disrupted gene expression signatures, and

activation of a p53-dependent apoptosis pathway (Jackson-Grusby et al. 2001). In the meantime, the *Dnmt1*^{loxP} allele has also been used to analyze the role of genomic methylation in other somatic cell types such as T cells (Lee et al. 2001), B cells (Cherry et al. 2000), hematopoietic stem and progenitor cells (Broske et al. 2009; Trowbridge et al. 2009), and cells of the central nervous system (Fan et al. 2001).

Conditional ablation of *Dnmt1* also leads to disrupted expression of many imprinted genes in somatic cells (Jackson-Grusby et al. 2001). In a clever model of transient *Dnmt1* ablation, the Jaenisch group could demonstrate a direct link between the loss of genomic imprinting and a higher incidence of malignant transformation, indicating that imprinting is essential for tumor suppression (Holm et al. 2005).

2.3.2.3 Hypomorphic *Dnmt1* Mice

Another option to study the role genomic hypomethylation in adult mice was made possible by a gradual methyltransferase knockdown through a hypomorphic *Dnmt1* allele (Tucker et al. 1996). This allele, termed *Dnmt1*^{chip} (chip=cDNA homologous insertion protocol), was created by knocking in a genomic/cDNA *Dnmt1* hybrid into the *Dnmt1*^{c} allele, resulting in functional *Dnmt1* expression at levels lower than those of the wild-type allele (Tucker et al. 1996). When the *Dnmt1*^{chip} allele was combined with a *Dnmt1*^{c} allele, expression of *Dnmt1* was reduced to approximately 10 % of wild-type levels, which was capable to rescue embryonic lethality and produce viable offspring (Gaudet et al. 2003). These animals show genomic hypomethylation but at a level substantially lower than that in mice with completely abolished *Dnmt1* expression. *Dnmt1*$^{c/chip}$ mice are smaller at birth and some develop T-cell tumors later in life by a mechanism that includes genomic instability and activation of the proto-oncogene c-myc (Gaudet et al. 2003; Eden et al. 2003). Consequently, this mouse provided the first purely genetic demonstration of a pro-oncogenic role of DNA hypomethylation. However, this effect appears to be tumor-type specific and developmental-stage specific since combining of the *Dnmt1*$^{c/chip}$ mouse with the *Apc*^{Min} allele showed that while DNA hypomethylation promoted early lesions in the colon and liver through induction of loss of heterozygosity, it suppressed later stages of intestinal tumorigenesis (Yamada et al. 2005).

2.3.2.4 *Dnmt3a* and *Dnmt3b* Knockout Mice

ES cells carrying a combined deletion in both genes, *Dnmt3a* and *Dnmt3b*, lack the capability to silence proviral DNA sequences by de novo methylation, whereas ES cells carrying deletions in either gene individually maintain normal de novo methylation capacity (Okano et al. 1999). *Dnmt3a* mice develop normally during embryogenesis and appear normal at birth and, however, become runted and die around 4 weeks of age. In contrast, no viable *Dnmt3b* mice can be recovered after birth because the embryos die of growth impairment and neural tube defects. Mice with a combined deficiency in both *Dnmt3a* and *Dnmt3b* suffer from even more severe embryonic defects which are similar to those of *Dnmt1* knockout mice (Okano et al. 1999). These results show that both *Dnmt3a* and *Dnmt3b* are important enzymes for de novo methylation and embryonic development.

2.3.2.5 Conditional *Dnmt3a* and *Dnmt3b* Knockout Mice

To study the role of de novo DNMTs in normal development and in the context of cancer, several conditional knockout mouse strains of *Dnmt3a* and *Dnmt3b* have been generated (Kaneda et al. 2004; Dodge et al. 2005; Lin et al. 2006; Nguyen et al. 2007; Tadokoro et al. 2007). These mice contain *lox*P sites flanking the exons that code for a catalytic domain of the corresponding enzyme. Breeding of *Dnmt3a* conditional knockout mice to transgenic lines expressing CRE recombinase at different stages of embryonic development allowed investigation of DNMT3A function in the establishment of the murine nervous system (Nguyen et al. 2007) and revealed its important role in imprinting (Kaneda et al. 2004). By a similar approach, conditional inactivation of *Dnmt3b* caused a decrease in DNA methylation levels, genomic instability, and spontaneous immortalization of mouse embryonic fibroblasts (Dodge et al. 2005). These findings suggest that Dnmt3 proteins can play an important role in cancer. This notion is also supported by colon-specific ablation of *Dnmt3b* in the $Apc^{Min/+}$ mouse, which inhibited the development of macroscopic intestinal tumors (Lin et al. 2006). *Dnmt3a* deficiency, in turn, was found to promote lung tumor progression as shown in the K-ras-induced lung cancer mouse model (Gao et al. 2011).

2.3.2.6 Inducible Dnmt Overexpression

A hallmark of most neoplasms is de novo methylation at promoter CpG islands, which silences the expression of selected tumor-suppressor genes (Baylin and Ohm 2006). To investigate the nature of this process, the Jaenisch lab has succeeded in generating mice which express doxycycline-inducible transgenes of *Dnmt3a* and *Dnmt3b* (Linhart et al. 2007). While no spontaneous tumors were reported in these mice following Dnmt3 overexpression upon doxycycline treatment, a twofold enhanced number of colon tumors was detected when the transgenes were crossed into the $Apc^{Min/+}$ intestinal neoplasia mouse model. The enhanced tumorigenesis was associated with a loss in imprinting and de novo methylation at selected tumor-suppressor loci (Linhart et al. 2007). Thus, these results provided evidence for a pro-oncogenic effect of increased DNMT expression through induced silencing of tumor-suppressor genes.

2.3.3 Genetic Targeting of Enzymes Involved in DNA Demethylation

2.3.3.1 *Tet* Knockout Mouse Models

Tet1 knockout mice have been created by flanking exon 4 with *lox*P sites which after CRE-mediated excision resulted in a truncated protein without a catalytic domain (Dawlaty et al. 2011). Despite the absence of enzymatic activity, $Tet1^{-/-}$ mice are viable and fertile and show partial loss of DNA methylation, which however is not severe enough to disturb embryonic or postnatal development (Dawlaty et al. 2011).

A more profound phenotype was observed in the case of *Tet2* deletion in mice, which has independently been conducted by several groups. To delete *Tet2* function, two different targeting approaches were applied: (1) gene-trap technology resulting in complete ablation of *Tet2* (Li et al. 2011) and (2) flanking exons 8–10 with *lox*P sites by gene targeting which together with excision by a CRE-deleter transgene resulted in a protein lacking a catalytic domain (Ko et al. 2011). *Tet2* null mice are born at the expected Mendelian ratios and are fertile. However, *Tet2* deletion is associated with a severe hematological phenotype which manifested in a reduction of 5hmC levels and accumulation of hematopoietic stem cells (HSCs) with skewed differentiation potential towards the myeloid lineage in the adult bone marrow (Ko et al. 2011; Li et al. 2011). Interestingly, with age a significant number of those mice develop lethal myeloid malignancies, phenotypically resembling human myeloid disorders such as chronic myelomonocytic leukemia (Li et al. 2011). Similar effects of *Tet2* ablation were observed by conditional deletion of *Tet2* exclusively in the hematopoietic compartment (Moran-Crusio et al. 2011).

2.4 Experimental Manipulations of Histone Methylation in the Context of Cancer in Mice

An increasing number of recent genomic studies have suggested alterations in histone modifications as an important factor in cancer formation. To prove the causal role of histone modifications in cancer, various mouse models that target writing and erasing enzymes have been generated. Here, we will focus on *Mll* mouse models as an example of the most frequently used system to model cancer (leukemia) in animals and to study the implication of the H3K4 methylation in leukemogenesis.

2.4.1 Mixed-Lineage Leukemia Gene Knockout and Overexpressing Mouse Models

Mixed-lineage leukemia (MLL) genes encode five different members of MLL proteins, whereby four of them (MLL1-4) have specificity to methylate H3K4. MLL family members play an important role in hematopoiesis and are frequent targets of gene rearrangement in human leukemias (Dimartino and Cleary 1999). Genetic lesions of the *Mll1 (=Mll)* gene are found in approximately 80 % of infant leukemias and 5–10 % of adult acute myeloid and lymphoid leukemias and more rarely in colorectal, pancreatic, brain, and breast cancers (Balakrishnan et al. 2007; Hess 2004; Huntsman et al. 1999; Krivtsov and Armstrong 2007; Sjoblom et al. 2006; Wang et al. 2011; Wood et al. 2007). Over 60 MLL-fusion products are known up to now, and some of them such as MLL-AF4, MLL-AF9, MLL-AF10, and MLL-ENL have been subject to intensive investigations.

To study the role of *Mll* in normal development and cancer, *Mll*-knockout mice were created by several different groups. These studies showed that *Mll* is important for embryonic development, because *Mll*$^{-/-}$ mice die during gestation (Yu et al. 1995). However, this phenotype appears not to depend on the methyltransferase activity of MLL as mice expressing a truncated MLL version lacking the SET domain are viable and fertile (Terranova et al. 2006). Inducible ablation in mice has further shown that MLL is crucial for proper self-renewal and quiescence of stem cells in the hematopoietic system (Jude et al. 2007). Furthermore, leukemogenic potential of MLL was studied by knock-in animals and retroviral overexpression of leukemic MLL-fusion products (Barabe et al. 2007; Chen et al. 2006; Collins et al. 2000; Corral et al. 1996; Forster et al. 2003; So et al. 2003; Wang et al. 2005; Zeisig et al. 2003). Both in vivo approaches and in vitro studies have demonstrated that *Mll* lesions can drive leukemia development by a mechanism that involves deregulation of homeobox (*Hox*) genes, which are important for HSC self-renewal and differentiation (Ayton and Cleary 2003; Horton et al. 2005; Krivtsov et al. 2006; Milne et al. 2005; Somervaille et al. 2009; Zeisig et al. 2003). Activation of *Hox* genes is strictly controlled during hematopoiesis (Argiropoulos and Humphries 2007) and their overexpression promotes leukemia induction (Kroon et al. 1998). *Mll* lesions deregulate *Hox* expression using epigenetic mechanisms which differ from the mechanism of *Hox* activation by wild-type MLL in HSCs. For example, partial tandem duplication of MLL (MLL-PTD), which frequently occurs in leukemia and was modelled in knock-in mice, induces expression of *Hoxa7* and *Hoxa9* genes by the establishment of H3/H4 acetylation and H3K4me2 marks on their promoters (Dorrance et al. 2006, 2008). The majority of MLL-fusion proteins studied so far in mice lose their H3K4-HMT domain due to gene rearrangement and therefore require additional factors to activate *Hox*-gene expression. In case of the most frequent MLL fusions (MLL-AF4, MLL-AF9, MLL-AF10, MLL-ENL), an interaction partner is DOTL1 (Okada et al. 2005), a methyltransferase which transfers the activating H3K79me mark to *Hox* promoters upon recruitment by MLL-fusion proteins (Guenther et al. 2008; Krivtsov et al. 2008; Milne et al. 2005; Mueller et al. 2007; Okada et al. 2005; Thiel et al. 2010).

2.5 Role of DNA Methylation in Normal and Cancerous Stem Cells

Because of a promising role in regenerative medicine, elucidation of the critical epigenetic mechanisms that control stem cell programs receives widespread attention. Analysis of ES cells and adult tissue stem cells with targeted mutations in DNA methyltransferase genes has demonstrated an important role of DNA methylation in the control of key stem cell programs. Ablation of *Dnmt1* results in severe, but not complete, demethylation in ES cells (Li et al. 1992). *Dnmt1*-deficient ES cells have a normal morphology and a normal self-renewal rate and do not undergo DNA damage-induced apoptosis, which is in stark contrast to the rapid cell death of *Dnmt1*-deficient mouse fibroblasts and human colon cancer cells (Jackson-Grusby et al. 2001; Chen et al. 2007). Of note, even combined deletion of *Dnmt1*, *Dnmt3a*, and *Dnmt3b*, leading to complete absence of detectable CpG methylation, does not affect ES cell viability and self-renewal (Tsumura et al. 2006), implying that in contrast to somatic cells, ES cells are protected against demethylation-provoked apoptosis. However, *Dnmt1*-ablated ES cells fail to develop when introduced into the germ line of mice, indicating that DNA methylation is required for their differentiation (Li et al. 1992; Lei et al. 1996).

While DNA methylation seems dispensable for self-renewal of ES cells in vitro, it is critical for self-renewal of somatic stem cells in vivo. Combined deletion of *Dnmt3a* and *Dnmt3b* results in a severely blocked self-renewal of HSCs that still retain differentiation capacities, whereas deletion of each gene individually did not show an effect in this study (Tadokoro et al. 2007). However, in a more recent study in which *Dnmt3a*-deficient HSCs were forced to divide by serial transplantations into recipient mice, they expanded due to enhanced self-renewal and disturbed differentiation (Challen et al. 2012). Mechanistically, *Dnmt3a* functions to promote differentiation by inactivating stem cell gene signatures upon differentiation signals.

Our group could recently show that conditional ablation of *Dnmt1* in HSCs leads to severe genomic demethylation, followed by a massive apoptosis-induced bone marrow pancytopenia and a rapid death of the animals (Broske et al. 2009). A similar role for *Dnmt1* in hematopoietic cells has been reported in a study by Stuart Orkin's group (Trowbridge et al. 2009). By analyzing *Dnmt1*$^{c/chip}$ mice, in which the stem cells are protected from apoptosis by the residual hypomorphic *Dnmt1* expression, we could further demonstrate a crucial requirement for DNA methylation in lineage-differentiation decision of HSCs. *Dnmt1*$^{c/chip}$ HSCs fail to suppress key myeloerythroid regulators and as a consequence can differentiate into myeloerythroid but not into lymphoid progeny (Broske et al. 2009; Vockentanz et al. 2010). Importantly, this finding has recently been confirmed and extended by showing that the genome of myeloid cells is less methylated than that of lymphocytes and that treatment of HSCs with a demethylating agent induces myeloid over lymphoid differentiation (Ji et al. 2010). Taken together, these results indicate that DNA methylation is an important epigenetic mechanism to equip HSCs with self-renewal capacity and multipotency (Fig. 2.1), a finding which has similarly been observed for epidermal and neuronal stem/progenitor cells (Fan et al. 2001; Sen et al. 2010; Trowbridge and Orkin 2010).

Since DNMTs have no DNA target sequence preferences other than CpGs, how can these enzymes be involved in the regulation of specific gene programs to orchestrate self-renewal and multipotency? The answer may lay in the important discovery that sequence-specific DNA interacting proteins can recruit DNMTs to their cognate-binding motifs to induce localized methylation at certain promoters. DNMTs have been shown to undergo direct protein-protein binding with the transcription factors PU.1 and c-MYC, the leukemia-associated transcription factor-fusions PML-RARA and AML-ETO, and the polycomb factor EZH2 (Suzuki et al. 2006; Brenner et al. 2005; Di et al. 2002; Liu et al. 2005; Viré et al. 2006). Another possible mechanism to position DNA methylation marks at specific gene regulatory regions came from genome-wide studies revealing that DNA methylation patterns correlate with histone methylation patterns, suggesting that particular histone modifications lead to the local recruitment of DNMTs (perhaps through DNMT3L) (Meissner et al. 2008).

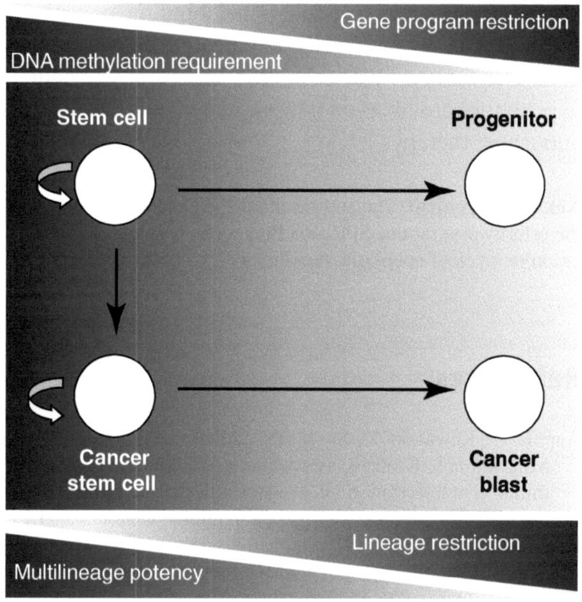

Fig. 2.1 A particular role for DNA methylation in stem cells. Stem cells are characterized by low expression of genes driving lineage differentiation but high expression of genes maintaining self-renewal. Recent studies in *Dnmt1*-mutant mice have shown that DNA methylation is an essential epigenetic program to protect self-renewal and multipotency in normal as well as leukemic stem cells by suppressing predominant lineage-specific genes

Increasing evidence indicates that many tumors are sustained by cancer stem cells (CSCs) whose self-renewal may be controlled by similar mechanisms that control normal stem cells (Weissman 2005; Passegue et al. 2003). We could show, using mouse models of leukemia, that the capacity of CSCs to self-renew and exert multilineage fate programs requires constitutive DNA methylation (Broske et al. 2009). This result is interesting because it suggests that altered DNA methylation may be an early event during leukemogenesis and that it may be possible to use demethylating chemicals to impair CSC function in cancer therapy (Trowbridge et al. 2012).

2.6 Outlook

Although intensive research on animal models has helped tremendously to better understand the functional role of DNA methylation in cancerogenesis, a number of questions remain still unanswered. Among the most important ones of these questions are the following: which genes are controlled by DNA methylation mechanisms in cancer cells, especially in CSCs; how these genes control neoplastic cell potential; and how we can properly correct their expression by DNA methylation-based therapy to selectively eradicate cancer cells? It may be helpful in this respect to not only concentrate efforts on the DNMTs alone but also include the proteins that cooperate with DNMTs to recruit DNA methylation activity to silence the expression of anticancer genes. A particular focus should therefore be put on deciphering global principles in the cooperation between DNA methylation with histone modifications and with functional binding patterns of transcription factors. The combination of genetically engineered mouse models with the rapidly evolving genomics tools provides a unique opportunity to address these important points and to push forward ideas on how we can manipulate epigenetic mechanisms to improve anticancer therapy.

Acknowledgement The authors thank the Deutsche Forschungsgemeinschaft for funding (within the priority programme SPP1463 Epigenetic regulation of normal haematopoiesis and its dysregulation in myeloid neoplasia; coordinators M. Lübbert, Freiburg, C. Plass, Heidelberg).

References

Aapola U, Kawasaki K, Scott HS, Ollila J, Vihinen M, Heino M, Shintani A, Kawasaki K, Minoshima S, Krohn K, Antonarakis SE, Shimizu N, Kudoh J, Peterson P (2000) Isolation and initial characterization of a novel zinc finger gene, DNMT3L, on 21q22.3, related to the cytosine-5-methyltransferase 3 gene family. Genomics 65:293–298

Aapola U, Lyle R, Krohn K, Antonarakis SE, Peterson P (2001) Isolation and initial characterization of the mouse Dnmt3l gene. Cytogenet Cell Genet 92:122–126

Adams RL (1990) DNA methylation. The effect of minor bases on DNA-protein interactions. Biochem J 265:309–320

Amir RE, Van den Veyver IB, Wan M, Tran CQ, Francke U, Zoghbi HY (1999) Rett syndrome is caused by mutations in X-linked MECP2, encoding methyl-CpG-binding protein 2. Nat Genet 23:185–188

Argiropoulos B, Humphries RK (2007) Hox genes in hematopoiesis and leukemogenesis. Oncogene 26:6766–6776

Ayton PM, Cleary ML (2003) Transformation of myeloid progenitors by MLL oncoproteins is dependent on Hoxa7 and Hoxa9. Genes Dev 17:2298–2307

Balakrishnan A, Bleeker FE, Lamba S, Rodolfo M, Daniotti M, Scarpa A, van Tilborg AA, Leenstra S, Zanon C, Bardelli A (2007) Novel somatic and germline mutations in cancer candidate genes in glioblastoma, melanoma, and pancreatic carcinoma. Cancer Res 67:3545–3550

Barabe F, Kennedy JA, Hope KJ, Dick JE (2007) Modeling the initiation and progression of human acute leukemia in mice. Science 316:600–604

Baylin SB, Ohm JE (2006) Epigenetic gene silencing in cancer – a mechanism for early oncogenic pathway addiction? Nat Rev Cancer 6:107–116

Bell AC, Felsenfeld G (2000) Methylation of a CTCF-dependent boundary controls imprinted expression of the Igf2 gene. Nature 405:482–485

Bernstein BE, Humphrey EL, Erlich RL, Schneider R, Bouman P, Liu JS, Kouzarides T, Schreiber SL (2002) Methylation of histone H3 Lys 4 in coding regions of active genes. Proc Natl Acad Sci U S A 99:8695–8700

Bernstein BE, Mikkelsen TS, Xie X, Kamal M, Huebert DJ, Cuff J, Fry B, Meissner A, Wernig M, Plath K, Jaenisch R, Wagschal A, Feil R, Schreiber SL, Lander ES (2006) A bivalent chromatin structure marks key developmental genes in embryonic stem cells. Cell 125:315–326

Bestor TH (1988) Cloning of a mammalian DNA methyltransferase. Gene 74:9–12

Bestor TH (1992) Activation of mammalian DNA methyltransferase by cleavage of a Zn binding regulatory domain. EMBO J 11:2611–2617

Bestor TH (2000) The DNA methyltransferases of mammals. Hum Mol Genet 9:2395–2402

Bird A (2002) DNA methylation patterns and epigenetic memory. Genes Dev 16:6–21

Bostick M, Kim JK, Esteve PO, Clark A, Pradhan S, Jacobsen SE (2007) UHRF1 plays a role in maintaining DNA methylation in mammalian cells. Science 317:1760–1764

Bourc'his D, Xu GL, Lin CS, Bollman B, Bestor TH (2001) Dnmt3L and the establishment of maternal genomic imprints. Science 294:2536–2539
Brenner C, Deplus R, Didelot C, Loriot A, Vire E, De SC, Gutierrez A, Danovi D, Bernard D, Boon T, Pelicci PG, Amati B, Kouzarides T, de LY, Di CL, Fuks F (2005) Myc represses transcription through recruitment of DNA methyltransferase corepressor. EMBO J 24:336–346
Broske AM, Vockentanz L, Kharazi S, Huska MR, Mancini E, Scheller M, Kuhl C, Enns A, Prinz M, Jaenisch R, Nerlov C, Leutz A, Andrade-Navarro MA, Jacobsen SE, Rosenbauer F (2009) DNA methylation protects hematopoietic stem cell multipotency from myeloerythroid restriction. Nat Genet 41:1207–1215
Cao R, Wang L, Wang H, Xia L, Erdjument-Bromage H, Tempst P, Jones RS, Zhang Y (2002) Role of histone H3 lysine 27 methylation in polycomb-group silencing. Science 298:1039–1043
Carr BI, Reilly JG, Smith SS, Winberg C, Riggs A (1984) The tumorigenicity of 5-azacytidine in the male Fischer rat. Carcinogenesis 5:1583–1590
Cedar H, Bergman Y (2009) Linking DNA methylation and histone modification: patterns and paradigms. Nat Rev Genet 10:295–304
Challen GA, Sun D, Jeong M, Luo M, Jelinek J, Berg JS, Bock C, Vasanthakumar A, Gu H, Xi Y, Liang S, Lu Y, Darlington GJ, Meissner A, Issa JP, Godley LA, Li W, Goodell MA (2012) Dnmt3a is essential for hematopoietic stem cell differentiation. Nat Genet 44:23–31
Chen W, Li Q, Hudson WA, Kumar A, Kirchhof N, Kersey JH (2006) A murine Mll-AF4 knock-in model results in lymphoid and myeloid deregulation and hematologic malignancy. Blood 108:669–677
Chen T, Hevi S, Gay F, Tsujimoto N, He T, Zhang B, Ueda Y, Li E (2007) Complete inactivation of DNMT1 leads to mitotic catastrophe in human cancer cells. Nat Genet 39:391–396
Cheng JC, Yoo CB, Weisenberger DJ, Chuang J, Wozniak C, Liang G, Marquez VE, Greer S, Orntoft TF, Thykjaer T, Jones PA (2004) Preferential response of cancer cells to zebularine. Cancer Cell 6:151–158
Cherry SR, Beard C, Jaenisch R, Baltimore D (2000) V(D)J recombination is not activated by demethylation of the kappa locus. Proc Natl Acad Sci U S A 97:8467–8472
Chuang LS, Ian HI, Koh TW, Ng HH, Xu G, Li BF (1997) Human DNA-(cytosine-5) methyltransferase-PCNA complex as a target for p21WAF1. Science 277:1996–2000
Claus R, Lübbert M (2003) Epigenetic targets in hematopoietic malignancies. Oncogene 22:6489–6496
Collins EC, Pannell R, Simpson EM, Forster A, Rabbitts TH (2000) Inter-chromosomal recombination of Mll and Af9 genes mediated by cre-loxP in mouse development. EMBO Rep 1:127–132
Comb M, Goodman HM (1990) CpG methylation inhibits proenkephalin gene expression and binding of the transcription factor AP-2. Nucleic Acids Res 18:3975–3982
Corral J, Lavenir I, Impey H, Warren AJ, Forster A, Larson TA, Bell S, McKenzie AN, King G, Rabbitts TH (1996) An Mll-AF9 fusion gene made by homologous recombination causes acute leukemia in chimeric mice: a method to create fusion oncogenes. Cell 85:853–861
Cortellino S, Xu J, Sannai M, Moore R, Caretti E, Cigliano A, Le CM, Devarajan K, Wessels A, Soprano D, Abramowitz LK, Bartolomei MS, Rambow F, Bassi MR, Bruno T, Fanciulli M, Renner C, Klein-Szanto AJ, Matsumoto Y, Kobi D, Davidson I, Alberti C, Larue L, Bellacosa A (2011) Thymine DNA glycosylase is essential for active DNA demethylation by linked deamination-base excision repair. Cell 146:67–79
Dawlaty MM, Ganz K, Powell BE, Hu YC, Markoulaki S, Cheng AW, Gao Q, Kim J, Choi SW, Page DC, Jaenisch R (2011) Tet1 is dispensable for maintaining pluripotency and its loss is compatible with embryonic and postnatal development. Cell Stem Cell 9:166–175
Dennis K, Fan T, Geiman T, Yan Q, Muegge K (2001) Lsh, a member of the SNF2 family, is required for genome-wide methylation. Genes Dev 15:2940–2944
Di Croce L, Raker VA, Corsaro M, Fazi F, Fanelli M, Faretta M, Fuks F, Lo CF, Kouzarides T, Nervi C, Minucci S, Pelicci PG (2002) Methyltransferase recruitment and DNA hypermethylation of target promoters by an oncogenic transcription factor. Science 295:1079–1082

Dimartino JF, Cleary ML (1999) Mll rearrangements in haematological malignancies: lessons from clinical and biological studies. Br J Haematol 106:614–626

Dodge JE, Okano M, Dick F, Tsujimoto N, Chen T, Wang S, Ueda Y, Dyson N, Li E (2005) Inactivation of Dnmt3b in mouse embryonic fibroblasts results in DNA hypomethylation, chromosomal instability, and spontaneous immortalization. J Biol Chem 280:17986–17991

Dong KB, Maksakova IA, Mohn F, Leung D, Appanah R, Lee S, Yang HW, Lam LL, Mager DL, Schubeler D, Tachibana M, Shinkai Y, Lorincz MC (2008) DNA methylation in ES cells requires the lysine methyltransferase G9a but not its catalytic activity. EMBO J 27:2691–2701

Dorrance AM, Liu S, Yuan W, Becknell B, Arnoczky KJ, Guimond M, Strout MP, Feng L, Nakamura T, Yu L, Rush LJ, Weinstein M, Leone G, Wu L, Ferketich A, Whitman SP, Marcucci G, Caligiuri MA (2006) Mll partial tandem duplication induces aberrant Hox expression in vivo via specific epigenetic alterations. J Clin Invest 116:2707–2716

Dorrance AM, Liu S, Chong A, Pulley B, Nemer D, Guimond M, Yuan W, Chang D, Whitman SP, Marcucci G, Caligiuri MA (2008) The Mll partial tandem duplication: differential, tissue-specific activity in the presence or absence of the wild-type allele. Blood 112:2508–2511

Eden A, Gaudet F, Waghmare A, Jaenisch R (2003) Chromosomal instability and tumors promoted by DNA hypomethylation. Science 300:455

Epsztejn-Litman S, Feldman N, Abu-Remaileh M, Shufaro Y, Gerson A, Ueda J, Deplus R, Fuks F, Shinkai Y, Cedar H, Bergman Y (2008) De novo DNA methylation promoted by G9a prevents reprogramming of embryonically silenced genes. Nat Struct Mol Biol 15:1176–1183

Espada J, Ballestar E, Fraga MF, Villar-Garea A, Juarranz A, Stockert JC, Robertson KD, Fuks F, Esteller M (2004) Human DNA methyltransferase 1 is required for maintenance of the histone H3 modification pattern. J Biol Chem 279:37175–37184

Esteve PO, Chin HG, Smallwood A, Feehery GR, Gangisetty O, Karpf AR, Carey MF, Pradhan S (2006) Direct interaction between DNMT1 and G9a coordinates DNA and histone methylation during replication. Genes Dev 20:3089–3103

Fan G, Beard C, Chen RZ, Csankovszki G, Sun Y, Siniaia M, Biniszkiewicz D, Bates B, Lee PP, Kuhn R, Trumpp A, Poon C, Wilson CB, Jaenisch R (2001) DNA hypomethylation perturbs the function and survival of CNS neurons in postnatal animals. J Neurosci 21:788–797

Feinberg AP, Ohlsson R, Henikoff S (2006) The epigenetic progenitor origin of human cancer. Nat Rev Genet 7:21–33

Feldman N, Gerson A, Fang J, Li E, Zhang Y, Shinkai Y, Cedar H, Bergman Y (2006) G9a-mediated irreversible epigenetic inactivation of Oct-3/4 during early embryogenesis. Nat Cell Biol 8:188–194

Flotho C, Claus R, Batz C, Schneider M, Sandrock I, Ihde S, Plass C, Niemeyer CM, Lübbert M (2009) The DNA methyltransferase inhibitors azacitidine, decitabine and zebularine exert differential effects on cancer gene expression in acute myeloid leukemia cells. Leukemia 23:1019–1028

Forster A, Pannell R, Drynan LF, McCormack M, Collins EC, Daser A, Rabbitts TH (2003) Engineering de novo reciprocal chromosomal translocations associated with Mll to replicate primary events of human cancer. Cancer Cell 3:449–458

Fuks F (2005) DNA methylation and histone modifications: teaming up to silence genes. Curr Opin Genet Dev 15:490–495

Fuks F, Hurd PJ, Deplus R, Kouzarides T (2003) The DNA methyltransferases associate with HP1 and the SUV39H1 histone methyltransferase. Nucleic Acids Res 31:2305–2312

Gao Q, Steine EJ, Barrasa MI, Hockemeyer D, Pawlak M, Fu D, Reddy S, Bell GW, Jaenisch R (2011) Deletion of the de novo DNA methyltransferase Dnmt3a promotes lung tumor progression. Proc Natl Acad Sci U S A 108:18061–18066

Gaudet F, Hodgson JG, Eden A, Jackson-Grusby L, Dausman J, Gray JW, Leonhardt H, Jaenisch R (2003) Induction of tumors in mice by genomic hypomethylation. Science 300:489–492

Ghoshal AK, Farber E (1984) The induction of liver cancer by dietary deficiency of choline and methionine without added carcinogens. Carcinogenesis 5:1367–1370

Glickman JF, Pavlovich JG, Reich NO (1997) Peptide mapping of the murine DNA methyltransferase reveals a major phosphorylation site and the start of translation. J Biol Chem 272:17851–17857
Goll MG, Kirpekar F, Maggert KA, Yoder JA, Hsieh CL, Zhang X, Golic KG, Jacobsen SE, Bestor TH (2006) Methylation of tRNAAsp by the DNA methyltransferase homolog Dnmt2. Science 311:395–398
Guenther MG, Lawton LN, Rozovskaia T, Frampton GM, Levine SS, Volkert TL, Croce CM, Nakamura T, Canaani E, Young RA (2008) Aberrant chromatin at genes encoding stem cell regulators in human mixed-lineage leukemia. Genes Dev 22:3403–3408
Guy J, Hendrich B, Holmes M, Martin JE, Bird A (2001) A mouse Mecp2-null mutation causes neurological symptoms that mimic Rett syndrome. Nat Genet 27:322–326
Hashimshony T, Zhang J, Keshet I, Bustin M, Cedar H (2003) The role of DNA methylation in setting up chromatin structure during development. Nat Genet 34:187–192
Hata K, Okano M, Lei H, Li E (2002) Dnmt3L cooperates with the Dnmt3 family of de novo DNA methyltransferases to establish maternal imprints in mice. Development 129:1983–1993
He YF, Li BZ, Li Z, Liu P, Wang Y, Tang Q, Ding J, Jia Y, Chen Z, Li L, Sun Y, Li X, Dai Q, Song CX, Zhang K, He C, Xu GL (2011) Tet-mediated formation of 5-carboxylcytosine and its excision by TDG in mammalian DNA. Science 333:1303–1307
Hendrich B, Bird A (1998) Identification and characterization of a family of mammalian methyl-CpG binding proteins. Mol Cell Biol 18:6538–6547
Hermann A, Goyal R, Jeltsch A (2004) The Dnmt1 DNA-(cytosine-C5)-methyltransferase methylates DNA processively with high preference for hemimethylated target sites. J Biol Chem 279:48350–48359
Hess JL (2004) MLL: a histone methyltransferase disrupted in leukemia. Trends Mol Med 10:500–507
Holm TM, Jackson-Grusby L, Brambrink T, Yamada Y, Rideout WM III, Jaenisch R (2005) Global loss of imprinting leads to widespread tumorigenesis in adult mice. Cancer Cell 8:275–285
Hong L, Schroth GP, Matthews HR, Yau P, Bradbury EM (1993) Studies of the DNA binding properties of histone H4 amino terminus. Thermal denaturation studies reveal that acetylation markedly reduces the binding constant of the H4 "tail" to DNA. J Biol Chem 268:305–314
Horton SJ, Grier DG, McGonigle GJ, Thompson A, Morrow M, De SI, Moulding DA, Kioussis D, Lappin TR, Brady HJ, Williams O (2005) Continuous MLL-ENL expression is necessary to establish a "Hox Code" and maintain immortalization of hematopoietic progenitor cells. Cancer Res 65:9245–9252
Hotchkiss RD (1948) The quantitative separation of purines, pyrimidines, and nucleosides by paper chromatography. J Biol Chem 175:315–332
Huang J, Fan T, Yan Q, Zhu H, Fox S, Issaq HJ, Best L, Gangi L, Munroe D, Muegge K (2004) Lsh, an epigenetic guardian of repetitive elements. Nucleic Acids Res 32:5019–5028
Huntsman DG, Chin SF, Muleris M, Batley SJ, Collins VP, Wiedemann LM, Aparicio S, Caldas C (1999) MLL2, the second human homolog of the Drosophila trithorax gene, maps to 19q13.1 and is amplified in solid tumor cell lines. Oncogene 18:7975–7984
Ikegami K, Iwatani M, Suzuki M, Tachibana M, Shinkai Y, Tanaka S, Greally JM, Yagi S, Hattori N, Shiota K (2007) Genome-wide and locus-specific DNA hypomethylation in G9a deficient mouse embryonic stem cells. Genes Cells 12:1–11
Ito S, D'Alessio AC, Taranova OV, Hong K, Sowers LC, Zhang Y (2010) Role of Tet proteins in 5mC to 5hmC conversion, ES-cell self-renewal and inner cell mass specification. Nature 466:1129–1133
Jackson JP, Lindroth AM, Cao X, Jacobsen SE (2002) Control of CpNpG DNA methylation by the KRYPTONITE histone H3 methyltransferase. Nature 416:556–560
Jackson-Grusby L, Beard C, Possemato R, Tudor M, Fambrough D, Csankovszki G, Dausman J, Lee P, Wilson C, Lander E, Jaenisch R (2001) Loss of genomic methylation causes p53-dependent apoptosis and epigenetic deregulation. Nat Genet 27:31–39
Jaenisch R (1997) DNA methylation and imprinting: why bother? Trends Genet 13:323–329
Ji H, Ehrlich LI, Seita J, Murakami P, Doi A, Lindau P, Lee H, Aryee MJ, Irizarry RA, Kim K, Rossi DJ, Inlay MA, Serwold T, Karsunky H, Ho L, Daley GQ, Weissman IL, Feinberg AP

(2010) Comprehensive methylome map of lineage commitment from haematopoietic progenitors. Nature 467:338–342

Jia D, Jurkowska RZ, Zhang X, Jeltsch A, Cheng X (2007) Structure of Dnmt3a bound to Dnmt3L suggests a model for de novo DNA methylation. Nature 449:248–251

Jones PA (1985) Effects of 5-azacytidine and its 2′-deoxyderivative on cell differentiation and DNA methylation. Pharmacol Ther 28:17–27

Jones PL, Veenstra GJ, Wade PA, Vermaak D, Kass SU, Landsberger N, Strouboulis J, Wolffe AP (1998) Methylated DNA and MeCP2 recruit histone deacetylase to repress transcription. Nat Genet 19:187–191

Jude CD, Climer L, Xu D, Artinger E, Fisher JK, Ernst P (2007) Unique and independent roles for MLL in adult hematopoietic stem cells and progenitors. Cell Stem Cell 1:324–337

Jüttermann R, Li E, Jaenisch R (1994) Toxicity of 5-aza-2′-deoxycytidine to mammalian cells is mediated primarily by covalent trapping of DNA methyltransferase rather than DNA demethylation. Proc Natl Acad Sci U S A 91:11797–11801

Kaneda M, Okano M, Hata K, Sado T, Tsujimoto N, Li E, Sasaki H (2004) Essential role for de novo DNA methyltransferase Dnmt3a in paternal and maternal imprinting. Nature 429:900–903

Ko M, Bandukwala HS, An J, Lamperti ED, Thompson EC, Hastie R, Tsangaratou A, Rajewsky K, Koralov SB, Rao A (2011) Ten-Eleven-Translocation 2 (TET2) negatively regulates homeostasis and differentiation of hematopoietic stem cells in mice. Proc Natl Acad Sci U S A 108:14566–14571

Kouzarides T (2007) Chromatin modifications and their function. Cell 128:693–705

Krivtsov AV, Armstrong SA (2007) MLL translocations, histone modifications and leukaemia stem-cell development. Nat Rev Cancer 7:823–833

Krivtsov AV, Twomey D, Feng Z, Stubbs MC, Wang Y, Faber J, Levine JE, Wang J, Hahn WC, Gilliland DG, Golub TR, Armstrong SA (2006) Transformation from committed progenitor to leukaemia stem cell initiated by MLL-AF9. Nature 442:818–822

Krivtsov AV, Feng Z, Lemieux ME, Faber J, Vempati S, Sinha AU, Xia X, Jesneck J, Bracken AP, Silverman LB, Kutok JL, Kung AL, Armstrong SA (2008) H3K79 methylation profiles define murine and human MLL-AF4 leukemias. Cancer Cell 14:355–368

Kroon E, Krosl J, Thorsteinsdottir U, Baban S, Buchberg AM, Sauvageau G (1998) Hoxa9 transforms primary bone marrow cells through specific collaboration with Meis1a but not Pbx1b. EMBO J 17:3714–3725

Lachner M, O'Carroll D, Rea S, Mechtler K, Jenuwein T (2001) Methylation of histone H3 lysine 9 creates a binding site for HP1 proteins. Nature 410:116–120

Laird PW, Jackson-Grusby L, Fazeli A, Dickinson SL, Jung WE, Li E, Weinberg RA, Jaenisch R (1995) Suppression of intestinal neoplasia by DNA hypomethylation. Cell 81:197–205

Lee PP, Fitzpatrick DR, Beard C, Jessup HK, Lehar S, Makar KW, Perez-Melgosa M, Sweetser MT, Schlissel MS, Nguyen S, Cherry SR, Tsai JH, Tucker SM, Weaver WM, Kelso A, Jaenisch R, Wilson CB (2001) A critical role for Dnmt1 and DNA methylation in T cell development, function, and survival. Immunity 15:763–774

Lehnertz B, Ueda Y, Derijck AA, Braunschweig U, Perez-Burgos L, Kubicek S, Chen T, Li E, Jenuwein T, Peters AH (2003) Suv39h-mediated histone H3 lysine 9 methylation directs DNA methylation to major satellite repeats at pericentric heterochromatin. Curr Biol 13:1192–1200

Lei H, Oh SP, Okano M, Jüttermann R, Goss KA, Jaenisch R, Li E (1996) De novo DNA cytosine methyltransferase activities in mouse embryonic stem cells. Development 122:3195–3205

Leonhardt H, Page AW, Weier HU, Bestor TH (1992) A targeting sequence directs DNA methyltransferase to sites of DNA replication in mammalian nuclei. Cell 71:865–873

Li E, Bestor TH, Jaenisch R (1992) Targeted mutation of the DNA methyltransferase gene results in embryonic lethality. Cell 69:915–926

Li Z, Cai X, Cai CL, Wang J, Zhang W, Petersen BE, Yang FC, Xu M (2011) Deletion of Tet2 in mice leads to dysregulated hematopoietic stem cells and subsequent development of myeloid malignancies. Blood 118:4509–4518

Liang G, Chan MF, Tomigahara Y, Tsai YC, Gonzales FA, Li E, Laird PW, Jones PA (2002) Cooperativity between DNA methyltransferases in the maintenance methylation of repetitive elements. Mol Cell Biol 22:480–491

Liang G, Lin JC, Wei V, Yoo C, Cheng JC, Nguyen CT, Weisenberger DJ, Egger G, Takai D, Gonzales FA, Jones PA (2004) Distinct localization of histone H3 acetylation and H3-K4 methylation to the transcription start sites in the human genome. Proc Natl Acad Sci U S A 101:7357–7362

Lin H, Yamada Y, Nguyen S, Linhart H, Jackson-Grusby L, Meissner A, Meletis K, Lo G, Jaenisch R (2006) Suppression of intestinal neoplasia by deletion of Dnmt3b. Mol Cell Biol 26:2976–2983

Linhart HG, Lin H, Yamada Y, Moran E, Steine EJ, Gokhale S, Lo G, Cantu E, Ehrich M, He T, Meissner A, Jaenisch R (2007) Dnmt3b promotes tumorigenesis in vivo by gene-specific de novo methylation and transcriptional silencing. Genes Dev 21:3110–3122

Lister R, Pelizzola M, Dowen RH, Hawkins RD, Hon G, Tonti-Filippini J, Nery JR, Lee L, Ye Z, Ngo QM, Edsall L, Antosiewicz-Bourget J, Stewart R, Ruotti V, Millar AH, Thomson JA, Ren B, Ecker JR (2009) Human DNA methylomes at base resolution show widespread epigenomic differences. Nature 462:315–322

Liu Y, Oakeley EJ, Sun L, Jost JP (1998) Multiple domains are involved in the targeting of the mouse DNA methyltransferase to the DNA replication foci. Nucleic Acids Res 26:1038–1045

Liu S, Shen T, Huynh L, Klisovic MI, Rush LJ, Ford JL, Yu J, Becknell B, Li Y, Liu C, Vukosavljevic T, Whitman SP, Chang KS, Byrd JC, Perrotti D, Plass C, Marcucci G (2005) Interplay of RUNX1/MTG8 and DNA methyltransferase 1 in acute myeloid leukemia. Cancer Res 65:1277–1284

Maiti A, Drohat AC (2011) Thymine DNA glycosylase can rapidly excise 5-formylcytosine and 5-carboxylcytosine: potential implications for active demethylation of CpG sites. J Biol Chem 286:35334–35338

Meissner A, Mikkelsen TS, Gu H, Wernig M, Hanna J, Sivachenko A, Zhang X, Bernstein BE, Nusbaum C, Jaffe DB, Gnirke A, Jaenisch R, Lander ES (2008) Genome-scale DNA methylation maps of pluripotent and differentiated cells. Nature 454:766–770

Metzger E, Schüle R (2007) The expanding world of histone lysine demethylases. Nat Struct Mol Biol 14:252–254

Metzger E, Wissmann M, Yin N, Muller JM, Schneider R, Peters AH, Gunther T, Buettner R, Schüle R (2005) LSD1 demethylates repressive histone marks to promote androgen-receptor-dependent transcription. Nature 437:436–439

Mikol YB, Hoover KL, Creasia D, Poirier LA (1983) Hepatocarcinogenesis in rats fed methyl-deficient, amino acid-defined diets. Carcinogenesis 4:1619–1629

Milne TA, Martin ME, Brock HW, Slany RK, Hess JL (2005) Leukemogenic MLL fusion proteins bind across a broad region of the Hox a9 locus, promoting transcription and multiple histone modifications. Cancer Res 65:11367–11374

Monk M, Boubelik M, Lehnert S (1987) Temporal and regional changes in DNA methylation in the embryonic, extraembryonic and germ cell lineages during mouse embryo development. Development 99:371–382

Moran-Crusio K, Reavie L, Shih A, Abdel-Wahab O, Ndiaye-Lobry D, Lobry C, Figueroa ME, Vasanthakumar A, Patel J, Zhao X, Perna F, Pandey S, Madzo J, Song C, Dai Q, He C, Ibrahim S, Beran M, Zavadil J, Nimer SD, Melnick A, Godley LA, Aifantis I, Levine RL (2011) Tet2 loss leads to increased hematopoietic stem cell self-renewal and myeloid transformation. Cancer Cell 20:11–24

Mueller D, Bach C, Zeisig D, Garcia-Cuellar MP, Monroe S, Sreekumar A, Zhou R, Nesvizhskii A, Chinnaiyan A, Hess JL, Slany RK (2007) A role for the MLL fusion partner ENL in transcriptional elongation and chromatin modification. Blood 110:4445–4454

Nan X, Ng HH, Johnson CA, Laherty CD, Turner BM, Eisenman RN, Bird A (1998) Transcriptional repression by the methyl-CpG-binding protein MeCP2 involves a histone deacetylase complex. Nature 393:386–389

Nguyen S, Meletis K, Fu D, Jhaveri S, Jaenisch R (2007) Ablation of de novo DNA methyltransferase Dnmt3a in the nervous system leads to neuromuscular defects and shortened lifespan. Dev Dyn 236:1663–1676

Norris DP, Patel D, Kay GF, Penny GD, Brockdorff N, Sheardown SA, Rastan S (1994) Evidence that random and imprinted Xist expression is controlled by preemptive methylation. Cell 77:41–51

Okada Y, Feng Q, Lin Y, Jiang Q, Li Y, Coffield VM, Su L, Xu G, Zhang Y (2005) hDOT1L links histone methylation to leukemogenesis. Cell 121:167–178

Okano M, Xie S, Li E (1998) Dnmt2 is not required for de novo and maintenance methylation of viral DNA in embryonic stem cells. Nucleic Acids Res 26:2536–2540

Okano M, Bell DW, Haber DA, Li E (1999) DNA methyltransferases Dnmt3a and Dnmt3b are essential for de novo methylation and mammalian development. Cell 99:247–257

Ooi SK, Qiu C, Bernstein E, Li K, Jia D, Yang Z, Erdjument-Bromage H, Tempst P, Lin SP, Allis CD, Cheng X, Bestor TH (2007) DNMT3L connects unmethylated lysine 4 of histone H3 to de novo methylation of DNA. Nature 448:714–717

Passegué E, Jamieson CH, Ailles LE, Weissman IL (2003) Normal and leukemic hematopoiesis: are leukemias a stem cell disorder or a reacquisition of stem cell characteristics? Proc Natl Acad Sci U S A 100(Suppl 1):11842–11849

Pfaffeneder T, Hackner B, Truss M, Munzel M, Muller M, Deiml CA, Hagemeier C, Carell T (2011) The discovery of 5-formylcytosine in embryonic stem cell DNA. Angew Chem Int Ed Engl 50:7008–7012

Pokholok DK, Harbison CT, Levine S, Cole M, Hannett NM, Lee TI, Bell GW, Walker K, Rolfe PA, Herbolsheimer E, Zeitlinger J, Lewitter F, Gifford DK, Young RA (2005) Genome-wide map of nucleosome acetylation and methylation in yeast. Cell 122:517–527

Prendergast GC, Ziff EB (1991) Methylation-sensitive sequence-specific DNA binding by the c-Myc basic region. Science 251:186–189

Qiu C, Sawada K, Zhang X, Cheng X (2002) The PWWP domain of mammalian DNA methyltransferase Dnmt3b defines a new family of DNA-binding folds. Nat Struct Biol 9:217–224

Santi DV, Norment A, Garrett CE (1984) Covalent bond formation between a DNA-cytosine methyltransferase and DNA containing 5-azacytosine. Proc Natl Acad Sci U S A 81:6993–6997

Sawada N, Poirier L, Moran S, Xu YH, Pitot HC (1990) The effect of choline and methionine deficiencies on the number and volume percentage of altered hepatic foci in the presence or absence of diethylnitrosamine initiation in rat liver. Carcinogenesis 11:273–281

Schilling E, El CC, Rehli M (2009) Allele-specific DNA methylation in mouse strains is mainly determined by cis-acting sequences. Genome Res 19:2028–2035

Schneider R, Bannister AJ, Myers FA, Thorne AW, Crane-Robinson C, Kouzarides T (2004) Histone H3 lysine 4 methylation patterns in higher eukaryotic genes. Nat Cell Biol 6:73–77

Schübeler D, MacAlpine DM, Scalzo D, Wirbelauer C, Kooperberg C, van LF, Gottschling DE, O'Neill LP, Turner BM, Delrow J, Bell SP, Groudine M (2004) The histone modification pattern of active genes revealed through genome-wide chromatin analysis of a higher eukaryote. Genes Dev 18:1263–1271

Sen GL, Reuter JA, Webster DE, Zhu L, Khavari PA (2010) DNMT1 maintains progenitor function in self-renewing somatic tissue. Nature 463:563–567

Sharif J, Muto M, Takebayashi S, Suetake I, Iwamatsu A, Endo TA, Shinga J, Mizutani-Koseki Y, Toyoda T, Okamura K, Tajima S, Mitsuya K, Okano M, Koseki H (2007) The SRA protein Np95 mediates epigenetic inheritance by recruiting Dnmtl to methylated DNA. Nature 450:908–912

Shi Y, Lan F, Matson C, Mulligan P, Whetstine JR, Cole PA, Casero RA, Shi Y (2004) Histone demethylation mediated by the nuclear amine oxidase homolog LSD1. Cell 119:941–953

Singal R, Ginder GD (1999) DNA methylation. Blood 93:4059–4070

Sjoblom T, Jones S, Wood LD, Parsons DW, Lin J, Barber TD, Mandelker D, Leary RJ, Ptak J, Silliman N, Szabo S, Buckhaults P, Farrell C, Meeh P, Markowitz SD, Willis J, Dawson D, Willson JK, Gazdar AF, Hartigan J, Wu L, Liu C, Parmigiani G, Park BH, Bachman KE,

Papadopoulos N, Vogelstein B, Kinzler KW, Velculescu VE (2006) The consensus coding sequences of human breast and colorectal cancers. Science 314:268–274

So CW, Karsunky H, Passegue E, Cozzio A, Weissman IL, Cleary ML (2003) MLL-GAS7 transforms multipotent hematopoietic progenitors and induces mixed lineage leukemias in mice. Cancer Cell 3:161–171

Somervaille TC, Matheny CJ, Spencer GJ, Iwasaki M, Rinn JL, Witten DM, Chang HY, Shurtleff SA, Downing JR, Cleary ML (2009) Hierarchical maintenance of MLL myeloid leukemia stem cells employs a transcriptional program shared with embryonic rather than adult stem cells. Cell Stem Cell 4:129–140

Stoner GD, Shimkin MB, Kniazeff AJ, Weisburger JH, Weisburger EK, Gori GB (1973) Test for carcinogenicity of food additives and chemotherapeutic agents by the pulmonary tumor response in strain a mice. Cancer Res 33:3069–3085

Suzuki M, Yamada T, Kihara-Negishi F, Sakurai T, Hara E, Tenen DG, Hozumi N, Oikawa T (2006) Site-specific DNA methylation by a complex of PU.1 and Dnmt3a/b. Oncogene 25:2477–2488

Tachibana M, Matsumura Y, Fukuda M, Kimura H, Shinkai Y (2008) G9a/GLP complexes independently mediate H3K9 and DNA methylation to silence transcription. EMBO J 27:2681–2690

Tadokoro Y, Ema H, Okano M, Li E, Nakauchi H (2007) De novo DNA methyltransferase is essential for self-renewal, but not for differentiation, in hematopoietic stem cells. J Exp Med 204:715–722

Tahiliani M, Koh KP, Shen Y, Pastor WA, Bandukwala H, Brudno Y, Agarwal S, Iyer LM, Liu DR, Aravind L, Rao A (2009) Conversion of 5-methylcytosine to 5-hydroxymethylcytosine in mammalian DNA by MLL partner TET1. Science 324:930–935

Tamaru H, Zhang X, McMillen D, Singh PB, Nakayama J, Grewal SI, Allis CD, Cheng X, Selker EU (2003) Trimethylated lysine 9 of histone H3 is a mark for DNA methylation in Neurospora crassa. Nat Genet 34:75–79

Tariq M, Saze H, Probst AV, Lichota J, Habu Y, Paszkowski J (2003) Erasure of CpG methylation in Arabidopsis alters patterns of histone H3 methylation in heterochromatin. Proc Natl Acad Sci U S A 100:8823–8827

Terranova R, Agherbi H, Boned A, Meresse S, Djabali M (2006) Histone and DNA methylation defects at Hox genes in mice expressing a SET domain-truncated form of Mll. Proc Natl Acad Sci U S A 103:6629–6634

Thiel AT, Blessington P, Zou T, Feather D, Wu X, Yan J, Zhang H, Liu Z, Ernst P, Koretzky GA, Hua X (2010) MLL-AF9-induced leukemogenesis requires coexpression of the wild-type Mll allele. Cancer Cell 17:148–159

Trowbridge JJ, Orkin SH (2010) DNA methylation in adult stem cells: new insights into self-renewal. Epigenetics 5:189–193

Trowbridge JJ, Snow JW, Kim J, Orkin SH (2009) DNA methyltransferase 1 is essential for and uniquely regulates hematopoietic stem and progenitor cells. Cell Stem Cell 5:442–449

Trowbridge JJ, Sinha AU, Zhu N, Li M, Armstrong SA, Orkin SH (2012) Haploinsufficiency of Dnmt1 impairs leukemia stem cell function through derepression of bivalent chromatin domains. Genes Dev 26:344–349

Tsumura A, Hayakawa T, Kumaki Y, Takebayashi S, Sakaue M, Matsuoka C, Shimotohno K, Ishikawa F, Li E, Ueda HR, Nakayama J, Okano M (2006) Maintenance of self-renewal ability of mouse embryonic stem cells in the absence of DNA methyltransferases Dnmt1, Dnmt3a and Dnmt3b. Genes Cells 11:805–814

Tucker KL, Talbot D, Lee MA, Leonhardt H, Jaenisch R (1996) Complementation of methylation deficiency in embryonic stem cells by a DNA methyltransferase minigene. Proc Natl Acad Sci U S A 93:12920–12925

Viré E, Brenner C, Deplus R, Blanchon L, Fraga M, Didelot C, Morey L, Van EA, Bernard D, Vanderwinden JM, Bollen M, Esteller M, Di CL, de LY, Fuks F (2006) The polycomb group protein EZH2 directly controls DNA methylation. Nature 439:871–874

Vockentanz L, Broske AM, Rosenbauer F (2010) Uncovering a unique role for DNA methylation in hematopoietic and leukemic stem cells. Cell Cycle 9:640–641

Wang J, Iwasaki H, Krivtsov A, Febbo PG, Thorner AR, Ernst P, Anastasiadou E, Kutok JL, Kogan SC, Zinkel SS, Fisher JK, Hess JL, Golub TR, Armstrong SA, Akashi K, Korsmeyer SJ (2005) Conditional MLL-CBP targets GMP and models therapy-related myeloproliferative disease. EMBO J 24:368–381

Wang XX, Fu L, Li X, Wu X, Zhu Z, Fu L, Dong JT (2011) Somatic mutations of the mixed-lineage leukemia 3 (MLL3) gene in primary breast cancers. Pathol Oncol Res 17:429–433

Weber M, Davies JJ, Wittig D, Oakeley EJ, Haase M, Lam WL, Schübeler D (2005) Chromosome-wide and promoter-specific analyses identify sites of differential DNA methylation in normal and transformed human cells. Nat Genet 37:853–862

Weissman I (2005) Stem cell research: paths to cancer therapies and regenerative medicine. JAMA 294:1359–1366

Wood LD, Parsons DW, Jones S, Lin J, Sjoblom T, Leary RJ, Shen D, Boca SM, Barber T, Ptak J, Silliman N, Szabo S, Dezso Z, Ustyanksky V, Nikolskaya T, Nikolsky Y, Karchin R, Wilson PA, Kaminker JS, Zhang Z, Croshaw R, Willis J, Dawson D, Shipitsin M, Willson JK, Sukumar S, Polyak K, Park BH, Pethiyagoda CL, Pant PV, Ballinger DG, Sparks AB, Hartigan J, Smith DR, Suh E, Papadopoulos N, Buckhaults P, Markowitz SD, Parmigiani G, Kinzler KW, Velculescu VE, Vogelstein B (2007) The genomic landscapes of human breast and colorectal cancers. Science 318:1108–1113

Xin Z, Tachibana M, Guggiari M, Heard E, Shinkai Y, Wagstaff J (2003) Role of histone methyltransferase G9a in CpG methylation of the Prader-Willi syndrome imprinting center. J Biol Chem 278:14996–15000

Yamada Y, Jackson-Grusby L, Linhart H, Meissner A, Eden A, Lin H, Jaenisch R (2005) Opposing effects of DNA hypomethylation on intestinal and liver carcinogenesis. Proc Natl Acad Sci U S A 102:13580–13585

Yoder JA, Bestor TH (1998) A candidate mammalian DNA methyltransferase related to pmt1p of fission yeast. Hum Mol Genet 7:279–284

Yokochi T, Robertson KD (2002) Preferential methylation of unmethylated DNA by Mammalian de novo DNA methyltransferase Dnmt3a. J Biol Chem 277:11735–11745

Yoo CB, Chuang JC, Byun HM, Egger G, Yang AS, Dubeau L, Long T, Laird PW, Marquez VE, Jones PA (2008) Long-term epigenetic therapy with oral zebularine has minimal side effects and prevents intestinal tumors in mice. Cancer Prev Res (Phila) 1:233–240

Yu BD, Hess JL, Horning SE, Brown GA, Korsmeyer SJ (1995) Altered Hox expression and segmental identity in Mll-mutant mice. Nature 378:505–508

Zeisig BB, Garcia-Cuellar MP, Winkler TH, Slany RK (2003) The oncoprotein MLL-ENL disturbs hematopoietic lineage determination and transforms a biphenotypic lymphoid/myeloid cell. Oncogene 22:1629–1637

Zhu JK (2009) Active DNA demethylation mediated by DNA glycosylases. Annu Rev Genet 43:143–166

Zhu D, Hensel J, Hilgraf R, Abbasian M, Pornillos O, Deyanat-Yazdi G, Hua XH, Cox S (2010) Inhibition of protein kinase CK2 expression and activity blocks tumor cell growth. Mol Cell Biochem 333:159–167

Epigenetic Regulation of Normal Hematopoietic Development

3

Pratima Chaurasia, Dmitriy Berenzon, and Ronald Hoffman

Abbreviations

5-AzaC	5-Azacytidine
5azaD	5-Aza-2′-deoxycytidine
CB	Cord blood
CFSE	Carboxyfluorescein diacetate succinimidyl ester
ChIP	Chromatin immunoprecipitation assay
CMA	Chromatin-modifying agents
DNMTI	DNA methyltransferase inhibitor
EPC	Erythroid progenitor cells
GPA	Glycophorin A
HDACI	Histone deacetylase inhibitor
HPC	Hematopoietic progenitor cells
HSC	Hematopoietic stem cells
LBH589	Panobinostat
LDS	Laser dye styryl–751
SAHA	Suberolylanilide hydroxamic acid
SRC	NOD-/SCID-repopulating cells
TP	Transfusion Product
TSA	Trichostatin A
VPA	Valproic acid

P. Chaurasia, PhD (✉) • R. Hoffman, MD
Division of Hematology/Medical Oncology, Department of Medicine, Tisch Cancer Institute, Mount Sinai School of Medicine, New York, NY 10029, USA
e-mail: pratima.chaurasia@mssm.edu; ronald.hoffman@mssm.edu

D. Berenzon, MD
Department of Hematology and Oncology, Wake Forest University School of Medicine, Winston Salem, NC 27157, USA
e-mail: dberenzo@wakehealth.edu

M. Lübbert, P.A. Jones (eds.), *Epigenetic Therapy of Cancer*,
DOI 10.1007/978-3-642-38404-2_3,

3.1 Introduction

Mammalian blood cell production ultimately originates from a pool of pluripotent hematopoietic stem cells (PHSC) which are capable of undergoing self-renewal or commitment to a variety of lineage-committed hematopoietic progenitor cells (HPC) which undergo progressive terminal differentiation resulting in the production of mature blood cells. There are several different ontogeny-related sources of HSC and HPC including fetal liver, cord blood (CB), bone marrow (BM), and peripheral blood (PB) which have distinctive functional characteristics. Since the DNA sequences of HSC, HPC, and terminally differentiated hematopoietic cells as well as the DNA sequence of different tissue sources of HSC/HPC remain constant throughout hematopoietic cell development, one can infer that epigenetic modifications likely play a pivotal role in defining these patterns of hematopoietic cell behavior. This conclusion is made with the caveat that such behavior patterns can also be influenced by the cytokine milieu and hematopoietic microenvironment in which particular hematopoietic cell populations are located.

3.1.1 Epigenetics and Hematopoietic Stem/Progenitor Cell Fate Decision

As a PHSC makes lineage-fate decisions along the path toward terminal differentiation, sequential changes in cell type and function occur (Humphries et al. 1985; Gubin et al. 1999; Grass et al. 2003; Anguita et al. 2004; Pal et al. 2004; Bottardi et al. 2005; Im et al. 2005; Martowicz et al. 2005, 2006; Iwasaki et al. 2006; Lamonica et al. 2006; Sieburg et al. 2006; Kim et al. 2007; Chaurasia et al. 2011; Giarratana et al. 2011; Ross et al. 2012). Such sequential changes are the result of modifications of histones leading to chromatin reorganization, altering transcription factor accessibility resulting ultimately in alterations in levels of transcription (Humphries et al. 1985; Gubin et al. 1999; Grass et al. 2003; Anguita et al. 2004; Pal et al. 2004; Bottardi et al. 2005; Im et al. 2005; Martowicz et al. 2005, 2006; Iwasaki et al. 2006; Lamonica et al. 2006; Sieburg et al. 2006; Kim et al. 2007; Bartels et al. 2010; Chaurasia et al. 2011; Elizalde et al. 2012). Studies of these processes have led to a greater understanding of how genetic networks orchestrate hematopoietic cell differentiation. GATA-1, for instance, is critical for terminal differentiation and maturation of erythroid cells whereas GATA-2 is required for maintenance and proliferation of HPC (Rice et al. 2007; Wozniak and Bresnick 2008). GATA-1 represses the expression of GATA-2 whereas GATA-2 activates GATA-1 expression thus providing evidence for a regulatory network of GATA factors controlling hematopoiesis. c-kit expression is another highly regulated event occurring during early erythropoiesis. GATA-1 and GATA-2 have opposing effects on c-kit expression by participating in the formation of chromatin loops (Apostolou and Thanos 2008; Jing et al. 2008). GATA-2 enhances c-kit transcription while an increase in GATA-1 protein level is associated with c-kit suppression and erythroid maturation (Apostolou and Thanos 2008; Jing et al. 2008). This displacement of

GATA-2 by GATA-1 results in the rearrangement of chromatin loops, clustering remote regulatory sites that affect not only gene activation but also gene repression. Such transcriptional events that are orchestrated by chromatin structure can be frequently reversed by implementation of a variety of strategies using small molecules capable of modifying chromatin structure (Gubin et al. 1999; Grass et al. 2003; Anguita et al. 2004; Pal et al. 2004; Bottardi et al. 2005; Im et al. 2005; Martowicz et al. 2005; Iwasaki et al. 2006; Lamonica et al. 2006; Martowicz et al. 2006; Kim et al. 2007; Rice et al. 2007; Chaurasia et al. 2011).

The organization of DNA into chromatin constitutes a means of regulating nuclear processes including transcription, replication, recombination, and DNA repair. The organization of DNA is dynamic, especially at the level of the nucleosome, which consists of DNA wrapped around a core histone octamer (two copies of each H2A, H2B, H3, and H4). Core histones are subjected to extensive posttranslational modifications including acetylation, methylation, phosphorylation, sumoylation, and ubiquitination (Kouzarides 2007; Lee et al. 2010). Such modifications serve as switches governing the accessibility of chromatin to DNA- and histone-binding factors. Epigenetic regulatory mechanisms constitute a fundamentally important mode of transcriptional control (Goll and Bestor 2005). The plasticity of epigenetic marks also allows for the exquisite fine-tuning of HSC gene expression necessary for critical processes such as symmetrical division, maintenance, self-renewal, fate determination, and terminal differentiation (Jaenisch and Bird 2003).

Several investigators have hypothesized that single or sequential histone modifications either act alone or sequentially define the "histone code." Histone codes can be recognized by nonhistone proteins, which form complexes which then determine the pattern of gene expression (Jenuwein and Allis 2001; Spotswood and Turner 2002; Lee et al. 2010). This hypothesis has been further extended to include the concept of "modification cassettes" and/or localized "binary switches." Modifications of adjacent amino acid sites within the specific neighborhood of a histone tail mediate specific cellular signals upon phosphorylation, methylation, or acetylation (Fischle et al. 2003). For instance, histone methylation at lysine and arginine residues is relatively stable and is thought to result in the transmission of epigenetic information which is retained throughout subsequent cycles of cell division.

Chromatin-modifying enzymes which influence gene expression include the DNA methyltransferases (DNMTs), histone acetyltransferases (HATs), histone deacetylases (HDACs), histone demethylases (HDMs), and histone methyltransferases (HMTs) which each play important roles in chromatin remodeling and regulation of gene expression (Kouzarides 2007; Lopez et al. 2009; Chaurasia et al. 2011). DNA methylation with the addition of a methyl group by DNMTs on cytosine-phosphate-guanine (CpG) dinucleotides within gene regulatory DNA sequences (Goll and Bestor 2005; Rice et al. 2007; Metivier et al. 2008) is an important mechanism resulting in gene silencing. It has become apparent that the effects of CpG island-promoter methylation on transcription may depend on other epigenetic events including recruitment of repressive complexes containing CpG-binding proteins (Zardo et al. 2008) or posttranslational modifications of histone tails resulting in condensation and inactivation of chromatin. DNMT1 preferentially targets hemimethylated DNA and is required for maintenance of methylation patterns during replication. Other DNMTs including DNMT3a and 3b are involved in de novo methylation during the differentiation of hematopoietic cells (Tadokoro et al. 2007). However, DNMT3L lacks canonical DNA methyltransferase motifs, but is otherwise closely related to the C-terminal domain of DNMT3a and DNMT3b which lead to de novo methylation. Crystallographic studies revealed that DNMT3L interacts with the catalytic domain of DNMT3a, indicating that DNMT3L provides the dual functions of binding the unmethylated histone tail and activating DNA methyltransferases (Jia et al. 2007). The impact of methylation on the features of murine HSC has been examined by several groups (Bachman et al. 2001; Robertson and Jones 2000; Fuks et al. 2000; Fuks 2005; Lessard and Crabtree 2010; Challen et al. 2011; Hogart et al. 2012). These studies indicate that distinct methylation threshold levels are required for HSC and HPC fate decisions and that cell differentiation or self-renewal programs require different doses of methylation. Ji and coworkers for instance have reported that myeloid commitment involves less global DNA methylation than lymphoid commitment. De novo DNA methylation is necessary for retention of HSC function, and DNMT1 is required for the creation of a gene expression pattern that defines a stem cell (Ji et al. 2010). By contrast, DNMT3a and DNMT3b are involved in de novo methylation during the differentiation of hematopoietic cells, while HSC deficient in DNMT3a-/b- progressively lose their replication potential but not their differentiation potential (Tadokoro et al. 2007). The DNMT also affect the degree of histone methylation contributes to the modulation of both permissive and nonpermissive chromatin states leading to either transcriptional activation or repression. For instance, histone H3 lysine 4 trimethylation or bimethylation (H3K4me3/2), H3 lysine 36 trimethylation (H3K36me3), and H3 lysine 79 trimethylation (H3K79me3) each results in a permissive/open chromatin structure leading to gene activation, while histone H3 lysine 20 (H3K20me3), lysine 27 (H3K27me3), and 9 (H3K9me3) trimethylation lead to a nonpermissive/closed chromatin structure and the eventual silencing of the genes (Rice et al. 2007; Zardo et al. 2008) (Fig. 3.1).

Histone acetylation status plays a critical role in defining the gene expression pattern of hematopoietic cells. The degree of histone acetylation is defined by the biological activities of HADC and HAT. There are 18 HDACs in humans which can be classified into three classes. Class I HDACs are localized to the nucleus, while class II HDACs are subcellular and may shuttle between the cytoplasm and the nucleus and have biological activities related to specific lineages (Dokmanovic et al. 2007; Martin et al. 2007; Smith 2008). Class III HDACs have homology to yeast Sir two group of deacetylases, are ubiquitously expressed, and have an absolute requirement for NAD^+ but are not affected by compounds that inhibit class I and II HDAC (Milne et al. 2007). Clearly the activities of HDACs are cell type and/or context dependent and therefore making broad predictions about the effects of functional inactivation of a single HDAC or class of HDAC at present impossible. Functional studies indicate that class I HDACs predominately regulate cell proliferation, apoptosis, and cell fate determination, while class II HDACs are more specifically involved in regulating cell migration and angiogenesis (Johnstone 2002; Wada et al.

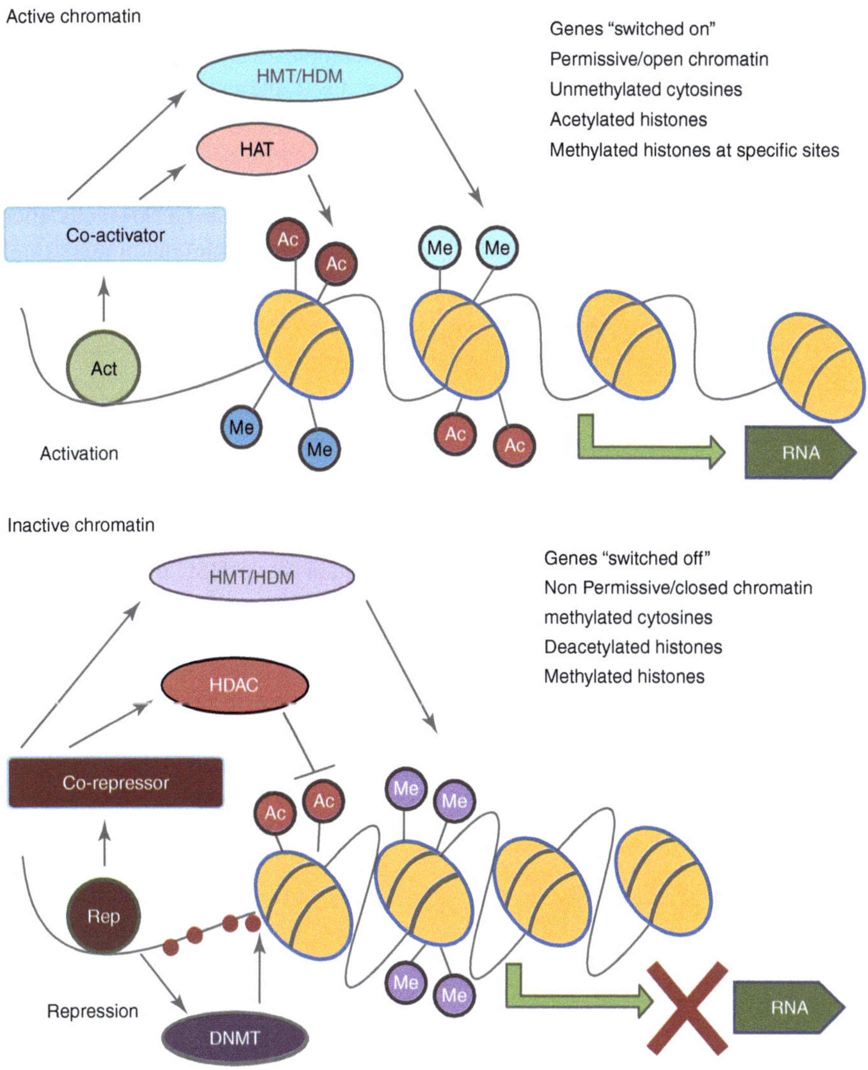

Fig. 3.1 Epigenetic regulation of gene expression. Gene transcription is associated with histone posttranslational modifications such as hyperacetylation (H3/H4Ac) and methylation at specific sites (H3K79me3, H3K36me3, H3K4me3, H4K4me2) in promoter regions of active chromatin. By contrast, the presence of methylated DNA and the deacetylated histones and methylated histones (H3K9me3, H3K27me3 or H3K20) can be associated with transcriptionally inactive chromatin. *HMT* histone methyltransferase, *HDM* histone demethylase, *HAT* histone acetylase *HDAC* histone deacetylase, *DNMT* DNA methyltransferase (Reproduced with permission Araki et al. (2007))

2009; Chaurasia et al. 2011; Kretsovali et al. 2012). Gene expression analyses have indicated that the expression of greater than 5–7 % of genes is altered following HDACI treatment. Histones are not the only targets of HDACs; a range of nuclear transcription factors and nonhistone proteins including p53, E2F, c-Myc, nuclear factor kappa B (NF-κB), hypoxia-inducible factor 1 (HIF-1), tubulin, Hsp90, as well as estrogen α-receptor and the androgen receptor complexes are targeted by HDACs, and their function is altered by their acetylation status (Lane and Chabner 2009). We also demonstrated that acetylation of histones is a highly dynamic and reversible process and that lysine residues on histones such as 9/14 and 27 are differentially modulated and create active marks on the chromatin structure leading to altered gene expression (Chaurasia et al. 2011). Regulatory regions in CD34+ cells after treatment with HDACI were significantly enriched for active chromatin marks and led to erythroid lineage commitment and differentiation particularly regulated by lineage-restricted transcription factors (Chaurasia et al. 2011).

3.1.2 Cord Blood Stem Cell Grafts

Allogeneic CB cells are an important alternative source of marrow-repopulating cells (MRC), which can serve as a stem cell graft for patients with hematological malignancies and blood-related genetic disorders (Cairo and Wagner 1997; Stanevsky et al. 2009). CB grafts frequently contain fewer HSC than marrow or mobilized peripheral blood grafts which leads to a higher incidence of graft failure and a more prolonged time for hematological reconstitution to occur (Migliaccio et al. 2000). The fixed number of HSC within a single CB unit has limited the use of this alternative source of stem cells in adults (Stanevsky et al. 2009). Numerous investigators have tried to increase the CB stem cell dose by culturing CB CD34+ cells ex vivo under a variety of conditions in order to shorten the time to engraftment and to make these grafts accessible to adult recipients. Such approaches have, to date, met with limited success (Stanevsky et al. 2009). We have hypothesized that the presently utilized in vitro culture conditions result in loss of the gene expression pattern needed to retain HSC function and the ability to undergo symmetrical division which is required for the expansion of the numbers of marrow-repopulating cells to occur. Several years ago we hypothesized that these obstacles to graft engineering could be overcome by the ex vivo use of CMA which would result in epigenetic effects that would overcome the influences of cell culture on HSC/HPC fate decisions (Milhem et al. 2004; Araki et al. 2006, 2007; Chaurasia et al. 2011). We have reported that the expansion of CB CD34+ cells in the presence of cytokines alone alters HSC function leading to the loss of functional HSC after prolonged culture and that the ex vivo addition of CMA to specific cytokine combinations can affect HSC fate decisions resulting in increased numbers of CB MRC (Milhem et al. 2004; Araki et al. 2006, 2007).

HSC can enjoy several fates. They may divide symmetrically into daughter cells which retain pluripotency leading to an increase in the absolute numbers of HSC or divide asymmetrically, resulting in the production of daughter cells with different potentials, one stem cell and another committed progenitor cell, leading to the maintenance of the number of HSC. Alternatively, an HSC population can produce two daughter cells that have undergone lineage commitment or directly undergo apoptosis, resulting in exhaustion of the HSC pool (Araki et al. 2006; Congdon and Reya 2008).

Any ex vivo strategy for HSC expansion must favor retention of the cellular program underlying symmetrical cell division which would lead to a net gain in HSC numbers. HSC express a promiscuous set of transcription factors and an open chromatin structure required to maintain their multipotentiality which is progressively altered as cells progress toward a particular lineage pathway. We hypothesize that differentiation may be mediated by stem cell DNA methylation, histone deacetylation, and histone methylation allowing the silencing of a large fraction of the genome, causing the transcriptional machinery to focus on those genes essential for the expression and maintenance of the differentiated blood lineage (Chaurasia et al. 2011). Recently, genome-wide analysis demonstrated that DNA methylation is notably altered during myeloid differentiation and identifies critical regions of the genome and transcription factor programs that contribute to hematopoiesis (Hogart et al. 2012). The chromatin structure which defines the epigenetic state of an HSC is likely altered in response to a variety of environmental cues during ex vivo culture of HSC, thereby reducing the numbers of functional HSC as well as HPC committed to the erythroid/megakaryocytic lineages (Araki et al. 2009).

3.1.3 Candidate DNA Methyltransferase Inhibitors and HDAC Inhibitors for Use in Graft Engineering

5-Azacytidine (5-AzaC, azacitidine) and 5 aza 2' deoxycytidine (5azaD, decitabine) are powerful inhibitors of DNA methylation but differ in their mechanism of action. 5-AzaC contains a ribose group and hence is phosphorylated by uridine-cytidine kinase. After phosphorylation it is subsequently incorporated into RNA, whereas decitabine which has a deoxyribose group is incorporated into DNA (Creusot et al. 1982). These different modes of action may account for divergence of methylation pattern and cytotoxicity profiles observed with the in vitro use of these two DNMT inhibitors (DNMTI) (Goffin and Eisenhauer 2002). In the presence of these analogs, a significant proportion of the DNA becomes hemimethylated. A second round of DNA synthesis in the presence of these drugs results in full double-stranded DNA demethylation leading to reactivation of silenced genes. This effect is not stable and is lost upon cessation of DNMTI treatment. In addition, methylation of specific residues on the histone H3 and H4 tails are known to be vital for determining chromatin structure. For instance, methylation of lysine 4 on H3 is associated with transcriptionally active euchromatin, on the other hand methylation of lysine 9 triggers transcriptional repression (Bannister et al. 2001; Nakayama et al. 2001; Jenuwein and Allis 2001; Jones and Baylin 2002; Clouaire and Stancheva 2008; Zardo et al. 2008).

During early hematopoiesis DNMT genes are constitutively expressed but are gradually downregulated as committed progenitors undergo differentiation. The expression of DNMTs is upregulated in leukemic cells and likely inducing greater degrees of leukemia cell-directed cytotoxicity with 5azaD treatment as compared to that achieved with normal cells (Jüttermann et al. 1994). By contrast there is very limited knowledge of the molecular effects of CMA on the fate of normal HSC and HPC (Saunthararajah et al. 2003; Gilbert et al. 2004; Milhem et al. 2004). Recently,

Challen and coworkers demonstrated that DNMT3a plays an important role in HSC differentiation and DNMT3a loss impairs HSC function after serial transplantation and simultaneously increases HSC numbers in the bone marrow (Challen et al. 2012).

Acetylation of histones is also essential to maintain an open, permissive chromatin conformation. That allows the binding of transcriptional factors, histone acetylases, and other regulatory coactivators to promote gene expression. Conversely, HDACs act to keep histone deacetylated and result in transcriptional silencing. Virtually all commercially available HDACI inhibit class I and II HDACs, although specific HDACI appear to selectively suppress specific HDAC or to affect biological processes to differing degrees (Dokmanovic et al. 2007; Martin et al. 2007; Smith 2008). The biological activities of histone deacetylases (HDACs) are not redundant (Dokmanovic et al. 2007; Martin et al. 2007). A number of in vitro studies have suggested that the treatment of primitive hematopoietic cells with HDAC inhibitors can alter HSC/HPC behavior suggesting that histone acetylation status influences cell fate decision (Milhem et al. 2004; De Felice et al. 2005; Araki et al. 2006, 2007; Bug et al. 2007; Lane and Chabner 2009; Bartels et al. 2010; Chaurasia et al. 2011; Elizalde et al. 2012). Most HDACIs currently in clinical development target multiple HDACs, and inhibition of specific HDACs may affect different molecular processes.

3.1.4 Effect of Chromatin-Modifying Agents on Ex Vivo Expansion of HSC

HSC are quiescent cells that are capable of exiting G_0/G_1 following exposure to early acting cytokines including stem cell factor (SCF), fms-like tyrosine kinase receptor-3 ligand (Flt-3), and thrombopoietin (TPO). There has been limited success in controlling HSC commitment and differentiation in vitro beyond HSCs undergoing a limited number of cell divisions. We have developed a system to assess the role of a DNMTI (5azaD) and a HDACI (TSA) in modifying CB and adult marrow HSC/HPC fate decisions (Milhem et al. 2004; Araki et al. 2006, 2007). In these studies we evaluated various cytokine combinations in order to determine optimal culture conditions for the expansion of numbers of CB NOD-/SCID-repopulating cells (SRC). The cytokine cocktail of SCF, Flt-3, and TPO provided the maximal expansion of numbers of CD34+CD90+ cells, colony-forming unit (CFU)-mix, CAFC, and SRC. In order to determine whether the pretreatment of CB CD34+ cells with 5azaD/TSA in vitro would result in further expansion of HSC, CB CD34+ cells were initially cultured in media supplemented with SCF, Flt-3, TPO, and IL-3. After 16 h, the cells were exposed to 5azaD (10^{-6} M). At 48 h, TSA was added and the cytokine cocktail was changed to a combination of SCF, FL, and TPO for an additional 7 days without IL-3 to minimize cellular differentiation. Following 9 days of culture, a 5.0-fold expansion of CD34+ cells was observed in the 5azaD-/TSA-pretreated CD34+ cells, while only a 2.6-fold expansion was observed in cultures exposed to cytokines alone. A 12.5-fold expansion of CD34+CD90+ cells was observed in the 5azaD-/TSA-treated cultures in

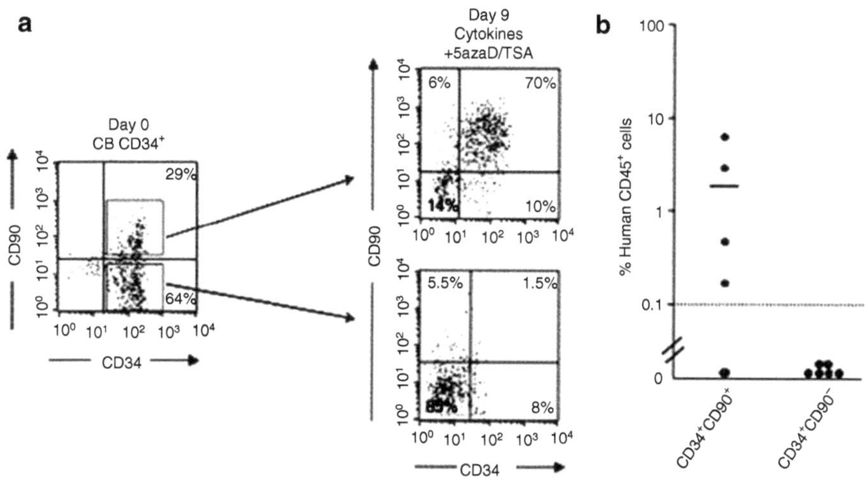

Fig. 3.2 Proliferation and marrow-repopulating potential of CD34+CD90+ cells of 5-aza-2-deoxycytidine (5azaD)-/trichostatin A (*TSA*)-treated culture. (**a**) CD34+ cord blood cells were sorted into two subpopulations, CD34+CD90+ cells and CD34+CD90-cells, using a FACSVantage and cultured in the presence of 5azaD/TSA. After 9 days of culture, expression of CD90 by CD34+ cells was examined. Results are representative of one of three independent experiments. (**b**) Nonobese diabetic (*NOD*)/SCID bone marrow engraftment was observed with the CD34+CD90+ cells, and CD34+CD90− cells were reisolated from the 5azaD/TSA cultures after 9 days. The percent of human hematopoietic cell chimerism in individual mice is plotted as dots and their mean values are indicated by horizontal bars (Reprinted with permission Araki et al. (2006))

comparison to the input cell number. In contrast, a 1.5-fold expansion of CB CD34+CD90+ cells was observed in the cultures containing cytokines alone, 35.4 % ± 5.8 % of the total cells in the cultures exposed to CMA co-expressed CD34+ and CD90+, while only 1.4 % ± 0.3 % of the cells in the cultures exposed to cytokines alone were CD34+CD90+ (Araki et al. 2006) (Fig. 3.2a). Although discordance between the phenotype and function of culture-expanded cells has been reported by numerous investigators, the co-expression of CD90 by CD34+ cells served as a reliable biomarker for the retention of marrow-repopulating potential following ex vivo culture. CB CD34+CD90+ and CD34+CD90− cell populations reisolated from 5azaD-/TSA-pretreated culture started with CD34+ cells after 9 days were transplanted in equal numbers into NOD/SCID mice. Four of five mice injected with the reisolated CD34+CD90+ cells pretreated with 5azaD/TSA had evidence of human multilineage hematopoietic cell engraftment. By contrast, an equivalent number of the reisolated CD34+CD90− cells pretreated with 5azaD/TSA were incapable of engrafting NOD/SCID mice (Fig. 3.2b). We found that elimination of IL-3 from the initial cytokine combination resulted in the abrogation of the expansion of HSC numbers. The pivotal effect of IL-3 is likely due to its ability to promote HSC cycling, which is crucial for the incorporation of 5azaD into the cell.

The cell division history of CB CD34+ cells following exposure to cytokines and CMA after in vitro culture was assessed using CFSE staining, a fluorescent

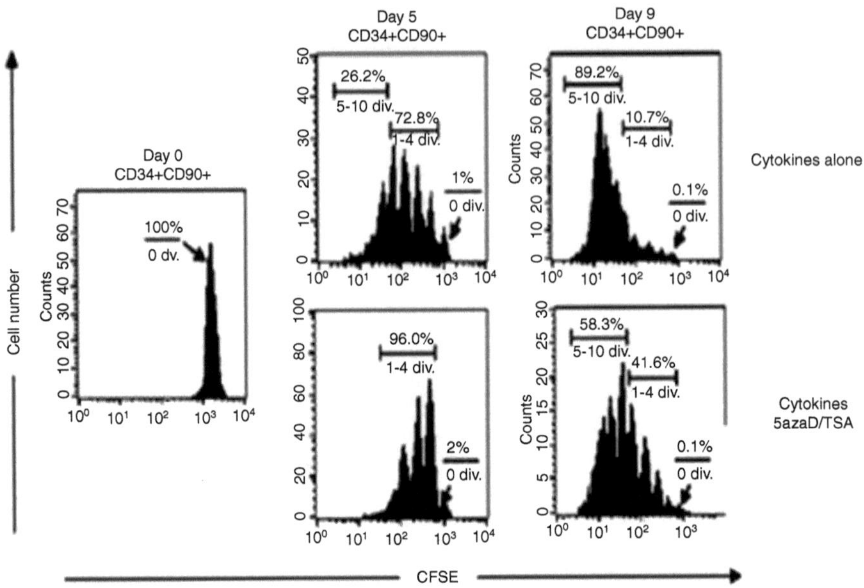

Fig. 3.3 The cell division history of CD34+CD90+ cells during ex vivo culture. CFSE-labeled CD34+ cells were cultured in the presence of cytokines with or without 5azaD/TSA treatment for 9 days. The panel shows a representative flow cytometric profile of CFSE fluorescence intensity after 5 and 9 days of culture. The *arrow* indicates the fraction of cells that have not undergone cell division (Reprinted with permission Araki et al. (2007))

cytoplasmic dye, which is equally distributed between daughter cells after each cell division. Irrespective of the treatment with the 5azaD/TSA, virtually no CD34+CD90+ cells (0.1 %) remained quiescent after 9 days of culture. In the absence of 5azaD/TSA treatment, about 73 % of the CD34+CD90+ cells had rapidly divided up to four times, and 26 % had divided five to ten times after 5 days of culture, whereas 5azaD-/TSA-treated cultures of CD34+CD90+ cells divided slowly with 98 % of the cells having divided only one to four times after 5 days. After 9 days of culture in the absence of 5azaD/TSA treatment, 90 % of CD34+CD90+ cells already had divided five to ten times, whereas in the presence of 5azaD/TSA treatment 42 % of CD34+CD90+ had divided one to four times and 58 % of CD34+CD90+ cells had undergone 5–10 cell divisions (Fig. 3.3).

These findings suggest that treatment with 5azaD/TSA is associated with CD34+CD90+ cell division occurring at a much slower rate than that observed in the presence of cytokines alone. To further examine the functional potential of CD34+CD90+ cells cultured in presence or absence of 5azaD/TSA, CD34+CD90+ cells were reisolated based on their cell division history after 9 days of culture and were transplanted into NOD/SCID mice following total body irradiation. When 5×10^4 CD34+CD90+ cells that had undergone 1–4 cell divisions after 5azaD/TSA treatment were injected into NOD/SCID mice, all mice displayed human multilineage hematopoietic cell engraftment after 8 weeks of transplantation (Fig. 3.4a).

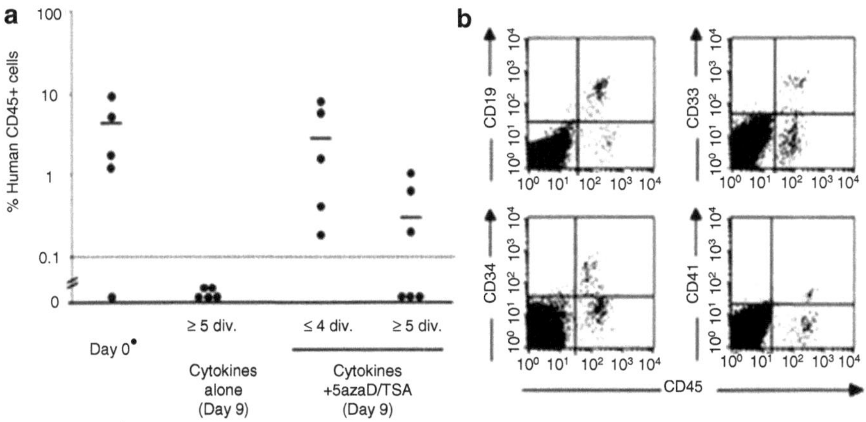

Fig. 3.4 The percentage of human cell chimerism following transplantation of reisolated CD34+CD90+ cells that have undergone five or more cell divisions following ex vivo culture. CD34+cells cultured in the presence of cytokines with or without 5azaD/TSA treatment were harvested after 9 days; the CD34+CD90+ cells that have undergone four or fewer divisions and five or more divisions were reisolated, then injected into NOD/SCID mice. (**a**) NOD/SCID engraftments achieved with CD34+CD90+ cells (≤4 divisions and ≥5 divisions). The percent of human hematopoietic cell chimerism is plotted as dots and their mean values indicated as horizontal bars. (**b**) Representative flow cytometric analysis of multilineage hematopoietic differentiation potential of engrafted human hematopoietic cells in NOD/SCID mice given transplants with reisolated CD34+CD90+ cells (≥5 divisions) is shown (Reprinted with permission Araki et al. (2006))

In addition, 50 % of mice receiving CD34+CD90+ cells treated with 5azaD/TSA in the culture that had undergone 5–10 cellular divisions still possessed evidence of human multilineage hematopoietic cell engraftment (Fig. 3.4a, b).

By contrast, when an equivalent number of CD34+CD90+ cells that had undergone 5–10 cellular divisions isolated from cultures receiving cytokines alone were transplanted, none of the recipient mice had any evidence of detectable human hematopoietic cell engraftment (Fig. 3.4a). Since 90 % of CD34+CD90+ cells in the cultures exposed to cytokines alone had undergone five or more cell divisions by day 9 (Fig. 3.3), only 0.15 % of the total CD34+CD90+ cells which had undergone 1–4 divisions remained making it impossible to directly assess the marrow-repopulating potential of this cell population. CD34+CD90+ cells that had undergone ≤4 and ≥5 divisions in the presence of 5azaD/TSA retained the ability both to engraft and to generate cells belonging to multiple lineages (Fig. 3.4a, b).

To evaluate whether 5azaD-/TSA-treated expanded CB cells still retain their self-renewal capacity after primary transplantation, BM cells from the primary NOD/SCID recipients were transplanted into secondary NOD/SCID recipients. Donor cell engraftment was achieved in five of six secondary mice receiving BM from primary mice engrafted with the cells treated with 5azaD/TSA (Table 3.1). Furthermore, these cells were capable of differentiating into cells belonging to multiple hematopoietic lineages in the secondary recipients.

Table 3.1 Secondary NOD/SCID mice repopulation of 5azaD/TSA treated ex vivo expanded cord blood cells

	Primary transplants		Secondary transplants	
	Human cell dose[a]	Primary mouse BM chimerism, % human	Human cell dose[b]	Secondary mouse BM chimerism, % human
No. 1	1.0×10^6	5.2	5.0×10^5	0.21
No. 2	1.0×10^6	13.1	1.4×10^6	1.5
No. 3	5.0×10^5	2.6	4.2×10^5	ND
No. 4	5.0×10^5	48.4	5.0×10^6	0.60
No. 5	5.0×10^5	11.2	1.4×10^6	0.20
No. 6	2.5×10^5	22.8	2.6×10^6	0.12

Murine BM from engrafted primary recipients was harvested, and unfractionated murine BM cells were injected into secondary NOD/SCID recipients. BM from primary and secondary recipients was stained for human CD45, CD71, CD19, CD33, CD34, and CD41 to assess multilineage human hematopoietic engraftment after 7 weeks of transplantation

ND indicates not detectable

[a]Cells injected in the primary mouse were cultured for 9 days pretreated with 5azaD/TSA (approximately 50 % of these cells express CD34)

[b]Cell dose is based on human CD45+ cells (Reprinted with permission Araki et al. 2007)

The frequency of SRC in the expanded cell product was quantitated using limiting dilution analysis. Increasing numbers (2,000, 5,000, 10,000, 20,000, 50,000) of primary CB CD34+CD90+ cells or the progeny of the same number of input CD34+CD90+ cells after 9 days of culture were transplanted into NOD/SCID mice (Fig. 3.5a). The frequency of SRC was 1 in 26,537 in primary CB CD34+CD90+ cells and 1 in 110,333 in cultures containing cytokines alone while frequency of SRC was 1 in 2,745 in the 5azaD-/TSA-treated cultures (Fig. 3.5b). Primary CB CD34+CD90+ cells, CD34+CD90+ cells from the 5azaD-/TSA-treated cultures, and cultures exposed to cytokines alone each retained the ability to differentiate into multiple hematopoietic cell lineages when transplanted into NOD/SCID mice.

3.1.5 Effect of HDAC Inhibitors on the Ability of CB CD34+ Cells to Generate Erythroid Progenitor Cells

The ex vivo generation of lineage-specific HPC and precursor cells including those belonging to the erythroid lineage has been associated with far greater success than that achieved with HSC expansion (Migliaccio et al. 2000; Neildez-Nguyen et al. 2002; Chang et al. 2006; Giarratana et al. 2005, 2011; Matsunaga et al. 2006; Miharada et al. 2006; Baek et al. 2008; Dorn et al. 2008; Fujimi et al. 2008; Chaurasia et al. 2011). There is presently a need for blood products with rare antigen profiles or for use in alloimmunized individuals. We have attempted to generate such products ex vivo using CMA.

We explored the ability of various HDACI including suberoylanilide hydroxamic acid (SAHA), TSA, valproic acid (VPA), and panobinostat (LBH589) to promote the in vitro generation of EPC. CB CD34+ cells in cultures supplemented with SCF, Flt-3, TPO, and IL-3 were exposed to several different HDACIs including SAHA,

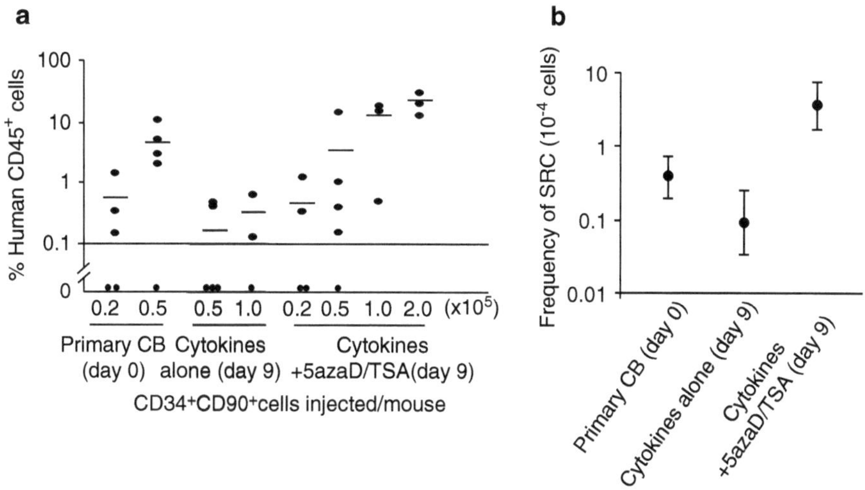

Fig. 3.5 Marrow-repopulating potential and cell division history of CD34+CD90+ cell population following ex vivo culture. (**a**) NOD/SCID engraftment was observed with transplantation of varying numbers of CD34+CD90+ cells calculated to be present in primary cord blood (*CB*) CD34+ cells (day 0) and varying numbers of CD34+CD90+ cells (day 9) calculated to be present after the culture. (**b**) Comparison of the frequency of SCID-repopulating cells (*SRC*) present in the primary CD34+CD90+ cells prior to day 0 and following culture in the presence or absence of 5azaD/TSA treatment on day 9. NOD/SCID mice were transplanted with increasing doses of CD34+CD90+ cells calculated to be present in the purified primary CB CD34+ cell fraction or the cellular products of 5azaD/TSA lacking (cytokines alone) or 5azaD-/TSA-treated cultures initiated with these numbers of CD34+CD90+ cells. Data from five independent limiting dilution experiments were pooled and analyzed by applying Poisson statistics according to the single-hit model (Reprinted with permission Araki et al. (2006))

VPA, TSA, and LBH589. The addition of each of the HDACIs promoted a greater degree of expansion of CD34+ and CD34+CD90+ cells as compared to cells exposed to cytokines. Cultures receiving cytokines alone experienced a 19.2±3.0-fold increase in the number of CD34+cells, while the addition of VPA resulted in the greatest degree of expansion of CD34+ cells (59.4±12.1-fold, $p=0.01$) as compared to LBH589 (48.9±10.9-fold), TSA (43.9±8.4-fold, $p=0.02$), and SAHA (39.5±5.4-fold, $p=0.02$). A 10.6±1.3-fold expansion of the numbers of CD34+CD90+ cells was observed in the presence of cytokines alone, while the greatest fold expansion of CD34+CD90+ cells was also observed in the VPA-containing cultures (66.7±4.7-fold, $p=0.02$) as compared to cultures containing LBH589 (51.5±5.3-fold), TSA (43.6±2.4-fold), or SAHA (25.9±1.6-fold).

The plating efficiency of cells exposed to cytokines alone was reduced by 50 % as compared to primary CB CD34+ cells while the plating efficiency of cells exposed to VPA and LBH589 were similar to that of the primary cells. Furthermore those cells exposed to cytokines alone generated far fewer EPC (BFU-E and CFU-mix) than primary CB CD34+ cells. The potential for each HDACI to increase the number of EPC within a whole CB collection was then examined. The addition of either VPA or LBH589 led to the generation of the greatest absolute numbers of

EPC (14.9×10^6 ($p=0.002$) and 12.9×10^6 ($p=0.01$)) which represented a 5,500- and 4,300-fold increase in the numbers, respectively, as compared to the number of EPC present in the primary CB collection (Chaurasia et al. 2011).

In order to determine if VPA treatment altered the differentiation program of CB CD34+ cells, an equivalent number of single primary CB CD34+ cells (Day0) and CD34+ reisolated from ex vivo cultures pretreated with cytokines alone or cytokines with VPA were analyzed for their ability to generate HPC. The plating efficiency of CD34+ cells reisolated from cultures containing cytokines alone was 66.6 % which was lower than that of primary CB 34+ cell (77.7 %). By contrast the plating efficiency of single CD34+ cells exposed to cytokines and VPA was 94.6 % indicating that HDACI treatment led to the generation of CD34+ cells that almost uniformly behave in vitro as fully functional HPC while treatment with cytokines alone led to considerable discordance between phenotype and function. The commitment patterns of the HPC from these various isolated cell populations were also dramatically different. Approximately 50 % of the HPC assayed from primary CB CD34+ cells were EPC while exposure to cytokines alone led to a shift in the commitment pattern resulting in far less EPC but a greater proportion of CFU-GM. By contrast, over 95 % of the CD34+ cells reisolated from cultures treated with cytokines and VPA were EPC. These data indicate that the addition of VPA preferentially promotes the decision of CD34+ cells to commit to the erythroid lineage thereby demonstrating the ability of CMA to alter CD34+ cell fate decisions (Chaurasia et al. 2011).

An increase in the H3 acetylation (AcH3K9) status of CD34+ cells reisolated from the VPA-treated cultures was observed as compared to CD34+ cells exposed to cytokines alone by using flow cytometric analyses. The CD34+ cells presented two distinct subpopulations based upon the levels of histone acetylation ($AcH3K9^{lo}$ and $AcH3K9^{hi}$). Both primary and VPA-treated CD34+ cells were characterized by a significant proportion of CD34+AcH3K9hi cells while this population was relatively diminished in cells exposed to cytokines alone, indicating that ex vivo exposure of CD34+ cells to cytokines alone leads to dramatic changes in their histone acetylation status which might be associated with terminal cell differentiation (Chaurasia et al. 2011).

The expression of phenotypic markers expressed by CD34+ cells exposed to cytokines alone or cytokines plus VPA were used to identify various cellular stages as a CD34+ cell differentiates to an EPC. The VPA-treated cells after 7 days contained the following phenotypes: CD71+ (69.8 ± 12.9 %) CD36+ (38.5 ± 8.6 %), GPA+ (12.8 ± 6.4 %), CD34+ (60 ± 6.7 %), and CD34+CD90+ (46 ± 6.1 %) cells on day 7, while on day 9 the number of CD34+ cells as well as CD34+CD90+ cells had declined (30.0 ± 5 %, 35.0 ± 6.7) while the percentage of CD71+ (71.7 ± 11.3 %), CD36+ (67.7 ± 10.2 %), and GPA+ (37.4 ± 7.3 %) cells had increased. The two additional days of incubation resulted in a 2.1-fold increase in the total number of nucleated cells and the appearance of greater number of EPC and erythroid precursor cells capable of further proliferation CD34+CD36+ (21.4 ± 4.2 % vs. 27.4 ± 3.5 %), CD36+GPA+ (19.8 ± 2.1 % vs. 33.9 ± 3.2 %), CD36+CD71+ (36.8 ± 1.3 % vs. 55.5 ± 5.3 %), CD71+GPA+ (19.2 ± 1.7 % vs. 31.3 ± 3.6 %), and CD34+CXCR4+ (19.8 ± 2.3 % vs. 29.8 ± 1.4 %). The day 9 EPC-transfusion product contained very limited numbers of CD19+ (1.4 ± 2.5 %), CD14+ (11.1 ± 3.1 %), or CD15+

(6.8 ± 2.5 %) cells which were not significantly increased as compared to the day 7 cultures. We also examined the expression of adhesion molecule CD49d (very late antigen (VLA)-4) and the chemokine receptor CXCR4 in ex vivo-generated cells. A greater number of both the CD34+ and CD34− cells expressed CXCR4 (49.8 %) and VLA-4(46.8 %), following the two additional days of cultures with SCF, IL-3, and EPO. Both CXCR4 and VLA-4 play pivotal roles in the trafficking and homing of hematopoietic cells to the BM.

In addition the cells after 7 days of incubation appeared as immature mononuclear cells with an agranular cytoplasm and prominent nucleoli, while by day 9 of culture, the cells were smaller with more compact nuclei and formed so-called erythroid islands formed by nucleated red cells surrounding with macrophages. These findings suggest that VPA treatment is capable of altering the fate of CB CD34+ cells and promoting their commitment to erythropoiesis.

Examination of the functional behavior of ex vivo expanded cells following their transfusion into sublethally irradiated NOD/SCID mice was performed by double staining the mouse blood with laser dye styryl–751(LDS), a nuclear dye, and human glycophorin (GPA) on serial days. Beginning on day 1, nucleated human red cells LDS+GPA+ (0.85 ± 2.35 %) were observed but there was no evidence of enucleated human red cells (LDS−GPA+). From day 3 until day 15 when the animals were sacrificed, however both human nucleated red cells and enucleated red cells were observed in the peripheral blood of NOD/SCID mice receiving the EPC-transfusion product. The greatest number of enucleated human red cells (12.4 ± 6.8 %) was observed 5 days after infusion of the expanded product. On day 12 when 6.8 ± 0.5 % of the cells in the PB were enucleated human red cells, the level of human CD14+ cells was only 0.4–0.8 % and CD19+ cells was 0.6–1.0 %. We confirmed the presence of human RBC in mice receiving the transfusion product by evaluating the expression of both human γ-globin and β-globin in the blood of these mice. These data strongly support the presence of circulating human erythroid precursors and their progressive differentiation into mature RBC in vivo (Fig. 3.6). The degree of human cell marrow and splenic engraftment was analyzed after 2 weeks. In the marrow, 7.4 % of the cells expressed hu-CD45+ while no evidence of human cell engraftment in the spleen was observed. The human cells present in the marrow were CD34+CD36− (2.0 %), CD34−CD36+ (1.8 %), CD34+CD36+ (2.7 %), CD36(4.5 %), and GPA+ (1.7 %); however, no evidence of CD33+, CD14+, CD19+, and CD41+ cells was noted. These data indicate the VPA-treated CD34+ cell product was capable of producing human erythroid cells which persisted for least 3 weeks in a xenogeneic transfusion model providing the rationale for further exploring the utility of such ex vivo-generated EPCs as a red cell transfusion product in man (Chaurasia et al. 2011).

3.1.6 Gene Reprogramming by Chromatin-Modifying Agents

HSC development, differentiation, and homeostasis are determined by transcriptional regulators that control gene expression under the influence of the signals from the microenvironment. Genes critical for early stem cell self-renewal and fate

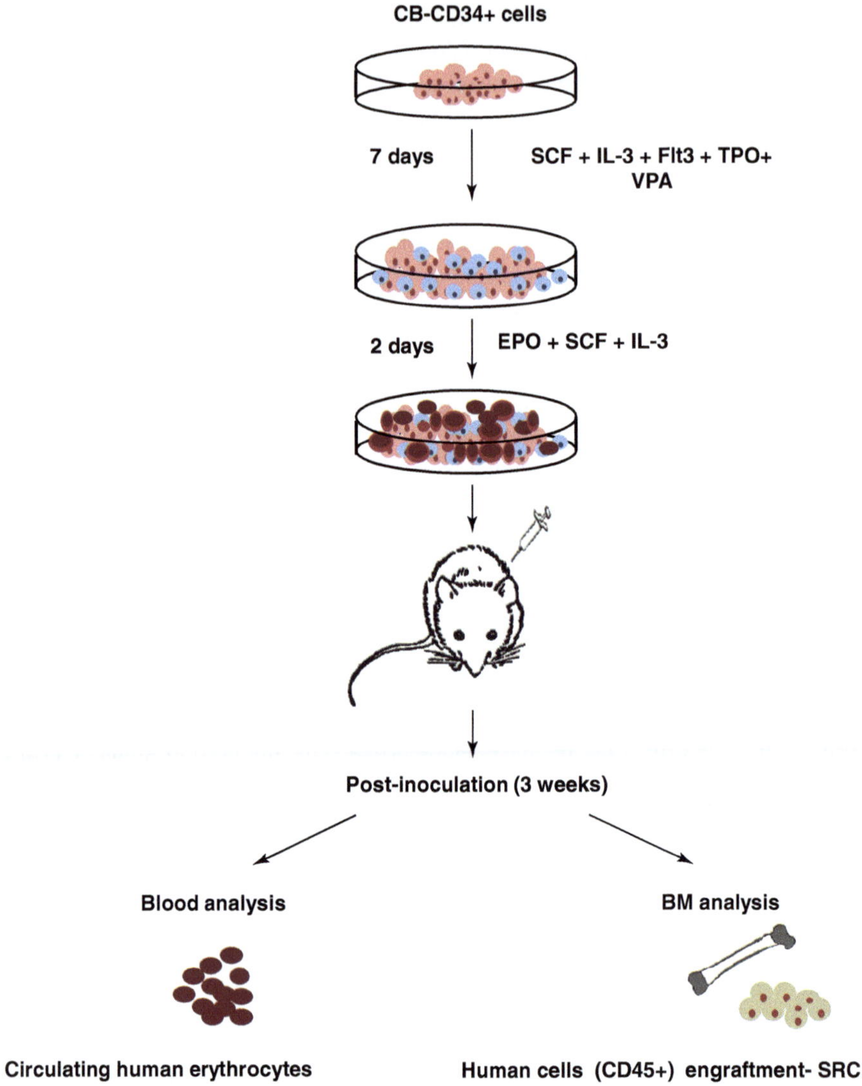

Fig. 3.6 Simplified view of ex vivo expansion of erythroid progenitor cells (EPC) and their functional behavior in NOD/SCID mice. Primary cord blood (*CB*)-CD34+ cells were treated with valproic acid (*VPA*) for a week in the presence of cytokines SCF, Flt-3, TPO, and IL-3 followed by an additional 2 days in the presence of SCF, erythropoietin (*EPO*), and IL-3 and to promote EPC expansion. After 9 days of culture, the EPC-transfusion product was infused into NOD/SCID mice. Evidence of circulating human erythroid cells was observed in the blood of NOD/SCID mice. Human hematopoietic cell chimerism (human CD45+ cells)-SRC was detected in the bone marrow of mice following 3 weeks of infusion of the EPC-transfusion product

decisions are likely activated in primitive cells while unnecessary and conflicting genes are concomitantly repressed. This balance involves the concerted actions of multiple transcriptional activators, repressors, and epigenetic modifiers. Recent studies have demonstrated that global chromatin modifiers influence stem cell fates. Among these modifiers, decitabine is a global hypomethylating agent, and treatment of HSC affects hundreds of genes that may favor cellular transformation.

Araki et al. have shown the altered transcription levels of several genes implicated in self-renewal of HSC occurred following treatment with 5azaD/TSA (Araki et al. 2007). A relatively higher level of transcripts for HOX4B, Bmi-1, and GATA-2 was shown in cultures treated with 5azaD/TSA as compared to cytokines alone. The transcription levels of the genes regulating cell cycle such as p21 and p27 were increased to a greater degree during the initial days of culture (day 5) as compared to day 9 cultures (Cheng et al. 2000; Araki et al. 2007). An increased level of GATA-2 mRNA was observed in primitive HSC/HPC. By contrast, a significant decrease in c-Myc expression was observed in 5azaD-/TSA-treated cells in comparison to the cells cultured in cytokines alone. These findings indicate that c-Myc expression does not define the HSC function following in vitro division but might affect in vivo HSC self-renewal, most likely by altering the interaction between an HSC and its niche within the marrow microenvironment (Wilson and Trumpp 2006). Interestingly, the expression of NOTCH1, which has been implicated in promoting stem cell expansion, was increased in cells exposed to cytokines alone but not to CMA. The expression of lineage-specific genes such as GATA-1 which plays a key role in the commitment of HSC to adult erythroid and megakaryocytic differentiation was increased almost to a similar level in CMA-containing cultures as well as cytokine-containing cultures, whereas MPO, a transcript associated with granulocytic differentiation, was increased in cultures exposed to cytokines alone as compared to cells cultured in the presence of 5azaD/TSA (Araki et al. 2007).

In studies exploring the use of VPA to promote the generation of an EPC-transfusion product, we observed alterations in the relative expression of a group of genes characteristic of both primitive HPC and erythroid commitment (Bmi1, Dnmt1, Ezh2, Smad5, Eklf, GATA1, GATA2, EpoR, and Pu.1). The molecular portrait of VPA-treated CD34+ cells was consistent with a population of EPC with higher expression of GATA2 and lower expression of GATA1 and Pu.1 (Chaurasia et al. 2011). A relatively higher expression of Bmi1, Dnmt1, and Ezh2 was observed, which is associated with maintenance and expansion of primitive HSC/HPC. Furthermore, the upregulation of Smad5 in the VPA-treated CD34+ cells is consistent with the presence of a primitive EPC population since the BMP/BMP receptor/Smad pathway directs the transcription factors Eklf and GATA1 during the earliest stages of erythroid development (Lohmann and Bieker 2008). These studies confirmed the hypothesis that treatment of CB CD34+ cells with different CMA can differentially alter the gene expression patterns of the ex vivo expanded cells.

3.1.7 The Potential Adverse Effects of Treatment with Chromatin-Modifying Agents to Expand Hematopoietic Stem/Progenitor Cells

One of the major obstacles to the use of CMA for HSC/HPC expansion is the theoretical possibility that the use of such agents might lead to nonspecific upregulation of genes which could ultimately result in a neoplastic transformation leading to leukemia arising from donor cells. CMA treatments have the potential to adversely affect oncogenes and/or tumor suppressor genes that result in leukemogenesis. There are, however, several compelling observations that suggest that this risk is not excessive. Epigenetic modifications produced by these CMA are nonspecific and reversible. Furthermore, DNMTIs and HDACIs have been extensively evaluated in a sizeable number of clinical trials with patients being treated for prolonged periods without evidence of chromosomal instability or evidence to date indicating that these agents result in secondary malignancies (Saunthararajah et al. 2008). Nevertheless, a careful safety assessment would be required before proceeding with clinical trials of HSC/HPC expanded in the presence of various CMA.

References

Anguita E, Hughes J, Heyworth C et al (2004) Globin gene activation during haemopoiesis is driven by protein complexes nucleated by GATA-1 and GATA-2. EMBO J 23(14): 2841–2852

Apostolou E, Thanos D (2008) Linking differential chromatin loops to transcriptional decisions. Mol Cell 29(2):154–156

Araki H, Mahmud N, Milhem M et al (2006) Expansion of human umbilical cord blood SCID-repopulating cells using chromatin-modifying agents. Exp Hematol 34(2):140–149

Araki H, Yoshinaga K, Boccuni P et al (2007) Chromatin-modifying agents permit human hematopoietic stem cells to undergo multiple cell divisions while retaining their repopulating potential. Blood 109(8):3570–3578

Araki H, Baluchamy S, Yoshinaga K et al (2009) Cord blood stem cell expansion is permissive to epigenetic regulation and environmental cues. Exp Hematol 37(9):1084–1095

Bachman KE, Rountree MR, Baylin SB (2001) Dnmt3a and Dnmt3b are transcriptional repressors that exhibit unique localization properties to heterochromatin. J Biol Chem 276(34):32282–32287

Baek EJ, Kim HS, Kim S et al (2008) In vitro clinical-grade generation of red blood cells from human umbilical cord blood CD34+ cells. Transfusion 48(10):2235–2245

Bannister AJ, Zegerman P, Partridge JF et al (2001) Selective recognition of methylated lysine 9 on histone H3 by the HP1 chromo domain. Nature 410(6824):120–124

Bartels M, Geest CR, Bierings M et al (2010) Histone deacetylase inhibition modulates cell fate decisions during myeloid differentiation. Haematologica 95(7):1052–1060

Bottardi S, Bourgoin V, Pierre-Charles N et al (2005) Onset and inheritance of abnormal epigenetic regulation in hematopoietic cells. Hum Mol Genet 14(4):493–502

Bug G, Schwarz K, Schoch C et al (2007) Effect of histone deacetylase inhibitor valproic acid on progenitor cells of acute myeloid leukemia. Haematologica 92(4):542–545

Cairo MS, Wagner JE (1997) Placental and/or umbilical cord blood: an alternative source of hematopoietic stem cells for transplantation. Blood 90(12):4665–4678

Challen GA, Sun D, Jeong M et al (2011) Dnmt3a is essential for hematopoietic stem cell differentiation. Nat Genet 44(1):23–31

Challen GA, Sun D, Jeong M et al (2012) Dnmt3a is essential for hematopoietic stem cell differentiation. Nat Genet 44:23–31

Chang AH, Stephan MT, Sadelain M (2006) Stem cell-derived erythroid cells mediate long-term systemic protein delivery. Nat Biotechnol 24(8):1017–1021

Chaurasia P, Berenzon D, Hoffman R (2011) Chromatin-modifying agents promote the ex vivo production of functional human erythroid progenitor cells. Blood 117(17):4632–4641

Cheng T, Rodrigues N, Dombkowski D et al (2000) Stem cell repopulation efficiency but not pool size is governed by p27(kip1). Nat Med 6(11):1235–1240

Clouaire T, Stancheva I (2008) Methyl-CpG binding proteins: specialized transcriptional repressors or structural components of chromatin? Cell Mol Life Sci 65(10):1509–1522

Congdon KL, Reya T (2008) Divide and conquer: how asymmetric division shapes cell fate in the hematopoietic system. Curr Opin Immunol 20(3):302–307

Creusot F, Acs G, Christman JK (1982) Inhibition of DNA methyltransferase and induction of friend erythroleukemia cell differentiation by 5-azacytidine and 5-aza-2′-deoxycytidine. J Biol Chem 257(4):2041–2048

De Felice L, Tatarelli C, Mascolo MG et al (2005) Histone deacetylase inhibitor valproic acid enhances the cytokine-induced expansion of human hematopoietic stem cells. Cancer Res 65(4):1505–1513

Dokmanovic M, Clarke C, Marks PA (2007) Histone deacetylase inhibitors: overview and perspectives. Mol Cancer Res 5(10):981–989

Dorn I, Lazar-Karsten P, Boie S, Ribbat J et al (2008) In vitro proliferation and differentiation of human CD34+ cells from peripheral blood into mature red blood cells with two different cell culture systems. Transfusion 48(6):1122–1132

Elizalde C, Fernández-Rueda J, Salcedo JM et al (2012) Histone deacetylase 3 modulates the expansion of human hematopoietic stem cells. Stem Cells Dev 21(14):2581–2591

Fischle W, Wang Y, Allis CD (2003) Binary switches and modification cassettes in histone biology and beyond. Nature 425(6957):475–479

Fujimi A, Matsunaga T, Kobune M et al (2008) Ex vivo large-scale generation of human red blood cells from cord blood CD34+ cells by co-culturing with macrophages. Int J Hematol 87(4):339–350

Fuks F (2005) DNA methylation and histone modifications: teaming up to silence genes. Curr Opin Genet Dev 15(5):490–495

Fuks F, Burgers WA, Brehm A et al (2000) DNA methyltransferase Dnmt1 associates with histone deacetylase activity. Nat Genet 24(1):88–91

Giarratana MC, Kobari L, Lapillonne H et al (2005) Ex vivo generation of fully mature human red blood cells from hematopoietic stem cells. Nat Biotechnol 23(1):69–74

Giarratana MC, Rouard H, Dumont A et al (2011) Proof of principle for transfusion of in vitro-generated red blood cells. Blood 118(19):5071–5079

Gilbert J, Gore SD, Herman JG et al (2004) The clinical application of targeting cancer through histone acetylation and hypomethylation. Clin Cancer Res 10(14):4589–4596

Goffin J, Eisenhauer E (2002) DNA methyltransferase inhibitors-state of the art. Ann Oncol 13(11):1699–1716

Goll MG, Bestor TH (2005) Eukaryotic cytosine methyltransferases. Annu Rev Biochem 74:481–514

Grass JA, Boyer ME, Pal S et al (2003) GATA-1-dependent transcriptional repression of GATA-2 via disruption of positive autoregulation and domain-wide chromatin remodeling. Proc Natl Acad Sci U S A 100(15):8811–8816

Gubin AN, Njoroge JM, Bouffard GG et al (1999) Gene expression in proliferating human erythroid cells. Genomics 59(2):168–177

Hogart A, Lichtenberg J, Ajay SS et al (2012) Genome-wide DNA methylation profiles in hematopoietic stem and progenitor cells reveal overrepresentation of ETS transcription factor binding sites. Genome Res 22:1407–1418

Humphries RK, Dover G, Young NS et al (1985) 5-Azacytidine acts directly on both erythroid precursors and progenitors to increase production of fetal hemoglobin. J Clin Invest 75(2):547–557

Im H, Grass JA, Johnson KD et al (2005) Chromatin domain activation via GATA-1 utilization of a small subset of dispersed GATA motifs within a broad chromosomal region. Proc Natl Acad Sci U S A 102(47):17065–17070

Iwasaki H, Mizuno S, Arinobu Y et al (2006) The order of expression of transcription factors directs hierarchical specification of hematopoietic lineages. Genes Dev 20(21):3010–3021

Jaenisch R, Bird A (2003) Epigenetic regulation of gene expression: how the genome integrates intrinsic and environmental signals. Nat Genet 33(Suppl):245–254
Jenuwein T, Allis CD (2001) Translating the histone code. Science 293(5532):1074–1080
Ji H, Ehrlich LI, Seita J et al (2010) Comprehensive methylome map of lineage commitment from haematopoietic progenitors. Nature 467(7313):338–342
Jia D, Jurkowska RZ, Zhang X et al (2007) Structure of Dnmt3a bound to Dnmt3L suggests a model for de novo DNA methylation. Nature 449(7159):248–251
Jing H, Vakoc CR, Ying L et al (2008) Exchange of GATA factors mediates transitions in looped chromatin organization at a developmentally regulated gene locus. Mol Cell 29(2):232–242
Johnstone RW (2002) Histone-deacetylase inhibitors: novel drugs for the treatment of cancer. Nat Rev Drug Discov 1:287–299
Jones PA, Baylin SB (2002) The fundamental role of epigenetic events in cancer. Nat Rev Genet 3(6):415–428
Jüttermann R, Li E, Jaenisch R (1994) Toxicity of 5-aza-2′-deoxycytidine to mammalian cells is mediated primarily by covalent trapping of DNA methyltransferase rather than DNA demethylation. Proc Natl Acad Sci U S A 91(25):11797–11801
Kim SI, Bultman SJ, Jing H et al (2007) Dissecting molecular steps in chromatin domain activation during hematopoietic differentiation. Mol Cell Biol 27(12):4551–4565
Kouzarides T (2007) Chromatin modifications and their function. Cell 128(4):693–705
Kretsovali A, Hadjimichael C, Charmpilas N (2012) Histone deacetylase inhibitors in cell pluripotency, differentiation, and reprogramming. Stem Cells Int 2012:184154
Lamonica JM, Vakoc CR, Blobel GA (2006) Acetylation of GATA-1 is required for chromatin occupancy. Blood 108(12):3736–3738
Lane AA, Chabner BA (2009) Histone deacetylase inhibitors in cancer therapy. J Clin Oncol 27(32):5459–5468
Lee JS, Smith E, Shilatifard A (2010) The language of histone crosstalk. Cell 142(5):682–685
Lessard JA, Crabtree GR (2010) Chromatin regulatory mechanisms in pluripotency. Annu Rev Cell Dev Biol 26:503–532
Lohmann F, Bieker JJ (2008) Activation of Eklf expression during hematopoiesis by Gata2 and Smad5 prior to erythroid commitment. Development 135(12):2071–2082
Lopez J, Percharde M, Coley HM et al (2009) The context and potential of epigenetics in oncology. Br J Cancer 100(4):571–577
Martin M, Kettmann R, Dequiedt F (2007) ClassIIa histone deacetylases: regulating the regulators. Oncogene 26(37):5450–5467
Martowicz ML, Grass JA, Boyer ME et al (2005) Dynamic GATA factor interplay at a multicomponent regulatory region of the GATA-2 locus. J Biol Chem 280(3):1724–1732
Martowicz ML, Grass JA, Bresnick EH (2006) GATA-1-mediated transcriptional repression yields persistent transcription factor IIB-chromatin complexes. J Biol Chem 281(49):37345–37352
Matsunaga T, Tanaka I, Kobune M et al (2006) Ex vivo large-scale generation of human platelets from cord blood CD34+ cells. Stem Cells 24(12):2877–2887
Metivier R, Gallais R, Tiffoche C et al (2008) Cyclical DNA methylation of a transcriptionally active promoter. Nature 452(7183):45–50
Migliaccio AR, Adamson JW, Stevens CE et al (2000) Cell dose and speed of engraftment in placental/umbilical cord blood transplantation: graft progenitor cell content is a better predictor than nucleated cell quantity. Blood 96(8):2717–2722
Miharada K, Hiroyama T, Sudo K et al (2006) Efficient enucleation of erythroblasts differentiated in vitro from hematopoietic stem and progenitor cells. Nat Biotechnol 24(10):1255–1256
Milhem M, Mahmud N, Lavelle D et al (2004) Modification of hematopoietic stem cell fate by 5aza 2′deoxycytidine and trichostatin A. Blood 103(11):4102–4110
Milne JC, Lambert PD, Schenk S et al (2007) Small molecule activators of SIRT1 as therapeutics for the treatment of type 2 diabetes. Nature 450(7170):712–716
Nakayama J, Rice JC, Strahl BD et al (2001) Role of histone H3 lysine 9 methylation in epigenetic control of heterochromatin assembly. Science 292(5514):110–113

Neildez-Nguyen TM, Wajcman H, Marden MC et al (2002) Human erythroid cells produced ex vivo at large scale differentiate into red blood cells in vivo. Nat Biotechnol 20(5):467–472

Pal S, Cantor AB, Johnson KD et al (2004) Coregulator-dependent facilitation of chromatin occupancy by GATA-1. Proc Natl Acad Sci U S A 101(4):980–985

Rice KL, Hormaeche I, Licht JD (2007) Epigenetic regulation of normal and malignant hematopoiesis. Oncogene 26(47):6697–6714

Robertson KD, Jones PA (2000) DNA methylation: past, present and future directions. Carcinogenesis 21(3):461–467

Ross K, Sedello AK, Todd GP et al (2012) Polycomb group ring finger 1 cooperates with Runx1 in regulating differentiation and self-renewal of hematopoietic cells. Blood 119(18):4152–4161

Saunthararajah Y, Hillery CA, Lavelle D et al (2003) Effects of 5-aza-2′-deoxycytidine on fetal hemoglobin levels, red cell adhesion, and hematopoietic differentiation in patients with sickle cell disease. Blood 102(12):3865–3870

Saunthararajah Y, Molokie R, Saraf S et al (2008) Clinical effectiveness of decitabine in severe sickle cell disease. Br J Haematol 141(1):126–129

Sieburg HB, Cho RH, Dykstra B et al (2006) The hematopoietic stem compartment consists of a limited number of discrete stem cell subsets. Blood 107(6):2311–2316

Smith CL (2008) A shifting paradigm: histone deacetylases and transcriptional activation. Bioessays 30(1):15–24

Spotswood HT, Turner BM (2002) An increasingly complex code. J Clin Invest 110(5):577–582

Stanevsky A, Goldstein G, Nagler A (2009) Umbilical cord blood transplantation: pros, cons and beyond. Blood Rev 23(5):199–204

Tadokoro Y, Ema H, Okano M et al (2007) De novo DNA methyltransferase is essential for self-renewal, but not for differentiation, in hematopoietic stem cells. J Exp Med 204(4):715–722

Wada T, Kikuchi J, Nishimura N et al (2009) Expression levels of histone deacetylases determine the cell fate of hematopoietic progenitors. J Biol Chem 284(44):30673–30683

Wilson A, Trumpp A (2006) Bone-marrow haematopoietic-stem-cell niches. Nat Rev Immunol 6(2):93–106

Wozniak RJ, Bresnick EH (2008) Epigenetic control of complex loci during erythropoiesis. Curr Top Dev Biol 82:55–83

Zardo G, Cimino G, Nervi C (2008) Epigenetic plasticity of chromatin in embryonic and hematopoietic stem/progenitor cells: therapeutic potential of cell reprogramming. Leukemia 22(8):1503–1518

4 Epigenetic Regulation of Globin Genes and Disturbances in Hemoglobinopathies

Yogen Saunthararajah, Donald Lavelle, and Joseph DeSimone

4.1 Introduction

Hemoglobin is composed of globin polypeptide chains and the iron-containing cofactor heme. In most species, different forms of hemoglobin, containing alternative combinations of globin polypeptide chains, accompany different stages of development. In humans, the globin genes are located in two clusters, the α-like and non-α-globin gene clusters, on chromosome 16 and chromosome 11, respectively; the products of these genes (two α- and two non-α-globin polypeptides) combine to form the hemoglobin tetramer. In humans, the developmental stage-specific hemoglobin tetramers are embryonic hemoglobins Gower 1 ($\zeta_2\varepsilon_2$), Portland 1 ($\zeta_2\gamma_2$), and Gower 2 ($\alpha_2\varepsilon_2$), fetal hemoglobin ($\alpha_2\gamma_2$), adult hemoglobin A ($\alpha_2\beta_2$), and adult hemoglobin A2 ($\alpha_2\delta_2$) (Fig. 4.1). This pattern of hemoglobin production is mostly regulated at the transcriptional level and requires coordinated transcription of α- and non-α-globin genes and silencing of alternative genes within each globin cluster (Higgs et al. 1989). The coordinated transcription activation and repression that occurs at the globin gene clusters is a valuable representation of the coordinated expression and repression of genes that must occur with differentiation and development in general. Hence, lessons from the discrete α- and non-α-globin gene cluster systems can provide widely relevant biological insights.

Y. Saunthararajah (✉)
Cleveland Clinic, Case Western Reserve University,
9500 Euclid Avenue, R40, Cleveland, OH 44195, USA
e-mail: saunthy@ccf.org

D. Lavelle
University of Illinois at Chicago, Jesse Brown VA Medical Center,
820 S. Damen Avenue, Chicago, IL 60612, USA

J. DeSimone
University of Illinois at Chicago, Sickle Cell Center,
MC712, 820 S. Wood Street, Suite 172, Chicago, IL 60612, USA

M. Lübbert, P.A. Jones (eds.), *Epigenetic Therapy of Cancer*,
DOI 10.1007/978-3-642-38404-2_4, © Springer-Verlag Berlin Heidelberg 2014

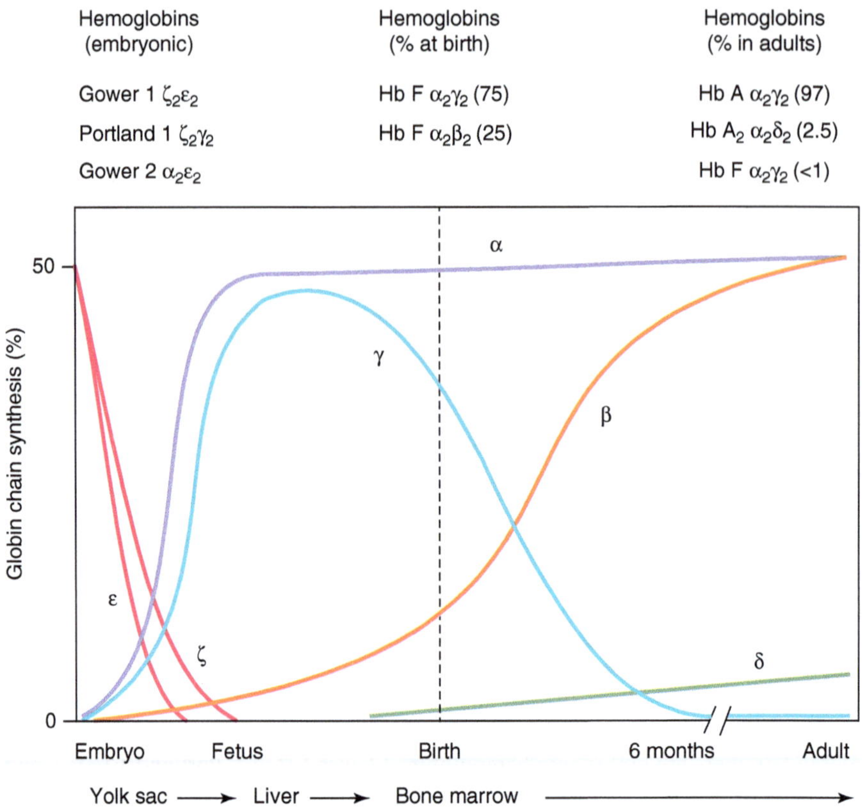

Fig. 4.1 The hemoglobin tetramers that are produced at different stages of human development (Figure from Steinberg (1994))

Diseases of the globin genes, dominated by the thalassemias and sickle cell disease, are the most common genetic diseases in man. Since these diseases involve mutations in specific adult globin genes but not others, understanding the mechanics of switching between different globin genes is of major significance in terms of understanding disease pathogenesis and for potential intervention. The coordinated activation and repression of globin genes ultimately must involve coordinated modification of chromatin. These chromatin changes and their potential therapeutic relevance are the main focus of this chapter: identification of chromatin-modifying enzymes that mediate the observed modifications in chromatin could potentially lead to therapy for the hemoglobinopathies, by inhibiting these enzymes to favor expression of non-mutated genes over mutated genes or to restore the balance between α- and non-α-globin gene expression. Globin gene locus-specific recruitment of chromatin-modifying enzymes is presumably driven by sequence-specific DNA-binding factors. Possibly, these DNA-binding factors can be targets of therapy with the intention of more locus-restricted effects than that possible with inhibition of globally functioning chromatin-modifying enzymes. The current state of knowledge remains ignorant regarding the nature and origin of the environmental signal or clock that sets the DNA-binding/chromatin-modifying machinery in motion to produce developmental globin gene switching. Nonetheless, the knowledge that is there may be sufficient to devise substantially more effective disease modifying strategies for the hemoglobinopathies than currently available.

4.2 Chromatin Changes Associated with Hemoglobin Switching

Globin genes in humans are located in two clusters, the α-like and the non-α-(or β-) gene clusters. The α-like cluster is located on chromosome 16: three α-like globin genes are arranged 5′–3′ in order of their developmental activation – *HBZ* (ζ), *HBA2* (α2), and *HBA1* (α1) (Higgs et al. 1989). The non-α (β)-cluster is located on chromosome 11: five non-α-globin genes are arranged 5′–3′ in order of their developmental activation – *HBE* (ε), *HBG2* (Gγ), *HBG1* (Aγ), *HBD* (δ), and *HBB* (β).

At the α-globin gene cluster, *HBZ* is silenced, and *HBA2* and *HBA1* activated, at the embryonic to fetal developmental transition (Fig. 4.1). HBA2 and HBA1 have sustained high expression through fetal and adult life. HBA2 is more expressed than HBA1; therefore, mutations of *HBA2* produce a more apparent α-thalassemia phenotype.

At the β (non-α)-globin cluster, *HBE* is silenced, and *HBG2* and *HBG1* activated at equal levels, at the embryonic to fetal transition. Then at the fetus to infant transition, *HBG2* and *HBG1* are silenced, and *HBB* is activated (Fig. 4.1). Globin genes are only expressed in erythroid cells. Therefore, one aspect of their transcription regulation is silencing in non-erythroid cells.

Both gene clusters have remote enhancers, which in the case of the β-cluster is commonly referred to as the β-globin locus control region (LCR). Here, we describe the chromatin status and changes associated with developmental stage-specific hemoglobin production at each globin gene cluster, including a description of sequence-specific DNA-binding factors implicated in driving these changes.

4.2.1 Chromatin and Chromatin-Modifying Enzymes at the α-Globin Gene Cluster

DNA Methylation: The α-globin cluster is located in a chromosome region which is rich in "housekeeping" (constitutively expressed) genes. Housekeeping genes are typically associated with unmethylated CpG islands (methylation is a DNA modification associated with silencing). This enrichment in housekeeping genes likely contributes to the unmethylated status of the DNA in this region, even in non-erythroid cells that do not express globin genes (Garrick et al. 2008b). All in all, DNA methylation does not appear to be involved in regulation of α-globin cluster genes.

Histone Modifications: In non-erythroid cells that do not express globin genes, the repression mark H3K27me3 (trimethylation of lysine 27 in histone 3) is highly enriched at the α-globin gene cluster (De Gobbi et al. 2007), suggesting a role for this mark, and the chromatin-modifying enzymes that place it, in silencing α-globin cluster genes. During erythroid differentiation of human CD34+ hematopoietic cells, the activation mark H3K4me2 was noted to progressively increase throughout the α-gene cluster, suggesting a role for this mark and the chromatin-modifying enzymes that place it, in activating α-globin cluster genes (Mahajan et al. 2009).

Higher-Order Chromatin Structure: Remote regulatory elements or enhancers (lying 50–70 kb upstream of the alpha-like genes) play a critical role in controlling α-globin gene expression (Hughes et al. 2005) and other genes on chromosome 16. The importance of DNA sequences cis-remote from the actual globin genes highlights the importance of higher-order chromatin structure in regulating globin genes. Competition for enhancers may play a role in reciprocal gene regulation, since deletion of putative competing genes increases expression of remaining genes (Lower et al. 2009).

Chromatin-Modifying Enzymes at the α-Globin Cluster: Consistent with the observed histone modifications, the Polycomb (PcG) proteins SUZ12 and EZH2 are associated with α-globin cluster genes, and depletion of EZH2 or SUZ12 by siRNA activated expression of α-globin genes even in non-erythroid cells. Histone deacetylases are also involved in repression of the α-globin cluster in non-erythroid cells (De Gobbi et al. 2007). Also consistent with observed histone modifications, histone deacetylase and histone methyltransferase enzymes, but not DNA methyltransferase enzymes, are associated with silenced α-globin genes (De Gobbi et al. 2007; Garrick et al. 2008a).

4.2.2 Chromatin and Chromatin-Modifying Enzymes at the β-Globin Gene Cluster

DNA Methylation: Unlike the α-globin cluster, the β-globin cluster resides in a gene-poor chromosomal neighborhood, with no housekeeping genes or associated CpG islands. Despite the paucity of CpG islands, the β-globin cluster was one of the first sites investigated for a correlation between DNA methylation and transcription (van der Ploeg and Flavell 1980). These studies showed that the CpGs in the promoters of β-cluster genes were unmethylated at developmental stages associated with expression and methylated at stages at which they were not expressed, or in non-erythroid cells. Studies of a transgenic human β-cluster also revealed methylation at the *HBG* promoters that correlated with postnatal suppression of fetal hemoglobin production (Goren et al. 2006). The nonhuman primate Papio anubis (baboon) demonstrates developmental globin switching similar to humans. In erythroid cells purified from baboon fetuses of varying gestational ages and from baboon adult bone marrow, DNA methylation changes at the *HBE* and *HBG* gene promoters inversely correlated with the stage-specific expression of these genes (Lavelle et al. 2006). In an evaluation of human *HBG* and *HBB* promoter methylation in primary human fetal liver and adult bone marrow erythroid cells, promoter methylation and gene expression were again inversely related (Lavelle et al. 2006). Other evidence for a role for DNA methylation in gene regulation of *HBG* at the β-globin gene cluster is a high local concentration of CpG residues in the 5′ *HBG* promoter (5 CpG in the first 105 bp) that is absent in the other β-like globin gene promoters, with phylogenetic footprinting studies demonstrating that acquisition of CpG residues in the 5′ *HBG* promoter was coincident with the recruitment of *HBG* to a fetal stage expression pattern during primate evolution (Tagle et al. 1988). DNA hypomethylation associated with β-globin gene activation is broad, since domains of hypomethylation spanning thousands of base pairs have been observed with developmental stage-specific gene activation at the β-globin gene cluster (Lathrop et al. 2009).

Histone Modifications: The human leukemia cell line K562 has been used as a model of the embryonic/fetal stage of erythroid development. In K562 cells, the LCR and the actively transcribed *HBG* are associated with active histone marks (H3Ac and H3K4me3). In contrast, the silent *HBB* in K562 had absent H3Ac and H3K9me3 (Kim et al. 2007). In chromatin immunoprecipitation analysis of erythroid cells purified from baboon fetuses and from baboon adult bone marrow, enrichment of H3Ac, H4Ac, and pol II at the promoters of developmentally active β-globin genes was observed. H3K4me2 and H3K79me2 were distributed around currently and previously active promoters. H3K36me2 was enriched at the silenced *HBE* promoter (Lavelle et al. 2006). At active β-globin genes, histones at promoters were less acetylated compared to histones over coding regions; histone hyperacetylation extended over tens of kilobases (Yin et al. 2007; Fromm et al. 2009). In an analysis of human primary fetal and bone marrow erythroblasts and human embryonic stem cell-derived primitive-like erythroblasts, the most expressed genes in both the fetal and embryonic cells were associated with the activation marks H3Ac and H3K4me2. At repressed *HBE* and *HBG* in adult erythroid cells, the repression mark H3K9me2 was noted (Lathrop et al. 2009).

In a comparison of histone acetylation and pol II binding at the LCR and β-globin genes in fetal and adult human erythroid cells, the LCR maintained similar acetylation levels at different developmental stages, whereas acetylation at individual gene loci correlated with transcription activation (Yin et al. 2007; Bottardi et al. 2003). In a study of the mouse *HBB* which is activated by HMBA treatment of the MEL cell line, the repression marks H3K9me2, K36me2, and K27me2 were removed from the LCR coincident with transcription initiation at *HBB*. The activation marks K9Ac, K36Ac, and K27Ac were noted after HMBA treatment but before transcription initiation (Kim and Kim 2010). Enrichment of H3K4me1 and depletion of H3K4me3 has been proposed as a signature for enhancers (Heintzman et al. 2007). Thus, the LCR appears to have a baseline pattern of active histone marks. These are supplemented, concurrent with removal of repression marks, upon HBB activation.

Therefore, the distribution of activation and repression histone marks at the β-globin gene cluster has some expected and some interesting characteristics that emphasize significant differences from the α-globin gene cluster.

Higher-Order Chromatin Structure: The remote enhancer that controls expression of the β-globin gene family, the β-LCR, was identified as a number of DNase hypersensitive sites (HS1–4) approximately 60 Kb from the β-globin gene cluster

(Grosveld et al. 1987; Tuan and London 1984). HS1–4 consist essentially of clusters of binding sites for DNA-binding factors. In transgenic experiments, linking HS1–4 to globin transgenes resulted in high expression of the β-globin genes, regardless of the position of integration of HS1–4. Therefore, the LCR was relatively "position independent" in its ability to regulate the globin locus (Li et al. 2002). The existence of a β-thalassemia caused by deletion of the LCR demonstrates its physiologic importance for high-level expression of β-globin genes (Forrester et al. 1990). Studies of erythroid cells lacking key DNA-binding factors such as GATA1 and NF-E2 demonstrate that specific transcription factors bind to the LCR and beta globin loci and recruit chromatin-modifying enzymes. Together, these transcription factors and the associated chromatin-modifying complexes most likely alter target promoters of β-globin cluster genes so that they become conducive to formation of an RNA pol II pre-initiation complex and transcription initiation. Consistent with this model, in a human chromosome with a large deletion that included the LCR, β-globin cluster chromatin in an erythroid background was silent and condensed (Forrester et al. 1990).

Since the LCR can be up to 60 kB distant from a target β-globin gene, higher-order chromatin structure, such as formation of loops, most likely brings the cis-distant β-globin loci into proximity with the LCR. This model is supported by studies that used methods such as chromosome conformation capture (3C) (Carter et al. 2002; Tolhuis et al. 2002). Proteins implicated in loop formation and bridging include GATA1, FOG-1, EKLF, BRG1, and LDB1/NL1 (Vakoc et al. 2005; Drissen et al. 2004; Song et al. 2007; Kim et al. 2009). A refinement of the above model is based on the observation that pol II, rather than being recruited to individual promoters, could be concentrated in subnuclear regions called transcription factories (Pombo et al. 2000; Kiefer et al. 2008) to which promoters which are to undergo high-level activation are recruited. Therefore, the LCR could produce high-level gene expression by influencing the subnuclear localization of β-globin genes such that they are taken to and retained in transcription factories (Kiefer et al. 2008).

Insulators: Insulators are DNA elements that protect genes from the influence of the surrounding DNA environment. Insulators can have a barrier function, blocking the spreading of heterochromatin into euchromatin, or, instead, an enhancer-blocking function, preventing an enhancer from activating a promoter. Insulators were characterized in the context of the chicken β-globin locus. In chickens, the protein CTCF is required for the enhancer-blocking activity of the insulator at the chicken β-globin locus (Bell et al. 1999). Although the human β-globin locus has sequences homologous to the chicken insulators, they may not have the same functional significance, probably because of differences between the overall chromatin environment of this locus between the species (Kiefer et al. 2008).

Intergenic Transcripts: Intergenic transcripts are produced from regions flanking active genes and distal enhancers and can be found throughout the β-globin locus in human erythroid cells, albeit at very low abundance compared to the gene transcripts (Ashe et al. 1997; Gribnau et al. 2000). The histone activation marks H3K4me2, H3K4me3, and H3Ac mark domains in the β-globin locus associated with high levels of intergenic transcription during S phase, suggesting a possible role for intergenic transcription in maintenance of these marks through cell division (Miles et al. 2007). Consistent with a role for intergenic transcripts in chromatin structure and transcription, deletion of an endogenous intergenic transcript promoter between *HBG* and *HBD* affected chromatin accessibility and transcription of downstream *HBB* (Gribnau et al. 2000).

Chromatin-Modifying Enzymes at the β-Globin Cluster: The histone methyltransferases MLL2, which adds activation marks (H3K4me3), and G9a, which adds repression marks (H3K9me2, H3K9me3), have been shown to localize to the β-globin locus, including the LCR and the β-globin genes (Hosey et al. 2010). The demethylase UTX has been implicated in antagonizing the corepressor function of G9a at *HBB* to facilitate expression of *HBB* during differentiation of adult erythroid cells. The histone-arginine methyltransferase PRMT5 (H4R3me2s) has been implicated in maintenance repression of *HBG* in human erythrocytes (Zhao et al. 2009). The histone deacetylase HDAC1 has also been implicated in maintenance of repression at *HBG* (Harju-Baker et al. 2008). In contrast to the α-globin cluster, the β-globin cluster is not enriched for H3K27me3 or the histone methyltransferase enzymes EZH2 and SUZ12 (De Gobbi et al. 2007).

The DNA methyltransferase enzyme DNMT3A, in conjunction with the histone methyltransferase PRMT5, has been implicated in DNA methylation and silencing of *HBG* (Zhao et al. 2009). The maintenance methyltransferase DNMT1 is involved in maintenance of the methylated status of *HBG* (Saunthararajah et al. 2003).

The histone acetyltransferase GCN5/PCAF has been identified as the enzyme responsible for the activation mark H3K9Ac at active *HBB* (Schiltz et al. 1999). PRMT1 creates the binding surface (H4R3me2s) for recruitment of the histone acetyltransferase PCAF that produces H3Ac to enable *HBB* activation (Li et al. 2010).

4.3 Transcription Factors Associated with Globin Gene Activation and Repression

The chromatin changes observed at the globin gene clusters during development are driven by DNA-binding factors, or possibly noncoding RNAs, that determine locus-specific changes in the recruitment of chromatin- modifying enzymes. A number of DNA-binding factors have been implicated in globin gene regulation (Sankaran et al. 2010). These are summarized in Table 4.1. In theory, targeting these DNA-binding factors could lead to more focused effects on globin gene expression than that possible with inhibition of presumably more globally functioning chromatin-modifying enzymes.

4.4 Chromatin Disturbances in the Hemoglobinopathies

The hemoglobinopathies are diseases in which the highly coordinated expression of α- and non-α-genes is disrupted (the thalassemias) or in which an abnormal β-globin peptide is produced (e.g., sickle cell disease). In a searchable database (HbVar

Table 4.1 DNA-binding factors with a role in regulating globin gene expression

Name of DNA-binding factor	Locus that is known to be targeted	Partnering proteins include	Activation and/or repression
GATA1	β-Globin cluster gene promoters, LCR	EKLF	Activation (Letting et al. 2003)
NF-E2	β-Globin cluster gene promoters, LCR	MLL component ASH2L (Kim et al. 2007), USF (Li et al. 2010)	Activation (Yung et al. 2001)
BCL11A	β-Globin cluster gene promoters, LCR	GATA1, FOG1, NuRD complex (Sankaran et al. 2010)	Repression of HBG (Sankaran et al. 2010)
SOX6	β-Globin cluster gene promoters (Yi et al. 2006)		Activation of early β-cluster genes
KLF1 (EKLF)	β-Globin cluster gene promoters, LCR (Miller and Bieker 1993)	CBP/p300, BRG1, SIN3A, HDAC1	Activation and repression
COUP-TF (ARP-1)	β-Globin cluster gene promoters	BCL11A? (Sankaran et al. 2010)	Repression
BRG1 (SWI/SNF)	β-Globin cluster gene promoters, LCR	GATA1, KLF1	Unknown

database), there are at least 395 mutations known to cause thalassemia (Giardine et al. 2007). These mutations are concentrated in the proximal promoters or distal enhancers of the α- and non-α-gene clusters (Giardine et al. 2007), highlighting the importance of these cis-elements and distal enhancers in regulation of both the α- and non-α-gene clusters. The mutation that causes the sickle β-globin variant (causing a glutamic acid to valine change at position six of the β-globin polypeptide) has arisen independently at multiple occasions during human evolution. The sickle mutation is one of more than 1,000 mutations that produce variant hemoglobins (Giardine et al. 2007). The extraordinarily high prevalence of these abnormalities reflects the survival advantage conferred on heterozygote infants and/or toddlers in malaria endemic zones.

In some individuals, fetal hemoglobin continues to be expressed at relatively high levels into adulthood. Like thalassemias and variant hemoglobin phenotypes, the hereditary persistence of fetal hemoglobin (HPFH) phenotypes is also informative of cis-elements and mechanisms involved in regulating globin gene expression. There are three genetic loci with a well-established role in variable adult fetal hemoglobin expression. These are single nucleotide polymorphisms (SNP) in the *HBG2* promoter (Xmn1-HBG2), in the *BCL11A* gene, and in an intergenic sequence on chromosome 6 located between the *HBS1L* and *MYB* genes (Gilman and Huisman 1985; Labie et al. 1985; Thein et al. 2007; Thein et al. 2007). The *BCL11A* SNP that is associated with high fetal hemoglobin expression is associated with low BCL11A expression (Sankaran et al. 2008). These genetic variants that account for a large proportion of interindividual variation in fetal hemoglobin expression may also play a role in variable responses to pharmacologic inducers of fetal hemoglobin (HbF) (Ma et al. 2007).

4.4.1 Therapeutic Implications

The growing understanding of the mechanics of globin gene switching should lead to more effective therapy for the hemoglobinopathies. The major focus is on activating *HBG*, since *HBG* is not mutated, and persistent HbF expression is clearly beneficial in patients with β-thalassemias or sickle cell disease (reviewed by Thein and Menzel 2009). For patients with α-thalassemias, one goal might be to increase activation of α-globin genes, or to turn down activation of β-globin genes, to restore a semblance of balance to α- and non-α-globin gene expression.

4.4.1.1 Therapy Based on Inhibition of Chromatin-Modifying Enzymes

Chromatin-modifying enzymes mediate globin gene repression, including *HBG* repression. Therefore, there has been extensive translational effort to evaluate the therapeutic potential of inhibiting chromatin-modifying enzymes to activate *HBG*. A major limitation in the interpretation and effective clinical translation of such studies is the complex or "dirty" mechanism of action of available drugs. The history of these studies is illustrative. The first studies set out to activate *HBG* by inhibiting the chromatin-modifying enzyme DNA methyltransferase 1 (DNMT1) with the cytosine analogue 5-azacytidine. 5-Azacytidine, after partial conversion in vivo into 5-aza-2′-deoxycytidine (decitabine), can incorporate into DNA and bind DNMT1, the maintenance DNA methyltransferase, culminating in the depletion of this key chromatin-modifying enzyme. Since DNA methylation was a chromatin modification associated with silencing of *HBG*, 5-azacytidine was evaluated in non-human primates, then in humans, for its ability to activate *HBG*, with very promising results. However, 5-azacytidine has other actions besides DNMT1 depletion, such as antimetabolite effects from RNA incorporation and the potential for causing DNA damage. These other actions suggested to some investigators that the observed effects on *HBG* activation could be recapitulated by nonspecific antimetabolite effects. Hence, it was proposed that drugs not directed at chromatin-modifying enzymes, but primarily antimetabolite in action, could be sufficient to produce clinically important HBG reactivation. Furthermore, some preclinical studies suggested that 5-azacytidine could increase the risk for cancer (Carr et al. 1984), deterring further studies with 5-azacytidine. Therefore, the antimetabolite hydroxyurea, which was available for oral administration and which had a long history of clinical use, was evaluated for its ability to activate *HBG*. To some extent validating the idea that antimetabolite effects were sufficient, these studies were successful and definitive, with important benefits demonstrated in a randomized controlled trial (Charache et al. 1995).

Currently, hydroxyurea remains the only drug that is approved by the United States Food and Drug Administration for disease modification of sickle cell disease. However, hydroxyurea has numerous limitations, most importantly, limited efficacy, both in terms of the proportion of patients who benefit from therapy and in terms of the magnitude of the *HBG* activation. Furthermore, even hydroxyurea-induced *HBG* expression is associated with local hypomethylation at *HBG*

(Platt et al. 1984), emphasizing that chromatin is still an important target. Since even hydroxyurea may have to activate *HBG* expression through epigenetic effects, it seems worthwhile to directly inhibit chromatin-modifying enzymes, rather than producing necessary epigenetic effects indirectly through poorly understood pathways downstream of antimetabolite-mediated cytostasis and cytotoxicity.

To avoid the clinical safety and efficacy issues and the mechanistic confusion that arose with the early use of 5-azacytidine as the drug to inhibit chromatin-modifying enzymes, it is necessary to use a drug or drugs that can target chromatin-modifying enzymes with minimal off-target effects such as antimetabolite-related cytotoxicity. Fortunately, the cytidine analogue decitabine can be repurposed for relatively exclusive depletion of DNMT1 which can be separated from off-target antimetabolite or cytotoxic DNA damaging effects (Covey et al. 1986; Schermelleh et al. 2007; Momparler and Goodman 1977; Jones and Taylor 1980; Creusot et al. 1982; Halaban et al. 2009; Saunthararajah et al. 2003): decitabine, like 5-azacytidine or cytarabine, is a cytidine analogue. However, the sugar moiety in decitabine is physiologic (Rogstad et al. 2009); hence after incorporation into the newly synthesized DNA strand during S phase, decitabine does not impede further chain elongation (Covey et al. 1986; Schermelleh et al. 2007). Therefore, at relatively low concentrations, the chromatin-modifying effects of decitabine that result from DNMT1 depletion can be separated from DNA damaging/cytotoxic effects that occur with higher concentrations (Covey et al. 1986; Schermelleh et al. 2007; Momparler and Goodman 1977; Jones and Taylor 1980; Creusot et al. 1982; Halaban et al. 2009; Saunthararajah et al. 2003). Furthermore, decitabine depletes DNMT1; since DNMT1 is a component of multi-protein complexes that modify histones as well as DNA, decitabine can produce broad chromatin relaxation (Haaf 1995). Using a clinical dose and schedule of decitabine that was rationalized to deplete DNMT1 without cytotoxicity, there were large increases in HbF in patients who did not have HbF elevations or clinical benefit with hydroxyurea therapy (Saunthararajah et al. 2003). Furthermore, the noncytotoxic, well-tolerated character of this dose and schedule has enabled effective treatment of severely ill patients with sickle cell disease who were not candidates for conventional hydroxyurea therapy (Saunthararajah et al. 2008).

To fully understand the mechanism by which decitabine activates *HBG*, it is necessary to review additional aspects of erythropoiesis and globin gene regulation, such as the "maturational globin switch."

4.4.1.2 The Maturational Globin Switch During Adult Erythropoiesis

During in vitro differentiation of adult erythroid cells, *HBG* promoters that are hyper-methylated in CD34+ hematopoietic stem and progenitor cells become hypomethylated. Then, as erythropoiesis proceeds, the *HBG* promoters are re-methylated. The period of promoter hypomethylation early in adult erythropoiesis correlates with transient *HBG* expression (Mabaera et al. 2007; Papayannopoulou et al. 1976; Kingsley et al. 2006). A similar maturational switch has been observed at the α-globin cluster (McGrath and Palis 2008).

These observations suggest that *HBG* activation by depleting DNMT1 is produced by preventing placement of repression marks at *HBG* during the maturational globin switch that occurs with progressive maturation of adult erythroid precursors, rather than by removal of repression marks that have already been placed (Hu et al. 2010).

4.4.1.3 Effects of Inhibitors of Chromatin-Modifying Enzymes on Cellular Differentiation

Inhibiting chromatin-modifying enzymes will affect corepressor/coactivator balance at multiple gene loci and, not surprisingly, shifts hematopoietic differentiation. Serendipitously, in the context of the hemoglobinopathies, one of these shifts in cell fate is an increase in erythropoiesis: a noncytotoxic but DNA hypomethylating dose and schedule of decitabine shifted hematopoietic differentiation towards the erythroid and megakaryocytic lineages, producing a direct increase in reticulocytes that was independent of fetal hemoglobin increases. This was most evident in in vitro studies with normal human cord-blood hematopoietic precursors, since there was no confounding effect from the survival advantage of F-reticulocytes in the context of erythroid precursors from patients with hemoglobinopathies (Milhem et al. 2004). As emphasized below, the changes in cell fate produced by DNMT1 depletion are baseline cell-context and differentiation-chronology dependent, since chromatin-modifying enzymes per se are not master determinants of cell fate.

4.4.1.4 A Model to Explain the Effects of Chromatin-Modifying Enzyme Inhibition on Globin Gene Expression

The preclinical and clinical results with decitabine optimized for noncytotoxic depletion of DNMT1 clearly demonstrate the potential of *HBG*-activating therapy based on inhibition of chromatin-modifying enzymes. It should be recognized that the cell fate/gene expression consequences of chromatin-modifying enzyme antagonism or depletion are cell-context dependent, since chromatin-modifying enzymes are not in themselves master regulators or determinants of cell fate. In other words, the ability of this strategy to activate *HBG* may be critically dependent not only on the cell but its stage of differentiation within a lineage. This is illustrated by the cell fate consequences of DNMT1 depletion: DNMT1 depletion by shRNA or by decitabine prevents repression of key stem cell driving genes by differentiation stimuli and thereby maintains self-renewal of normal hematopoietic stem cells even in the presence of pharmacologic dosage of differentiation stimuli (Hu et al. 2010; Milhem et al. 2004). As expected, depletion of DNMT1 after the repression of the stem cell driving factors does not produce a reversion to a stem cell phenotype and may even accelerate progressive maturation (Hu et al. 2010). Thus, key drivers of the baseline cell state must be repressed if the cell is to execute a cell fate transition. This consideration also explains why other drugs that antagonize the epigenetic machinery of transcription repression (e.g., histone deacetylase inhibitors) maintain normal HSC self-renewal (Milhem et al. 2004; De Felice et al. 2005; Bug et al. 2005; Young et al. 2004; Lee et al. 2004; Araki et al. 2006; Suzuki et al. 2004; Chung et al. 2009). These observations emphasize that the gene expression consequences of depleting DNMT1 depend critically on the baseline cellular context. Interestingly, the *HBG* promoter is transiently hypomethylated accompanied by transient *HBG* expression during normal adult erythropoiesis (Mabaera et al. 2007). Taken together with the context-dependent consequences of DNMT1 depletion as discussed above, these findings suggest that instead of "reactivating" expression of *HBG*, the mechanism of action of DNMT1 depletion by decitabine might relate to preventing repression of *HBG* after its activation in the course of progressive maturation of adult erythroid precursors. This working model also explains the preservation of coordinated gene expression during therapy, that is, inhibiting chromatin-modifying enzymes does not result in an uncoordinated increase in the expression of multiple globin genes from the same cluster.

To summarize, the data with decitabine demonstrates that disrupting the chromatin-modifying enzyme network that is involved in transcription repression need not be lethal to cells and can produce clinically important increases in HbF. Furthermore, the effects of such therapy include an increase in erythropoiesis that is separate from improved red cell survival from increased HbF. As such, efforts should continue to develop this line of translational and clinical research. Table 4.2 summarizes chromatin-modifying enzyme strategies to increase HbF.

4.4.1.5 Globin Gene-Specific Therapy

The strategies based on inhibition of DNA methyltransferase or histone deacetylase activity as outlined above have global effects on the cell. A better understanding on the locus-specific role of specific chromatin-modifying enzymes or DNA-binding factors could in theory lead to therapy that is more selective for a particular globin gene locus. As an example, knockdown of G9a caused activation of *HBE* and repression of *HBB* in differentiating murine erythroid cells (murine cells do not have *HBG*) (Chaturvedi et al. 2009). Unlike the result with G9a, knocking down EZH2 (H3K27me3) did not lead to reactivation of *HBE* in the murine erythroid cells (Chaturvedi et al. 2009). Therefore, the histone methyltransferase G9a, but not the histone methyltransferase EZH2, appeared to have a functional and potentially a therapeutic target role in terms of *HBE* and possibly *HBG* reactivation.

PcG members EZH2 and SUZ12 could have an important role in repressing genes that are associated with unmethylated CpG islands or in repression of genes that are embedded in gene-dense regions that contain surrounding actively transcribed genes (i.e., in regions of euchromatin). Histone deacetylases, but not DNA methyltransferases, appear to be associated with such localized repression (Garrick et al. 2008a). This suggests that histone deacetylase inhibitors could in theory have a role in increasing expression of α-globin cluster genes.

Chromatin-modifying enzymes are recruited to specific loci, at least initially, by sequence-specific DNA-binding factors. Therefore, sequence-specific DNA-binding

Table 4.2 Available drugs that inhibit chromatin-modifying enzymes with a possible role in activating HBG expression

Name of agent	Chromatin-modifying enzyme inhibited	Other molecular effects	Stage of development
Cytidine analogue decitabine	DNMT1 (DNMT1 depletion may also disrupt multi-protein complexes that contain DNMT1 and mediate histone methylation)	Can damage DNA and induce apoptosis, separation of these effects from DNMT1 depletion is feasible.	Clinical phase 2 (Saunthararajah et al. 2003) (FDA approved for other indications)
Cytosine analogue 5-azacytidine	DNMT1 (DNMT1 depleted as per decitabine)	Can damage DNA and RNA and induce apoptosis; separation of these effects from DNMT1 depletion may be less feasible than with decitabine	Clinical phase 2 (FDA approved for other indications)
Short-chain fatty acid butyrate and its derivatives	Histone deacetylase class I, IIa	In addition to histone acetylation, affects acetylation status of proteins involved in cell cycle, splicing, nuclear transport and actin nucleation (Choudhary et al. 2009), which can result in apoptosis	Clinical phases 1 and 2
Short-chain fatty acid valproic acid	Histone deacetylase class I, IIa	As above	Preclinical (FDA approved for other indications)
Benzamide (entinostat, MS-275)	Histone deacetylases 1, 2, 3, 8	As above	Preclinical (in clinical trials for other indications)
Hydroxamate (vorinostat, suberoylanilide hydroxamic acid, SAHA)	Histone deacetylase class I, II	As above	Preclinical (FDA approved for other indications)
Thalidomide and other "IMiDs"	Not known if it directly inhibits chromatin-modifying enzymes; however, *HBG* activation associated with increased H4 acetylation (Aerbajinai et al. 2007)	Poorly understood, but multiple effects including effects on cytokines involved in inflammation and angiogenesis	Preclinical (FDA approved for other indications)

factors, as listed in Table 4.1, could also be molecular targets of therapy that aims to produce more locus-specific effects in globin gene expression. For example, the inverse correlation between BCL11A and *HBG* expression suggests that inhibiting BCL11A is a potential therapy for β-hemoglobinopathies (Sankaran et al. 2008).

Conclusion

The developmental changes in globin gene expression are a fascinating representation of the coordinated activation and repression of genes that defines development and differentiation. In addition to valuable scientific lessons, studies of globin gene switching illuminate a path towards more effective disease modification of the hemoglobinopathies, the most common genetic diseases in man. Current therapy has not exploited the improved understanding of the mechanisms of globin gene switching, but such therapy is within grasp. Although chromatin-modifying enzymes are unlikely to drive globin gene switching, these enzymes are necessary mediators of actions likely initiated by sequence-specific DNA-binding factors. Importantly, chromatin-modifying enzymes such as DNMT1 can be safely depleted from cells using drugs which are available for clinical use. This approach maintains expression of *HBG*, which is otherwise only transiently expressed during a maturational switch that occurs during progressive maturation of adult erythroid precursors. The hemoglobinopathies were the first diseases for which a molecular basis was characterized. It seems likely that the molecular lessons of the decades since will soon lead to rational, mechanism-based therapy.

References

Aerbajinai W, Zhu J, Gao Z, Chin K, Rodgers GP (2007) Thalidomide induces gamma-globin gene expression through increased reactive oxygen species-mediated p38 MAPK signaling and histone H4 acetylation in adult erythropoiesis. Blood 110:2864–2871

Araki H, Mahmud N, Milhem M, Nunez R, Xu M, Beam CA, Hoffman R (2006) Expansion of human umbilical cord blood SCID-repopulating cells using chromatin-modifying agents. Exp Hematol 34:140–149

Ashe HL, Monks J, Wijgerde M, Fraser P, Proudfoot NJ (1997) Intergenic transcription and transinduction of the human beta-globin locus. Genes Dev 11:2494–2509

Bell AC, West AG, Felsenfeld G (1999) The protein CTCF is required for the enhancer blocking activity of vertebrate insulators. Cell 98:387–396

Bottardi S, Aumont A, Grosveld F, Milot E (2003) Developmental stage-specific epigenetic control of human beta-globin gene expression is potentiated in hematopoietic progenitor cells prior to their transcriptional activation. Blood 102:3989–3997

Bug G, Gul H, Schwarz K, Pfeifer H, Kampfmann M, Zheng X, Beissert T, Boehrer S, Hoelzer D, Ottmann OG, Ruthardt M (2005) Valproic acid stimulates proliferation and self-renewal of hematopoietic stem cells. Cancer Res 65:2537–2541

Carr BI, Reilly JG, Smith SS, Winberg C, Riggs A (1984) The tumorigenicity of 5-azacytidine in the male Fischer rat. Carcinogenesis 5:1583–1590

Carter D, Chakalova L, Osborne CS, Dai YF, Fraser P (2002) Long-range chromatin regulatory interactions in vivo. Nat Genet 32:623–626

Charache S, Terrin ML, Moore RD, Dover GJ, Barton FB, Eckert SV, McMahon RP, Bonds DR (1995) Effect of hydroxyurea on the frequency of painful crises in sickle cell anemia. Investigators of the multicenter study of hydroxyurea in sickle cell anemia. N Engl J Med 332:1317–1322

Chaturvedi CP, Hosey AM, Palii C, Perez-Iratxeta C, Nakatani Y, Ranish JA, Dilworth FJ, Brand M (2009) Dual role for the methyltransferase G9a in the maintenance of beta-globin gene transcription in adult erythroid cells. Proc Natl Acad Sci U S A 106:18303–18308

Choudhary C, Kumar C, Gnad F, Nielsen ML, Rehman M, Walther TC, Olsen JV, Mann M (2009) Lysine acetylation targets protein complexes and co-regulates major cellular functions. Science 325:834–840

Chung YS, Kim HJ, Kim TM, Hong SH, Kwon KR, An S, Park JH, Lee S, Oh IH (2009) Undifferentiated hematopoietic cells are characterized by a genome-wide undermethylation dip around the transcription start site and a hierarchical epigenetic plasticity. Blood 114:4968–4978

Covey JM, D'Incalci M, Tilchen EJ, Zaharko DS, Kohn KW (1986) Differences in DNA damage produced by incorporation of 5-aza-2′-deoxycytidine or 5,6-dihydro-5-azacytidine into DNA of mammalian cells. Cancer Res 46:5511–5517

Creusot F, Acs G, Christman JK (1982) Inhibition of DNA methyltransferase and induction of friend erythroleukemia cell differentiation by 5-azacytidine and 5-aza-2′-deoxycytidine. J Biol Chem 257:2041–2048

De Felice L, Tatarelli C, Mascolo MG, Gregorj C, Agostini F, Fiorini R, Gelmetti V, Pascale S, Padula F, Petrucci MT, Arcese W, Nervi C (2005) Histone deacetylase inhibitor valproic acid enhances the cytokine-induced expansion of human hematopoietic stem cells. Cancer Res 65:1505–1513

De Gobbi M, Anguita E, Hughes J, Sloane-Stanley JA, Sharpe JA, Koch CM, Dunham I, Gibbons RJ, Wood WG, Higgs DR (2007) Tissue-specific histone modification and transcription factor binding in alpha globin gene expression. Blood 110:4503–4510

Drissen R, Palstra RJ, Gillemans N, Splinter E, Grosveld F, Philipsen S, de Laat W (2004) The active spatial organization of the beta-globin locus requires the transcription factor EKLF. Genes Dev 18:2485–2490

Forrester WC, Epner E, Driscoll MC, Enver T, Brice M, Papayannopoulou T, Groudine M (1990) A deletion of the human beta-globin locus activation region causes a major alteration in chromatin structure and replication across the entire beta-globin locus. Genes Dev 4: 1637–1649

Fromm G, de Vries C, Byron R, Fields J, Fiering S, Groudine M, Bender MA, Palis J, Bulger M (2009) Histone hyperacetylation within the beta-globin locus is context-dependent and precedes high-level gene expression. Blood 114:3479–3488

Garrick D, De Gobbi M, Lynch M, Higgs DR (2008a) Switching genes on and off in haemopoiesis. Biochem Soc Trans 36:613–618

Garrick D, De Gobbi M, Samara V, Rugless M, Holland M, Ayyub H, Lower K, Sloane-Stanley J, Gray N, Koch C, Dunham I, Higgs DR (2008b) The role of the polycomb complex in silencing alpha-globin gene expression in nonerythroid cells. Blood 112:3889–3899

Giardine B, van Baal S, Kaimakis P, Riemer C, Miller W, Samara M, Kollia P, Anagnou NP, Chui DH, Wajcman H, Hardison RC, Patrinos GP (2007) HbVar database of human hemoglobin variants and thalassemia mutations: 2007 update. Hum Mutat 28:206

Gilman JG, Huisman TH (1985) DNA sequence variation associated with elevated fetal G gamma globin production. Blood 66:783–787

Goren A, Ram O, Amit M, Keren H, Lev-Maor G, Vig I, Pupko T, Ast G (2006) Comparative analysis identifies exonic splicing regulatory sequences – the complex definition of enhancers and silencers. Mol Cell 22:769–781

Gribnau J, Diderich K, Pruzina S, Calzolari R, Fraser P (2000) Intergenic transcription and developmental remodeling of chromatin subdomains in the human beta-globin locus. Mol Cell 5:377–386

Grosveld F, van Assendelft GB, Greaves DR, Kollias G (1987) Position-independent, high-level expression of the human beta-globin gene in transgenic mice. Cell 51:975–985

Haaf T (1995) The effects of 5-azacytidine and 5-azadeoxycytidine on chromosome structure and function: implications for methylation-associated cellular processes. Pharmacol Ther 65:19–46

Halaban R, Krauthammer M, Pelizzola M, Cheng E, Kovacs D, Sznol M, Ariyan S, Narayan D, Bacchiocchi A, Molinaro A, Kluger Y, Deng M, Tran N, Zhang W, Picardo M, Enghild JJ (2009) Integrative analysis of epigenetic modulation in melanoma cell response to decitabine: clinical implications. PLoS One 4:e4563

Harju-Baker S, Costa FC, Fedosyuk H, Neades R, Peterson KR (2008) Silencing of Agamma-globin gene expression during adult definitive erythropoiesis mediated by GATA-1-FOG-1-Mi2 complex binding at the −566 GATA site. Mol Cell Biol 28:3101–3113

Heintzman ND, Stuart RK, Hon G, Fu Y, Ching CW, Hawkins RD, Barrera LO, Van Calcar S, Qu C, Ching KA, Wang W, Weng Z, Green RD, Crawford GE, Ren B (2007) Distinct and predictive chromatin signatures of transcriptional promoters and enhancers in the human genome. Nat Genet 39:311–318

Higgs DR, Vickers MA, Wilkie AO, Pretorius IM, Jarman AP, Weatherall DJ (1989) A review of the molecular genetics of the human alpha-globin gene cluster. Blood 73:1081–1104

Hosey AM, Chaturvedi CP, Brand M (2010) Crosstalk between histone modifications maintains the developmental pattern of gene expression on a tissue-specific locus. Epigenetics 5

Hu Z, Negrotto S, Gu X, Mahfouz R, Ng KP, Ebrahem Q, Copelan E, Singh H, Maciejewski JP, Saunthararajah Y (2010) Decitabine maintains hematopoietic precursor self-renewal by preventing repression of stem cell genes by a differentiation-inducing stimulus. Mol Cancer Ther 9:1536–1543

Hughes JR, Cheng JF, Ventress N, Prabhakar S, Clark K, Anguita E, De Gobbi M, de Jong P, Rubin E, Higgs DR (2005) Annotation of cis-regulatory elements by identification, subclassification, and functional assessment of multispecies conserved sequences. Proc Natl Acad Sci U S A 102:9830–9835

Jones PA, Taylor SM (1980) Cellular differentiation, cytidine analogs and DNA methylation. Cell 20:85–93

Kiefer CM, Hou C, Little JA, Dean A (2008) Epigenetics of beta-globin gene regulation. Mutat Res 647:68–76

Kim K, Kim A (2010) Sequential changes in chromatin structure during transcriptional activation in the beta globin LCR and its target gene. Int J Biochem Cell Biol 42:1517–1524

Kim A, Kiefer CM, Dean A (2007) Distinctive signatures of histone methylation in transcribed coding and noncoding human beta-globin sequences. Mol Cell Biol 27:1271–1279

Kim SI, Bresnick EH, Bultman SJ (2009) BRG1 directly regulates nucleosome structure and chromatin looping of the alpha globin locus to activate transcription. Nucleic Acids Res 37:6019–6027

Kingsley PD, Malik J, Emerson RL, Bushnell TP, McGrath KE, Bloedorn LA, Bulger M, Palis J (2006) "Maturational" globin switching in primary primitive erythroid cells. Blood 107:1665–1672

Labie D, Dunda-Belkhodja O, Rouabhi F, Pagnier J, Ragusa A, Nagel RL (1985) The −158 site 5′ to the G gamma gene and G gamma expression. Blood 66:1463–1465

Lathrop MJ, Hsu M, Richardson CA, Olivier EN, Qiu C, Bouhassira EE, Fiering S, Lowrey CH (2009) Developmentally regulated extended domains of DNA hypomethylation encompass highly transcribed genes of the human beta-globin locus. Exp Hematol 37:807–813

Lavelle D, Vaitkus K, Hankewych M, Singh M, DeSimone J (2006) Developmental changes in DNA methylation and covalent histone modifications of chromatin associated with the epsilon-, gamma-, and beta-globin gene promoters in Papio anubis. Blood Cells Mol Dis 36:269–278

Lee JH, Hart SR, Skalnik DG (2004) Histone deacetylase activity is required for embryonic stem cell differentiation. Genesis 38:32–38

Letting DL, Rakowski C, Weiss MJ, Blobel GA (2003) Formation of a tissue-specific histone acetylation pattern by the hematopoietic transcription factor GATA-1. Mol Cell Biol 23:1334–1340

Li Q, Peterson KR, Fang X, Stamatoyannopoulos G (2002) Locus control regions. Blood 100:3077–3086

Li X, Hu X, Patel B, Zhou Z, Liang S, Ybarra R, Qiu Y, Felsenfeld G, Bungert J, Huang S (2010) H4R3 methylation facilitates beta-globin transcription by regulating histone acetyltransferase binding and H3 acetylation. Blood 115:2028–2037

Lower KM, Hughes JR, De Gobbi M, Henderson S, Viprakasit V, Fisher C, Goriely A, Ayyub H, Sloane-Stanley J, Vernimmen D, Langford C, Garrick D, Gibbons RJ, Higgs DR (2009) Adventitious changes in long-range gene expression caused by polymorphic structural variation and promoter competition. Proc Natl Acad Sci U S A 106:21771–21776

Ma Q, Wyszynski DF, Farrell JJ, Kutlar A, Farrer LA, Baldwin CT, Steinberg MH (2007) Fetal hemoglobin in sickle cell anemia: genetic determinants of response to hydroxyurea. Pharmacogenomics J 7:386–394

Mabaera R, Richardson CA, Johnson K, Hsu M, Fiering S, Lowrey CH (2007) Developmental- and differentiation-specific patterns of human gamma- and beta-globin promoter DNA methylation. Blood 110:1343–1352

Mahajan MC, Karmakar S, Newburger PE, Krause DS, Weissman SM (2009) Dynamics of alpha-globin locus chromatin structure and gene expression during erythroid differentiation of human CD34(+) cells in culture. Exp Hematol 37:1143–1156

McGrath K, Palis J (2008) Ontogeny of erythropoiesis in the mammalian embryo. Curr Top Dev Biol 82:1–22

Miles J, Mitchell JA, Chakalova L, Goyenechea B, Osborne CS, O'Neill L, Tanimoto K, Engel JD, Fraser P (2007) Intergenic transcription, cell-cycle and the developmentally regulated epigenetic profile of the human beta-globin locus. PLoS One 2:e630

Milhem M, Mahmud N, Lavelle D, Araki H, DeSimone J, Saunthararajah Y, Hoffman R (2004) Modification of hematopoietic stem cell fate by 5aza 2′deoxycytidine and trichostatin A. Blood 103:4102–4110

Miller IJ, Bieker JJ (1993) A novel, erythroid cell-specific murine transcription factor that binds to the CACCC element and is related to the Kruppel family of nuclear proteins. Mol Cell Biol 13:2776–2786

Momparler RL, Goodman J (1977) In vitro cytotoxic and biochemical effects of 5-aza-2′-deoxycytidine. Cancer Res 37:1636–1639

Papayannopoulou TH, Brice M, Stamatoyannopoulos G (1976) Stimulation of fetal hemoglobin synthesis in bone marrow cultures from adult individuals. Proc Natl Acad Sci U S A 73:2033–2037

Platt OS, Orkin SH, Dover G, Beardsley GP, Miller B, Nathan DG (1984) Hydroxyurea enhances fetal hemoglobin production in sickle cell anemia. J Clin Invest 74:652–656

Pombo A, Jones E, Iborra FJ, Kimura H, Sugaya K, Cook PR, Jackson DA (2000) Specialized transcription factories within mammalian nuclei. Crit Rev Eukaryot Gene Expr 10:21–29

Rogstad DK, Herring JL, Theruvathu JA, Burdzy A, Perry CC, Neidigh JW, Sowers LC (2009) Chemical decomposition of 5-aza-2′-deoxycytidine (decitabine): kinetic analyses and identification of products by NMR, HPLC, and mass spectrometry. Chem Res Toxicol 22:1194–1204

Sankaran VG, Menne TF, Xu J, Akie TE, Lettre G, Van Handel B, Mikkola HK, Hirschhorn JN, Cantor AB, Orkin SH (2008) Human fetal hemoglobin expression is regulated by the developmental stage-specific repressor BCL11A. Science 322:1839–1842

Sankaran VG, Xu J, Orkin SH (2010) Advances in the understanding of haemoglobin switching. Br J Haematol 149:181–194

Saunthararajah Y, Hillery CA, Lavelle D, Molokie R, Dorn L, Bressler L, Gavazova S, Chen YH, Hoffman R, DeSimone J (2003) Effects of 5-aza-2′-deoxycytidine on fetal hemoglobin levels, red cell adhesion, and hematopoietic differentiation in patients with sickle cell disease. Blood 102:3865–3870

Saunthararajah Y, Molokie R, Saraf S, Sidhwani S, Gowhari M, Vara S, Lavelle D, DeSimone J (2008) Clinical effectiveness of decitabine in severe sickle cell disease. Br J Haematol 141:126–129

Schermelleh L, Haemmer A, Spada F, Rosing N, Meilinger D, Rothbauer U, Cardoso MC, Leonhardt H (2007) Dynamics of Dnmt1 interaction with the replication machinery and its role in postreplicative maintenance of DNA methylation. Nucleic Acids Res 35:4301–4312

Schiltz RL, Mizzen CA, Vassilev A, Cook RG, Allis CD, Nakatani Y (1999) Overlapping but distinct patterns of histone acetylation by the human coactivators p300 and PCAF within nucleosomal substrates. J Biol Chem 274:1189–1192

Song SH, Hou C, Dean A (2007) A positive role for NLI/Ldb1 in long-range beta-globin locus control region function. Mol Cell 28:810–822

Steinberg MH (1994) Hemoglobinopathies and thalassemias. In: Stein JH (ed) Internal medicine, 4th edn. Mosby-Year Book, St. Louis, p 852

Suzuki M, Harashima A, Okochi A, Yamamoto M, Nakamura S, Motoda R, Yamasaki F, Orita K (2004) 5-Azacytidine supports the long-term repopulating activity of cord blood CD34(+) cells. Am J Hematol 77:313–315

Tagle DA, Koop BF, Goodman M, Slightom JL, Hess DL, Jones RT (1988) Embryonic epsilon and gamma globin genes of a prosimian primate (Galago crassicaudatus). Nucleotide and amino acid sequences, developmental regulation and phylogenetic footprints. J Mol Biol 203:439–455

Thein SL, Menzel S (2009) Discovering the genetics underlying foetal haemoglobin production in adults. Br J Haematol 145:455–467

Thein SL, Menzel S, Peng X, Best S, Jiang J, Close J, Silver N, Gerovasilli A, Ping C, Yamaguchi M, Wahlberg K, Ulug P, Spector TD, Garner C, Matsuda F, Farrall M, Lathrop M (2007) Intergenic variants of HBS1L-MYB are responsible for a major quantitative trait locus on chromosome 6q23 influencing fetal hemoglobin levels in adults. Proc Natl Acad Sci U S A 104:11346–11351

Tolhuis B, Palstra RJ, Splinter E, Grosveld F, de Laat W (2002) Looping and interaction between hypersensitive sites in the active beta-globin locus. Mol Cell 10:1453–1465

Tuan D, London IM (1984) Mapping of DNase I-hypersensitive sites in the upstream DNA of human embryonic epsilon-globin gene in K562 leukemia cells. Proc Natl Acad Sci U S A 81:2718–2722

Vakoc CR, Letting DL, Gheldof N, Sawado T, Bender MA, Groudine M, Weiss MJ, Dekker J, Blobel GA (2005) Proximity among distant regulatory elements at the beta-globin locus requires GATA-1 and FOG-1. Mol Cell 17:453–462

van der Ploeg LH, Flavell RA (1980) DNA methylation in the human gamma delta beta-globin locus in erythroid and nonerythroid tissues. Cell 19:947–958

Yi Z, Cohen-Barak O, Hagiwara N, Kingsley PD, Fuchs DA, Erickson DT, Epner EM, Palis J, Brilliant MH (2006) Sox6 directly silences epsilon globin expression in definitive erythropoiesis. PLoS Genet 2:e14

Yin W, Barkess G, Fang X, Xiang P, Cao H, Stamatoyannopoulos G, Li Q (2007) Histone acetylation at the human beta-globin locus changes with developmental age. Blood 110:4101–4107

Young JC, Wu S, Hansteen G, Du C, Sambucetti L, Remiszewski S, O'Farrell AM, Hill B, Lavau C, Murray LJ (2004) Inhibitors of histone deacetylases promote hematopoietic stem cell self-renewal. Cytotherapy 6:328–336

Yung R, Kaplan M, Ray D, Schneider K, Mo RR, Johnson K, Richardson B (2001) Autoreactive murine Th1 and Th2 cells kill syngeneic macrophages and induce autoantibodies. Lupus 10:539–546

Zhao Q, Rank G, Tan YT, Li H, Moritz RL, Simpson RJ, Cerruti L, Curtis DJ, Patel DJ, Allis CD, Cunningham JM, Jane SM (2009) PRMT5-mediated methylation of histone H4R3 recruits DNMT3A, coupling histone and DNA methylation in gene silencing. Nat Struct Mol Biol 16:304–311

DNA Methylation Abnormalities in Hematopoietic Disorders: Biological Significance and Methodological Approaches

5

Rainer Claus, Maximilian Schmutz, Gabriele Greve, and Lars Bullinger

5.1 Epigenetic Modifications in Hematopoietic Disorders

5.1.1 Introduction

Developmental steps in normal and malignant hematopoiesis are well understood and have been a prime example for deciphering complex developmental pathways. All mature blood cell types originate from hematopoietic stem cells (HSCs) in a strongly regulated differentiation process thereby gradually losing the potential for self-renewal. This sophisticated system is highly sensitive for any kind of interference that might cause alterations on a genetic level. Mutational events either might enhance the proliferation of undifferentiated precursors (class I mutation) or might block defined differentiation steps (class II mutation), thus resulting in the subversion of affected cells into leukemic cells (Gilliland 2001).

Recent work revealed that leukemic diseases are not limited to this widely accepted framework of acquiring either a proliferative stimulus or a block in

R. Claus, MD (✉) • G. Greve
Department of Medicine, Division of Hematology/Oncology,
University of Freiburg Medical Center, Hugstetterstr. 55, 79106 Freiburg, Germany
e-mail: rainer.claus@uniklinik-freiburg.de; gabriele.greve@uniklinik-freiburg.de

M. Schmutz
Division of Epigenomics and Cancer Risk Factors,
German Cancer Research Center, Im Neuenheimer Feld 280, 69120 Heidelberg, Germany
e-mail: m.schmutz@dkfz.de

L. Bullinger, MD
Department of Internal Medicine III,
University of Ulm, Albert-Einstein-Allee 23, 89081 Ulm, Germany
e-mail: lars.bullinger@uniklinik-ulm.de

M. Lübbert, P.A. Jones (eds.), *Epigenetic Therapy of Cancer*,
DOI 10.1007/978-3-642-38404-2_5, © Springer-Verlag Berlin Heidelberg 2014

differentiation (Shih et al. 2012). This view is supported by the fact that a large portion of leukemia patients does not harbor class I or II mutations. Moreover, recent studies identified additional classes of mutations involving the epigenetic machinery, such as perturbations in elements regulating DNA methylation or posttranslational histone modifications.

These disturbances in epigenetic regulators seem to be both a crucial and common event in malignant hematopoietic transformation. The perturbations in epigenetic regulators do not only occur additionally to class I or class II mutations but do possess the potential to elicit myeloid transformation.

5.1.2 The Role of DNA Methylation Events in Normal Hematopoiesis

Epigenetic alterations include modifications of the DNA and the histone proteins and do not change the genetic code but have the ability to alter gene expression either *in cis* or *in trans.* They can be transmitted to daughter cells through mitosis (Jones and Baylin 2002). In general, each of the "epigenetic pathways" includes enzymes that perform the modification ("writers"), enzymes that alter or revert the modification ("editors" and "erasers"), and enzymes that recognize the modification ("readers"). Since noncoding RNAs also regulate expression of protein-coding genes, they are included in the list of epigenetic alterations and reviewed elsewhere (Guil and Esteller 2012).

Modifications of the DNA include 5-methylcytosine (5mC), 5-hydroxymethylcytosine (5hmC), 5-formylcytosine (5fC), and 5-carboxylcytosine (5caC) (He et al. 2011; Ito et al. 2011) and have been investigated in the context of normal developmental processes (Reik et al. 2001), X-chromosome inactivation (Brockdorff 2011), and genomic imprinting (Barlow 2011).

During the process of differentiation, precursor cells continuously lose the ability to give rise to alternative pathways. DNA methylation patterns are established early in embryonic development and are controlled by *de* novo DNA methyltransferases (DNMT3A/B) as well as by maintenance transferases (DNMT1) that require hemi-methylated DNA as a substrate (Chen and Li 2006). Interestingly, it still remains unclear how specific methylation patterns are established: either a specific recruitment machinery exists allowing for specific genes to be targeted by *de* novo DNA methylases in a sequence-specific context or a progressive methylation of inactive genes takes place, defined by an absence of transcription factor binding in specific lineages. A probable decomposition can be envisioned by combining both approaches.

On a par with changes in expression of genes during hematopoietic differentiation into specific lineages are distinct patterns of DNA methylation (Ji et al. 2010). This results in demethylation and concomitant activation of genes required for specific lineage commitment. In contrast, genes required for maintaining a stem or progenitor state such as *MEIS1* or *HOXA9* are methylated and thus silenced with advancing steps in differentiation (Faber et al. 2009; Borgel et al. 2010).

5.1.3 Aberrant Promoter Methylation in Malignant Hematopoiesis

In hematopoietic malignancies, DNA methylation patterns as well as the transcription factor network are subverted towards leukemic cell survival (Baylin and Ohm 2006). Tumor suppressor genes, for example, are well known to be inactivated by DNA hypermethylation (Rush and Plass 2002). Especially changes in promoter methylation have been described to play a crucial role in the gene expression levels of growth factor receptors during normal myeloid development and leukemogenesis (Lübbert et al. 1997). DNA methylation changes in non-promoter regions such as gene bodies or gene 3′ regions are frequently observed; however, their functional impact is not as clear.

First evidence for aberrant DNA methylation in myeloid leukemia came from studies of the human *calcitonin* gene promoter (Baylin et al. 1987). Since then, candidate approaches have identified a large variety of hypermethylated genes in AML, some of which were shown to have a prognostic impact (Melki et al. 1999; Claus et al. 2006).

For example, estrogen receptor (*ER*) methylation has been associated with improved overall survival (Toyota et al. 1999), while the prognostic significance of promoter hypermethylation in genes like *CDH1* (E-Cadherin), *HIC1* (hypermethylated in cancer 1), *DAPK1*, and *CEBPA* remains controversially discussed (Issa et al. 1996, 1997; Herman et al. 1997; Plass et al. 1999; Melki et al. 2000; Chim et al. 2001; Seedhouse et al. 2003; Voso et al. 2004; Galm et al. 2005; Shimamoto et al. 2005; Agrawal et al. 2007; Hackanson et al. 2008).

Furthermore, *CDKN2B* (encoding p15), the prime example for silencing of a tumor suppressor gene by aberrant hypermethylation in cancer (Galm et al. 2004; Rosu-Myles and Wolff 2008), is also frequently found hypermethylated in myeloid leukemia and MDS (Cameron et al. 1999; Daskalakis et al. 2002; Christiansen et al. 2003; Shimamoto et al. 2005). In addition, transient *p15* methylation has also been described in myeloid development (Sakashita et al. 2001).

5.1.4 Global DNA Methylation Analyses in Acute Myeloid Leukemia

First approaches to comprehensively characterize the extent of aberrant DNA methylation in myeloid blasts were conducted using restriction landmark genomic scanning (RLGS), which for the first time allowed to simultaneously interrogate hundreds to thousands of CpG-dense areas in promoter regions of genes. RLGS-based genome scans in acute myeloid leukemia (AML) revealed that up to 8.3 % of all CpG islands (CGI) (this equals more than 2,000 CGIs in a human genome) show increased DNA methylation and thereby are epigenetically altered (Rush et al. 2001; Raval et al. 2002). This was a surprisingly high number of candidate genes and exceeded by far the estimated number of potential tumor suppressor genes. Furthermore, it became also clear that DNA methylation patterns of different AML samples show striking similarities and are non-random. On the other hand comparisons of DNA methylation patterns between different malignant entities revealed significant differences suggesting characteristic tumor-type-specific methylation events (Costello et al. 2000).

A first study integrating promoter microarray DNA methylation and SNP (single-nucleotide polymorphism) karyotyping analysis in myelodysplastic syndrome (MDS) and AML demonstrated that the average methylation and the number of aberrantly methylated CpG sites were significantly greater in high-risk MDS/AML as compared to low-risk MDS (Jiang et al. 2009). Furthermore, it was shown that aberrant methylation might cooperate with chromosome deletions to silence tumor suppressor genes. Thus, the progression of aberrant DNA methylation might reflect the dominant role of epigenetic events for the silencing of tumor suppressor genes and clonal variation in MDS evolution to AML.

Similarly, using the HELP (H*pa*II tiny fragment Enrichment by Ligation-mediated PCR) method, the distribution of DNA methylation of 14,000 promoters was compared in MDS and secondary AML patients (Figueroa et al. 2009). Here, MDS and AML cases also displayed extensive aberrant DNA methylation involving thousands of genes, which tended to affect particular chromosomal regions and included prominent genes linked to the WNT and MAPK signaling pathways. Interestingly, MDS and secondary AML showed distinct epigenetic features that distinguished them from *de* novo AML.

In line with these initial reports, the first large genome-wide study of primary AML cells comprising a cohort of 344 newly diagnosed AML patients provided many additional insights (Figueroa et al. 2010b). Unsupervised data analysis of HELP-based microarray data revealed several distinct methylation patterns, which correlated well with known cytogenetically defined AML subgroups. This important observation reflects the differences underlying, e.g., the t(15;17), inv(16), t(8;21), or t(11q23) AML subgroups, which are not only characterized by distinct gene expression patterns but are also known to influence the epigenetic machinery in hematopoietic cells. In line with the study by Gebhard and colleagues (Gebhard et al. 2006), there was only a partial overlap of the aberrantly methylated and expressed genes in each AML subgroup (Figueroa et al. 2010b). This further confirms that epigenetic deregulation can have a significant biological impact in AML, thereby influencing gene expression profiles in general.

In addition, the fact that not all methylated genes were found repressed at the expression level suggests that (1) the detected DNA methylation was incomplete (and thus insufficient to inactivate gene expression), (2) the targeted region does not directly influence expression, (3) the promoter DNA methylation associated transcriptional repression can be overcome by other mechanisms, and (4) the aberrant gene expression in leukemia is influenced by many factors.

Accordantly, the observed methylation patterns were also significantly enriched for genes belonging to distinct pathways. For example, enrichment of p53 signaling and DNA damage response pathway members pointed to distinct pathogenic differences between the respective methylation-defined clusters, thereby providing an optimal starting point to further dissect leukemia biology.

5.1.5 Mutations in DNA Methylation Pathways

Genetic defects were identified in enzymes that are involved in the establishment and removal of DNA methylation patterns, such as in DNMT3A, IDH1/2, and TET2. These mutations affect – like in a chain reaction – global gene expression patterns by altering promoter DNA methylation, which highlights the tight interconnection of genetic events leading to genome-wide epigenetic reprogramming.

5.1.5.1 DNMT3A

The *de* novo methyltransferase DNMT3A is a member of the mammalian family of methyltransferases and was first described in 2010 to be somatically mutated in patients suffering from AML (Ley et al. 2010; Yamashita et al. 2010). The presence of this mutation implies a critical role for aberrant epigenetic gene regulation in AML pathogenesis. Subsequent studies revealed *DNMT3A* mutations in about 20 % of adult AML cases and showed a correlation with an increased risk of disease relapse (Thol et al. 2011; Yan et al. 2011; Gaidzik et al. 2013). Moreover, these patients often harbor *NPM1, FLT3* and *IDH1* mutations (Ley et al. 2010).

For MDS, only a single study, correlating a mutation in *DNMT3A* with an unfavorable prognosis, exists (Walter et al. 2011). No prognostic correlation for myeloproliferative neoplasms (MPN) has been demonstrated, so far. The majority of *DNMT3A* mutations either results in a truncated product or occurs at a single amino acid R882 presumably resulting in decreased catalytic function (Gowher et al. 2006; Yamashita et al. 2010). Clinically, patients with *DNMT3A* mutations typically present with high white blood cell counts. Interestingly, haploinsufficiency also leads to an effectual perturbation since the remaining allele is not mutated in the vast majority of cases (Ley et al. 2010). Possibly a dominant-negative effect on the wild-type enzyme can be considered as the actual mechanism. Although it has been demonstrated that *DNMT3A* mutations lead to considerable loss of its enzymatic activity, fundamentally altered DNA methylation patterns could not be observed in AML patients harboring this mutation.

5.1.5.2 TET2

Ten-eleven translocation (TET) proteins (TET1, TET 2 and TET3) are involved in the conversion of 5mC and based on this function play a central role in demethylation of genomic DNA. TET proteins catalyze the oxidation of 5mC, which leads to 5hmC (Tahiliani et al. 2009; Ito et al. 2010), and through further oxidation by TET proteins to 5fC and 5caC (Ito et al. 2011). Consecutive steps in active demethylation require the removal of 5fC and 5caC by either thymine DNA glycosylase (TDG), a protein involved in base excision repair (BER), or deamination mediated by AID/APOBEC followed by BER.

Since loss of 5mC is a hallmark of almost all cancers, this pathway plays a key role in the establishment of DNA methylation patterns and possibly other epigenetic marks. *TET* gene mutations have been discovered in MPN, MDS, AML, and T-cell lymphoma (Quivoron et al. 2011). *TET1* is a known fusion partner with mixed lineage leukemia (MLL) in rare translocations t(10;11) found in AML (Abdel-Wahab et al. 2009). TET2 and TET3 have been discovered due to their functional homology. Mutations in *TET2* are frequent in AML (66 mutations in 783 AML samples, 7.6 %) including missense, frameshift and nonsense mutations (Gaidzik et al. 2012) and more rarely found in solid tumors (COSMIC database). Mutation rates in MPN are higher (>20 %), but the numbers of tested samples are smaller and thus these figures may be biased (Pronier and Delhommeau 2012).

Interestingly, mutations in *TET2* are mutually exclusive with *isocitrate dehydrogenase* (*IDH1* and *IDH2*) mutations. It was hypothesized that activating *IDH1/2* mutants, frequently found in AML and glioblastoma, are producing 2-hydroxyglutarate which is structurally similar to α-ketoglutarate, the substrate for TET proteins, and thus 2-hydroxyglutarate might act as an inhibitor of TET protein activity. Most striking, but in line with the known function of these proteins, cases with mutations in these enzymes are characterized by distinct DNA methylation patterns, both in AML (Figueroa et al. 2010a) and in glioblastoma (Noushmehr et al. 2010; Sturm et al. 2012; Turcan et al. 2012), further substantiating the role of these enzymes in epigenetic programming.

As implied by their prominent role in DNA demethylation, *IDH1/2*- and *TET2*-mutant AML cases have myeloid blasts with specific DNA methylation signatures and a considerable tendency towards global hypermethylation (Figueroa et al. 2010a).

Considering a role of *DNMT3A* and *TET2* mutations in the context of clonal evolution, much remains to be unraveled since recent studies in patient samples found no consistent pattern of mutation acquisition between antecedent MDS and secondary AML (Fernandez-Mercado and Yib 2012). Although recent studies suggested that *DNMT3A* mutations can occur as rather early events (Krönke et al. 2013). Already recent studiey suggested that DNMT3A mutations can occur as rather early events.

5.2 Technologies and Methods for the Assessment of DNA Methylation

5.2.1 Principles for Capturing DNA Methylation

The detection of methylated cytosines is primarily based on three principles forming the basis of the various assays described in literature. The methylation status of a given cytosine can be approached by (1) digestion with methylation-specific restriction enzymes, by (2) precipitation with methylation-specific antibodies and proteins, and (3) by bisulfite modification.

The first category takes advantage of methylation-specific restriction enzymes which typically cleave methylated CpG sites at a lower rate than they cleave unmethylated sites. However, the presence of CpG dinucleotides in the enzyme recognition sites limit the detection capabilities by restriction enzymes.

Another principle is based on abundantly available proteins within the epigenetic machinery itself. These proteins specifically bind DNA containing methylated cytosines thus allowing the enrichment of methylated sequences in various assays and reducing genomic complexity.

The last category represents a method for analyzing DNA methylation in both a sensitive and quantitative manner by relying on inorganic bisulfite. This chemical compound reliably converts unmethylated cytosine to uracil sparing methylated cytosine which is not transformed (Clark et al. 1994). Transforming epigenetic information into a sequence context on the one hand allows further processing by methods broadly applied in molecular biology, e.g., PCR, but on the other hand increases the methodological burden by reducing the complexity of the genome and thus turning primer design into a more challenging task. Bisulfite treatment of genomic DNA generates strands which are no longer complementary to each other but rather are distinguished by two different strands, one being rich in guanine and the other being rich in cytosine. However, despite this caveats, bisulfite-based methods still represent the most powerful tools for methylation analysis.

Taking advantage of these basic principles, various assays have been developed for candidate-based DNA methylation assessment. In recent years a switch towards genome-wide screening methods has reached a new scale of high-throughput analyses, allowing an integrated approach of understanding disease complexity. The following section provides a brief overview of commonly used methods for site-specific and global DNA methylation analyses.

5.2.2 Site-Specific Methylation Analysis

5.2.2.1 Bisulfite Sequencing

Bisulfite sequencing is considered the "gold standard" of DNA methylation analysis. PCR amplifies bisulfite-converted DNA by using methylation insensitive primers which do exclude CpG dinucleotides in their recognition sites before continuing with subsequent sequencing steps and finally comparing the results with the genomic counterpart. This traditional method has been advanced to a quantitative level of assessment, furthermore allowing a higher throughput of samples by the introduction of pyrosequencing technique (Colella et al. 2003; Tost et al. 2003). This method is a direct sequencing approach based on the detection of emitted light during the synthesis of the complementary strand. Quantification accuracy as well as reliability is dependent on the sequencing length, thereby imposing the disadvantage of limiting the size of analyzable sequencing stretches to a maximum of 150 bp.

5.2.2.2 MSP

An easily conductible and cost-effective assay is the methylation-specific PCR (MSP) (Herman et al. 1996). Developed in the 1990s, it has been a landmark in translating research results into clinically applicable tools. A striking example is the application of MSP for the evaluation of the methylation status of the *MGMT* promoter in glioblastoma patients (Hegi et al. 2005). Epigenetic silencing of this DNA repair gene by promoter methylation has been associated with better response to alkylating agents and longer survival of patients with glioblastoma. Moreover, MSP has served as a powerful technique for the identification of numerous target genes for aberrant DNA methylation in virtually all malignancies. Hypermethylation of *CDKN2B* (encoding p15) and *CDKN2A* (encoding p16) in hematopoietic malignancies including AML was first detected by MSP (Herman et al. 1997).

In practice, two primer sets containing three or more CpG dinucleotides are designed both for a methylated and an unmethylated bisulfite-converted target sequence. Subsequently a gel electrophoresis of each reaction is used for the detection of the PCR products, qualitatively indicating the methylation state. In combination with nested PCR approaches MSP can reach a very high sensitivity (Palmisano et al. 2000). Quantitative PCR approaches in combination with MSP have tried to enable quantification of DNA methylation levels. Nevertheless, MSP is suffering from a broad variety of critical disadvantages such as a tremendous variability of results due to assay conditions (e.g., primer design, annealing temperature and cycle number) and a high number of false positive results (Claus et al. 2012c).

5.2.2.3 MALDI-TOF

This recent approach is based on mass spectrometry and allows quantitative analyses on a high-throughput scale. High sensitivity and reproducibility of quantitative measurements as well as a high resolution of CpG sites are major advantages of this technology. The Matrix-assisted laser desorption ionization – time of flight (MALDI-TOF) mass spectrometry uses an elegant strategy for methylation analyses by either applying single-nucleotide primer extension or base-specific cleavage (Ehrich et al. 2005). The latter one involves PCR amplification of target regions after bisulfite-conversion of genomic DNA and subsequent base-specific cleavage of single-stranded RNA copies. These products are then analyzed by MALDI-TOF mass spectrometry. Detected signal shifts of specific cleavage products represent methylation events at single CpGs or small groups of CpGs (CpG units). Signal intensity is correlated with the degree of methylation.

In conclusion, there has been a vast expansion of high-throughput quantitative assays, in particular pyrosequencing and MALDI-TOF enabling more reliable high resolution, quantitative DNA methylation analyses in large sample sets (Claus et al. 2012a).

5.2.3 Global Methylation Analysis

Although the techniques mentioned above are suited well for the verification of the methylation status in candidate genes, they are not sufficient to display the entire methylome. Therefore it is essential for the comprehensive understanding of cancer (epi)genome alterations to apply genome-wide screening methods. The following section provides a brief overview of strategies for approaching this task. The methylome comprises 2.8 × 10^7 CpG dinucleotides rendering the attempt to covering this number entirely into a challenging endeavor. Therefore, many first-generation genome-wide screening assays focus on capturing a representative part of the genome by complexity reduction.

First assays such as differential methylation hybridization (DMH) (Huang et al. 1999) and restriction landmark genomic scanning (RLGS) (Plass et al. 1999) focused specifically on CpG island sequences and revealed valuable information on overall CpG island methylation frequency resulting in the identification of many tumor suppressors affected by aberrant methylation events. Methylated CpG island amplification (MCA) was successfully used to identify methylated sequences in particular in colon cancer (Toyota et al. 1999). Over the last few years, novel technologies allowing more comprehensive genome-wide screening options have successfully entered the field. In particular, microarray and next-generation sequencing (NGS) techniques have facilitated extensive genome-wide analyses (Esteller 2007).

At present, most comprehensive second-generation approaches still include forms of reduction in genomic complexity by sequence enrichment. A variety of enzymatic assays are available to distinguish between methylated and unmethylated states at CpG sites. Microarray-based integrated analysis of methylation by isoschizomers (MIAMI) (Hatada et al. 2006) and *Hpa*II tiny fragment enrichment by ligation-mediated PCR (HELP) (Khulan et al. 2006) use the methylation-sensitive restriction enzyme *Hpa*II and the methylation-independent *Msp*I that both recognize the identical sequence are two prime examples. In *Msp*I-reduced representation bisulfite sequencing (RRBS), genomic DNA is cut with *Msp*I which favors GC-rich regions (recognition site 5′-C^CGG-3′), subsequently bisulfite-treated followed by PCR amplification and sequenced using NGS technology (Meissner et al. 2005, 2008).

Complexity reduction can likewise successfully be achieved by affinity purification using antibodies or recombinant proteins with high affinity for methylated DNA. A commonly used approach is termed methyl-DNA immunoprecipitation (MeDIP) using antibodies against single-stranded methyl-DNA (Weber et al. 2005). Alternatively, recombinant human proteins or protein complexes that bind with high affinity to double-stranded methylated DNA are applied, such as MBD2 (MCIp) (Gebhard et al. 2006) or MBD2/MBD3L1 (MIRA) (Rauch et al. 2006). Subsequently after complexity reduction, the enriched sequences are most often subjected to either hybridization onto high-density oligonucleotide microarrays or to NGS approaches (Yalcin et al. 2013).

Different commercial microarray platforms ranging from whole genome tiling to selective representation of CpG islands, promoter sequences, or distinct chromosomal regions are currently available. In comparison, NGS platforms are not restricted in sequence detection and thus constitute superior alternatives to microarray analysis for the combination with enrichment technologies (Ball et al. 2009; Deng et al. 2009). However, the number of reads (sequencing depths) to cover the majority of information present in the enriched DNA fragments is still a matter of debate which is currently approached by bioinformatical saturation approaches.

The major advantage of NGS-based approaches is the unrestricted and more unbiased character of identifying enriched regions including stretches that might not be represented on commonly used microarray platforms (e.g., enhancer sequences, which are incompletely covered on promoter CpG island arrays). Furthermore NGS can be applied to enriched and subsequently bisulfite-treated samples for detection of specific methylation patterns. Providing a sufficient read coverage, multiplexing of several samples in one sequencing reaction by nucleotide bar coding allows highly efficient experimental designs. Costs of NGS assays have dramatically decreased by now, highlighting the option of large-scale setups involving whole genome bisulfite sequencing. This approach might bridge the gap between unbiased screening and high-resolution candidate analysis, allowing the generation of comprehensive genome-wide single-base-resolution maps of DNA methylation (Lister et al. 2009). Although provided with powerful tools, deciphering the epigenome remains a challenging task (Laird 2010).

5.2.4 Clinical Impact of DNA Methylation Analysis

In past decades cancer has been termed a "genetic disease" which accounts for the insights into chromosomal aberrations that have been increasingly discovered and characterized. However, epigenetics' contribution to carcinogenesis is well accepted today, and there has been a vast expansion in research activities on this particular field. Although a major focus has been put on cancer, research on methylation is likewise evolving in other diseases such as autoimmune disorders (Klein and Gay 2013), cardiovascular diseases (Zhao et al. 2012), and psychiatric disorders (Kinoshita et al. 2013).

Various examples can be consulted on how the assessment of methylation can be brought into a context in clinical hemato-oncology. The analysis of aberrant methylation offers a new way not only for disease stratification and identification of novel drug targets but also for early detection of disease, for prediction of treatment response, and last but not least for basic research on the understanding of disease (Bullinger et al. 2010; Patel et al. 2012). As an example, site-specific methylation patterns proved to be predictive biomarkers for overall survival in hematopoietic diseases such as AML and chronic lymphatic leukemia (CLL) (Figueroa et al. 2010b; Claus et al. 2012b).

Conclusion

New data suggests that the commonly accepted two-hit model of malignant myeloid transformation has to be updated by accounting for mutations in epigenetic modifiers. In contrast to somatic mutations, epigenetic perturbations can potentially be reversed thus offering targets of clinical importance (Goldberg et al. 2007). A refinement of AML classification has recently been possible by generating comprehensive methylation profiles – due to refined detection methods – allowing for a subclassification of patients according to a core set of genes enriched by distinct patterns of methylation. These findings emphasize the importance of aberrant epigenetic regulation in the pathogenesis of myeloid leukemogenesis (Bullinger et al. 2004).

References

Abdel-Wahab O, Mullally A et al (2009) Genetic characterization of TET1, TET2, and TET3 alterations in myeloid malignancies. Blood 114(1):144–147

Agrawal S, Hofmann WK et al (2007) The C/EBPdelta tumor suppressor is silenced by hypermethylation in acute myeloid leukemia. Blood 109(9):3895–3905

Ball MP, Li JB et al (2009) Targeted and genome-scale strategies reveal gene-body methylation signatures in human cells. Nat Biotechnol 27(4):361–368

Barlow DP (2011) Genomic imprinting: a mammalian epigenetic discovery model. Annu Rev Genet 45:379–403

Baylin SB, Ohm JE (2006) Epigenetic gene silencing in cancer – a mechanism for early oncogenic pathway addiction? Nat Rev Cancer 6(2):107–116

Baylin SB, Fearon ER et al (1987) Hypermethylation of the 5′ region of the calcitonin gene is a property of human lymphoid and acute myeloid malignancies. Blood 70(2):412–417

Borgel J, Guibert S et al (2010) Targets and dynamics of promoter DNA methylation during early mouse development. Nat Genet 42(12):1093–1100

Brockdorff N (2011) Chromosome silencing mechanisms in X-chromosome inactivation: unknown unknowns. Development 138(23):5057–5065

Bullinger L, Döhner K et al (2004) Use of gene-expression profiling to identify prognostic subclasses in adult acute myeloid leukemia. N Engl J Med 350(16):1605–1616

Bullinger L, Ehrich M et al (2010) Quantitative DNA methylation predicts survival in adult acute myeloid leukemia. Blood 115(3):636–642

Cameron EE, Baylin SB et al (1999) p15(INK4B) CpG island methylation in primary acute leukemia is heterogeneous and suggests density as a critical factor for transcriptional silencing. Blood 94(7):2445–2451

Chen T, Li E (2006) Establishment and maintenance of DNA methylation patterns in mammals. Curr Top Microbiol Immunol 301:179–201

Chim CS, Tam CY et al (2001) Methylation of p15 and p16 genes in adult acute leukemia: lack of prognostic significance. Cancer 91(12):2222–2229

Christiansen DH, Andersen MK et al (2003) Methylation of p15INK4B is common, is associated with deletion of genes on chromosome arm 7q and predicts a poor prognosis in therapy-related myelodysplasia and acute myeloid leukemia. Leukemia 17(9):1813–1819

Clark SJ, Harrison J et al (1994) High sensitivity mapping of methylated cytosines. Nucleic Acids Res 22(15):2990–2997

Claus R, Fliegauf M et al (2006) Inhibitors of DNA methylation and histone deacetylation independently relieve AML1/ETO-mediated lysozyme repression. J Leukoc Biol 80(6):1462–1472

Claus R, Hackanson B et al (2012a) Quantitative analyses of DAPK1 methylation in AML and MDS. Int J Cancer 131(2):E138–E142

Claus R, Lucas DM et al (2012b) Quantitative DNA methylation analysis identifies a single CpG dinucleotide important for ZAP-70 expression and predictive of prognosis in chronic lymphocytic leukemia. J Clin Oncol 30(20):2483–2491

Claus R, Wilop S et al (2012c) A systematic comparison of quantitative high-resolution DNA methylation analysis and methylation-specific PCR. Epigenetics 7(7):772–780

Colella S, Shen L et al (2003) Sensitive and quantitative universal pyrosequencing methylation analysis of CpG sites. Biotechniques 35(1):146–150

Costello JF, Fruhwald MC et al (2000) Aberrant CpG-island methylation has non-random and tumour-type-specific patterns. Nat Genet 24(2):132–138

Daskalakis M, Nguyen TT et al (2002) Demethylation of a hypermethylated P15/INK4B gene in patients with myelodysplastic syndrome by 5-Aza-2′-deoxycytidine (decitabine) treatment. Blood 100(8):2957–2964

Deng J, Shoemaker R et al (2009) Targeted bisulfite sequencing reveals changes in DNA methylation associated with nuclear reprogramming. Nat Biotechnol 27(4):353–360

Ehrich M, Nelson MR et al (2005) Quantitative high-throughput analysis of DNA methylation patterns by base-specific cleavage and mass spectrometry. Proc Natl Acad Sci U S A 102(44):15785–15790

Esteller M (2007) Cancer epigenomics: DNA methylomes and histone-modification maps. Nat Rev Genet 8(4):286–298

Faber J, Krivtsov AV et al (2009) HOXA9 is required for survival in human MLL-rearranged acute leukemias. Blood 113(11):2375–2385

Fernandez-Mercado M, Yib BH (2012) Mutation patterns of 16 genes in primary and secondary acute myeloid leukemia (AML) with normal cytogenetics. PLoS One 7(8):e42334

Figueroa ME, Skrabanek L et al (2009) MDS and secondary AML display unique patterns and abundance of aberrant DNA methylation. Blood 114(16):3448–3458

Figueroa ME, Abdel-Wahab O et al (2010a) Leukemic IDH1 and IDH2 mutations result in a hypermethylation phenotype, disrupt TET2 function, and impair hematopoietic differentiation. Cancer Cell 18(6):553–567

Figueroa ME, Lugthart S et al (2010b) DNA methylation signatures identify biologically distinct subtypes in acute myeloid leukemia. Cancer Cell 17(1):13–27

Gaidzik VI, Paschka P et al (2012) TET2 mutations in acute myeloid leukemia (AML): results from a comprehensive genetic and clinical analysis of the AML study group. J Clin Oncol 30(12):1350–1357

Gaidzik VI, Schlenk RF et al (2013) Clinical impact of DNMT3A mutations in younger adult patients with acute myeloid leukemia: results of the AML Study Group (AMLSG). Blood 121(23):4769–4777

Galm O, Wilop S et al (2004) DNA methylation changes in multiple myeloma. Leukemia 18(10):1687–1692

Galm O, Wilop S et al (2005) Clinical implications of aberrant DNA methylation patterns in acute myelogenous leukemia. Ann Hematol 84(Suppl 1):39–46

Gebhard C, Schwarzfischer L et al (2006) Genome-wide profiling of CpG methylation identifies novel targets of aberrant hypermethylation in myeloid leukemia. Cancer Res 66(12):6118–6128

Gilliland DG (2001) Hematologic malignancies. Curr Opin Hematol 8:189–191

Goldberg AD, Allis CD et al (2007) Epigenetics: a landscape takes shape. Cell 128(4):635–638

Gowher H, Loutchanwoot P et al (2006) Mutational analysis of the catalytic domain of the murine Dnmt3a DNA-(cytosine C5)-methyltransferase. J Mol Biol 357(3):928–941

Guil S, Esteller M (2012) Cis-acting noncoding RNAs: friends and foes. Nat Struct Mol Biol 19(11):1068–1075

Hackanson B, Bennett KL et al (2008) Epigenetic modification of CCAAT/enhancer binding protein alpha expression in acute myeloid leukemia. Cancer Res 68(9):3142–3151

Hatada I, Fukasawa M et al (2006) Genome-wide profiling of promoter methylation in human. Oncogene 25(21):3059–3064

He YF, Li BZ et al (2011) Tet-mediated formation of 5-carboxylcytosine and its excision by TDG in mammalian DNA. Science 333(6047):1303–1307

Hegi ME, Diserens AC et al (2005) MGMT gene silencing and benefit from temozolomide in glioblastoma. N Engl J Med 352(10):997–1003

Herman JG, Graff JR et al (1996) Methylation-specific PCR: a novel PCR assay for methylation status of CpG islands. Proc Natl Acad Sci U S A 93(18):9821–9826

Herman JG, Civin CI et al (1997) Distinct patterns of inactivation of p15INK4B and p16INK4A characterize the major types of hematological malignancies. Cancer Res 57(5):837–841

Huang TH, Perry MR et al (1999) Methylation profiling of CpG islands in human breast cancer cells. Hum Mol Genet 8(3):459–470

Issa JP, Zehnbauer BA et al (1996) The estrogen receptor CpG island is methylated in most hematopoietic neoplasms. Cancer Res 56(5):973–977

Issa JP, Zehnbauer BA et al (1997) HIC1 hypermethylation is a late event in hematopoietic neoplasms. Cancer Res 57(9):1678–1681

Ito S, D'Alessio AC et al (2010) Role of Tet proteins in 5mC to 5hmC conversion, ES-cell self-renewal and inner cell mass specification. Nature 466(7310):1129–1133

Ito S, Shen L et al (2011) Tet proteins can convert 5-methylcytosine to 5-formylcytosine and 5-carboxylcytosine. Science 333(6047):1300–1303

Ji H, Ehrlich LI et al (2010) Comprehensive methylome map of lineage commitment from haematopoietic progenitors. Nature 467(7313):338–342

Jiang Y, Dunbar A et al (2009) Aberrant DNA methylation is a dominant mechanism in MDS progression to AML. Blood 113(6):1315–1325

Jones PA, Baylin SB (2002) The fundamental role of epigenetic events in cancer. Nat Rev Genet 3(6):415–428

Khulan B, Thompson RF et al (2006) Comparative isoschizomer profiling of cytosine methylation: the HELP assay. Genome Res 16(8):1046–1055

Kinoshita M, Numata S et al (2013) DNA methylation signatures of peripheral leukocytes in schizophrenia. Neuromolecular Med 15(1):95–101

Klein K, Gay S (2013) Epigenetic modifications in rheumatoid arthritis, a review. Curr Opin Pharmacol S1471–4892(13):00011–00018

Krönke J, Bullinger L (2013) Clonal evolution in relapsed NPM1-mutated acute myeloid leukemia. Blood 122(1):100–108

Laird PW (2010) Principles and challenges of genomewide DNA methylation analysis. Nat Rev Genet 11(3):191–203

Ley TJ, Ding L et al (2010) DNMT3A mutations in acute myeloid leukemia. N Engl J Med 363(25):2424–2433

Lister R, Pelizzola M et al (2009) Human DNA methylomes at base resolution show widespread epigenomic differences. Nature 462(7271):315–322

Lübbert M, Mertelsmann R et al (1997) Cytosine methylation changes during normal hematopoiesis and in acute myeloid leukemia. Leukemia 11(Suppl 1):S12–S18

Meissner A, Gnirke A et al (2005) Reduced representation bisulfite sequencing for comparative high-resolution DNA methylation analysis. Nucleic Acids Res 33(18):5868–5877

Meissner A, Mikkelsen TS et al (2008) Genome-scale DNA methylation maps of pluripotent and differentiated cells. Nature 454(7205):766–770

Melki JR, Vincent PC et al (1999) Concurrent DNA hypermethylation of multiple genes in acute myeloid leukemia. Cancer Res 59(15):3730–3740

Melki JR, Vincent PC et al (2000) Hypermethylation of E-cadherin in leukemia. Blood 95(10):3208–3213

Noushmehr H, Weisenberger DJ et al (2010) Identification of a CpG island methylator phenotype that defines a distinct subgroup of glioma. Cancer Cell 17(5):510–522

Palmisano WA, Divine KK et al (2000) Predicting lung cancer by detecting aberrant promoter methylation in sputum. Cancer Res 60(21):5954–5958

Patel JP et al (2012) Prognostic relevance of integrated genetic profiling in acute myeloid leukemia. N Engl J Med 366(12):1079–1089

Plass C, Yu F et al (1999) Restriction landmark genome scanning for aberrant methylation in primary refractory and relapsed acute myeloid leukemia; involvement of the WIT-1 gene. Oncogene 18(20):3159–3165

Pronier E, Delhommeau F (2012) Role of TET2 mutations in myeloproliferative neoplasms. Curr Hematol Malig Rep 7(1):57–64

Quivoron C et al (2011) TET2 inactivation results in pleiotropic hematopoietic abnormalities in mouse and is a recurrent event during human lymphomagenesis. Cancer Cell 20:25–38

Rauch T, Li H et al (2006) MIRA-assisted microarray analysis, a new technology for the determination of DNA methylation patterns, identifies frequent methylation of homeodomain-containing genes in lung cancer cells. Cancer Res 66(16):7939–7947

Raval A, Rush LJ et al (2002) Aberrant DNA methylation in chronic lymphocytic leukemia: a role in pathogenesis? Blood 100(11):379a

Reik W, Dean W et al (2001) Epigenetic reprogramming in mammalian development. Science 293(5532):1089–1093

Rosu-Myles M, Wolff L (2008) p15Ink4b: dual function in myelopoiesis and inactivation in myeloid disease. Blood Cells Mol Dis 40(3):406–409

Rush LJ, Plass C (2002) Alterations of DNA methylation in hematologic malignancies. Cancer Lett 185(1):1–12

Rush LJ, Dai Z et al (2001) Novel methylation targets in de novo acute myeloid leukemia with prevalence of chromosome 11 loci. Blood 97(10):3226–3233

Sakashita K, Koike K et al (2001) Dynamic DNA methylation change in the CpG island region of p15 during human myeloid development. J Clin Invest 108(8):1195–1204

Seedhouse CH, Das-Gupta EP et al (2003) Methylation of the hMLH1 promoter and its association with microsatellite instability in acute myeloid leukemia. Leukemia 17(1):83–88

Shih AH, Abdel-Wahab O et al (2012) The role of mutations in epigenetic regulators in myeloid malignancies. Nat Rev Cancer 12(9):599–612

Shimamoto T, Ohyashiki JH et al (2005) Methylation of p15(INK4b) and E-cadherin genes is independently correlated with poor prognosis in acute myeloid leukemia. Leuk Res 29(6):653–659

Sturm D, Witt H et al (2012) Hotspot mutations in H3F3A and IDH1 define distinct epigenetic and biological subgroups of glioblastoma. Cancer Cell 22(4):425–437

Tahiliani M, Koh KP et al (2009) Conversion of 5-methylcytosine to 5-hydroxymethylcytosine in mammalian DNA by MLL partner TET1. Science 324(5929):930–935

Thol F, Damm F et al (2011) Incidence and prognostic influence of DNMT3A mutations in acute myeloid leukemia. J Clin Oncol 29(21):2889–2896

Tost J, Dunker J et al (2003) Analysis and quantification of multiple methylation variable positions in CpG islands by pyrosequencing. Biotechniques 35(1):152–156

Toyota M, Ho C et al (1999) Identification of differentially methylated sequences in colorectal cancer by methylated CpG island amplification. Cancer Res 59(10):2307–2312

Turcan S, Rohle D et al (2012) IDH1 mutation is sufficient to establish the glioma hypermethylator phenotype. Nature 483(7390):479–483

Voso MT, Scardocci A et al (2004) Aberrant methylation of DAP-kinase in therapy-related acute myeloid leukemia and myelodysplastic syndromes. Blood 103(2):698–700

Walter MJ, Ding L et al (2011) Recurrent DNMT3A mutations in patients with myelodysplastic syndromes. Leukemia 25(7):1153–1158

Weber M, Davies JJ et al (2005) Chromosome-wide and promoter-specific analyses identify sites of differential DNA methylation in normal and transformed human cells. Nat Genet 37(8):853–862

Yalcin A, Kreutz C et al (2013) MeDIP coupled with a promoter tiling array as a platform to investigate global DNA methylation patterns in AML cells. Leuk Res 37(1):102–111

Yamashita Y, Yuan J et al (2010) Array-based genomic resequencing of human leukemia. Oncogene 29(25):3723–3731

Yan XJ, Xu J et al (2011) Exome sequencing identifies somatic mutations of DNA methyltransferase gene DNMT3A in acute monocytic leukemia. Nat Genet 43(4):309–315

Zhao J, Forsberg CW et al (2012) MAOA promoter methylation and susceptibility to carotid atherosclerosis: role of familial factors in a monozygotic twin sample. BMC Med Genet 13:100

Epigenetic Modifications Mediated by the AML1/ETO and MLL Leukemia Fusion Proteins

6

Jesús Duque-Afonso, Michael Lübbert, and Michael L. Cleary

6.1 Acute Myeloid Leukemia

Acute myeloid leukemia (AML) is a clonal hematological neoplasia characterized by an increase of immature myeloid precursors in the bone marrow and a block in their differentiation. It is frequently accompanied by hematopoietic insufficiency and leukocytosis. The molecular etiology of AML involves accumulated genetic damage in the form of chromosomal aberrations or mutations that result in the activation of oncogenes or inactivation of tumor suppressor genes (Löwenberg et al. 1999).

Chromosomal translocations play important roles in the etiology of human leukemias by generating oncogenic fusion proteins, many of which have features of chimeric transcription factors (Cleary 1991). This chapter focuses on the pathobiology of AML1/ETO and MLL fusion proteins, which together constitute the most common chimeric transcription factors in AML and function in part through epigenetic mechanisms that lead to deregulated gene expression by aberrant recruitment of chromatin-modifying enzymes and DNA methyltransferases.

J. Duque-Afonso, MD
Department of Hematology/Oncology, University Medical Center Freiburg, University of Freiburg, Hugstetterstr. 55, Freiburg D-79106, Germany

Department of Pathology, Stanford University Medical Center, 300 Pasteur Dr., Stanford, CA 94305-5324, USA
e-mail: jduque@stanford.edu

M. Lübbert, MD, PhD
Department of Hematology/Oncology, University Medical Center Freiburg, University of Freiburg, Hugstetterstr. 55, Freiburg D-79106, Germany
e-mail: michael.luebbert@uniklinik-freiburg.de

M.L. Cleary, MD (✉)
Department of Pathology, Stanford University Medical Center, 300 Pasteur Dr., Stanford, CA 94305-5324, USA
e-mail: mcleary@stanford.edu

M. Lübbert, P.A. Jones (eds.), *Epigenetic Therapy of Cancer*,
DOI 10.1007/978-3-642-38404-2_6, © Springer-Verlag Berlin Heidelberg 2014

6.2 The Leukemia-Specific Fusion Protein AML1/ETO

6.2.1 Clinical Characteristics of AML1/ETO-Positive Leukemias

The most common chromosomal translocation in AML is the t(8;21), which results in the fusion protein AML1/ETO. It is present in 12–15 % of AMLs overall and in 40 % of AML M2 according to the French American British (FAB) classification (Walker et al. 1994). Translocations affecting the *AML1* gene on chromosome 21 along with those affecting the *CBFB* gene on chromosome 16 define the core binding factor (CBF) leukemias, since they disrupt alternative subunits of this essential hematopoietic transcription complex. Clinically, they are associated with a relatively favorable prognosis (Schlenk et al. 2004; Marcucci et al. 2005). The CBF complex functions as a key transcriptional regulator of hematopoiesis, coordinately activating the transcription of several crucial genes during myelopoiesis and lymphopoiesis.

6.2.2 The Hematopoietic Transcription Factor AML1 (RUNX1)

AML1 (also known as RUNX1 or CBFA2 or PEBP2α) is a 21 kDa protein that forms part of the CBF complex together with the CBFβ (PEBP2β) subunit. AML1 binds DNA through residues in the runt homology domain (RHD), which recognizes the consensus sequence TGT/cGGT in promoters of its target genes (Meyers et al. 1993; Otto et al. 2003). The CBFβ subunit interacts with the RHD domain of AML1, increasing CBF transcriptional activity (Ogawa et al. 1993; Tahirov et al. 2001) and protecting the CBF complex from proteolytic degradation through ubiquitination (Huang et al. 2001). The CBF complex interacts with the multifunctional transcriptional coactivators p300 and CREB-binding protein (CBP), thus recruiting histone acetyltransferases through the proline-serine-threonine (PST) domain at the C-terminus of AML1 and activating the transcription of its target genes (Kitabayashi et al. 1998).

The crucial role of the CBF complex for hematopoiesis was shown in knockout mice. Mice deficient for the AML1 subunit die at day E12.5 due to lethal intracranial hemorrhage and lack fetal liver hematopoiesis (Okuda et al. 1996). The phenotype of *Cbfβ* knockout mice is very similar to *Aml1* knockout mice (Wang et al. 1996), showing the importance of the CBF complex during the early stages of hematopoiesis.

6.2.3 The ETO Protein

The *ETO* gene (also known as *RUNX1T1* or *MTG8*) codes for a 60 kDa protein that contains four conserved domains with homology to the *Drosophila* protein nervy (NHRs, nervy homology regions). *ETO* knockout mice show gastrointestinal defects but no hematological abnormalities (Calabi et al. 2001). Three of the nervy homology domains (NHR1, NHR3, and NHR4) interact with a corepressor complex comprised of SMRT, N-CoR, and Sin3A (Lutterbach et al. 1998; Wang et al. 1998; Amann et al. 2001; Hildebrand et al. 2001). The remaining NHR2 domain mediates tetramerization of ETO (Liu et al. 2006) and is thought to interact with mSin3b (Dhanda et al. 2008). The NHR1 domain also interacts with E-box transcription factors HEB and E2A (Zhang et al. 2004; Wei et al. 2007), illustrating the complex protein interactions mediated by ETO.

6.2.4 The Leukemic Fusion Protein AML1/ETO

The t(8;21) fuses the *N*-terminal portion of *AML1* encoded on chromosome 21 to almost the entire *ETO* gene encoded on chromosome 8, forming the AML1/ETO chimeric fusion protein (Miyoshi et al. 1991; Erickson et al. 1992). Recently, an alternatively spliced isoform of AML1/ETO that contains an extra exon (exon 9a) but lacks NHR3 and NHR4 of ETO was found to be more leukemogenic in mouse models than the full-length AML1/ETO (Yan et al. 2006) (Fig. 6.1). AML1/ETO contains the RHD domain of AML1 that interacts with target DNA and the CBFβ subunit. It also contains the NHRs of ETO, which recruit corepressor complexes containing histone deacetylases and DNA methyltransferases, thus dysregulating expression of AML1 target genes (Fig. 6.2).

AML1/ETO is known to cooperate with activating mutations in tyrosine kinase receptors, such as the stem cell factor receptor C-KIT, to induce leukemia (Becker et al. 2008; Chevalier et al. 2010; Wang et al. 2011a). Therefore, in addition to epigenetic deregulation of gene transcription, activated proliferative signaling pathways are necessary to induce leukemia in AML1/ETO-bearing cells (Müller et al. 2008) consistent with the two-hit model of leukemogenesis (Kelly and Gilliland 2002).

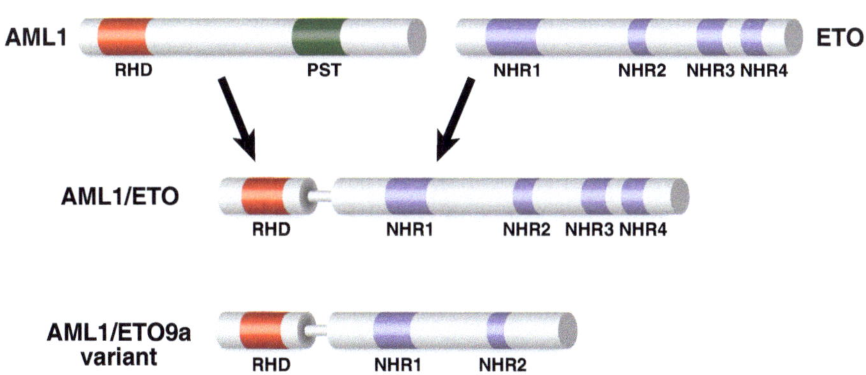

Fig. 6.1 Schematic representations of the AML1 protein, AML1/ETO fusion protein, and the AML1/ETO9a fusion variant. Representative functional domains are shown as colored boxes. *Abbreviations*: *RHD* runt homology domain, *PST* proline-serine-threonine domain, *NHR* nervy homology domain

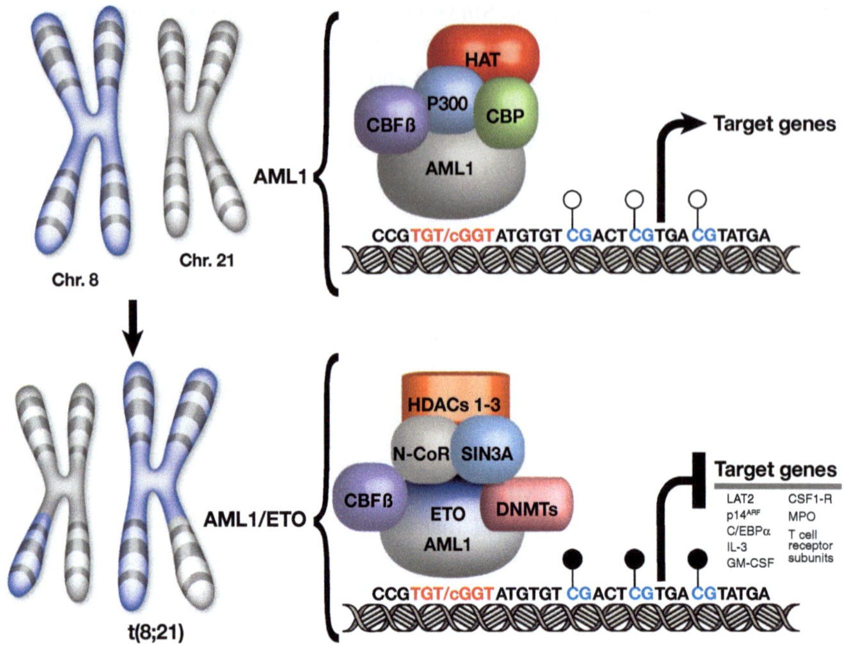

Fig. 6.2 Functional representation and protein interactions of AML1 and AML1/ETO proteins. The t(8;21) fuses the *AML1* gene from chromosome 21 with the *ETO* gene on chromosome 8. AML1 is a key transcription factor of hematopoiesis that binds the DNA consensus sequence TGT/cGGT on target promoters through the runt homology domain (RHD). CBFβ stabilizes AML1 and protects it from degradation. Histone acetyltransferases (HATs) are recruited via p300 and CBP proteins, activating gene transcription through histone acetylation. AML1/ETO retains the capacity of DNA binding and dimerization with CBFβ. However, the ETO moiety interacts with a corepressor complex constituted by N-CoR and SIN3A proteins, which recruits histone deacetylases (HDACs). HDACs alter the conformation of histones around the promoters of AML1/ETO target genes, to prevent transcription. DNA methyltransferases (DNMTs) are recruited directly or indirectly to AML1/ETO target genes, thus contributing to gene silencing

6.2.5 AML1 and AML1/ETO Target Genes

Many target genes of AML1 and AML1/ETO have been described. They provide insights into the oncogenic potential of AML1/ETO and may explain features of AML1/ETO-positive cells. Some of these genes are implicated in the regulation of hematopoiesis and encode cytokines such as IL3 (Cameron et al. 1994; Uchida et al. 1997; Liu et al. 2005), MIP-α (Bristow and Shore 2003), or GM-CSF (Frank et al. 1995); cytokine receptors such as M-CSF-R (Zhang et al. 1994) and G-CSF-R (Shimizu et al. 2000); or adaptor molecules, e.g., LAT2 (Fliegauf et al. 2004; Duque-Afonso et al. 2011a, b). AML1/ETO also influences cell cycle regulation of myeloid cells through downregulating the expression of $p14^{arf}$ (Linggi et al. 2002) or upregulating $p21^{waf1}$ (Alcalay et al. 2003; Peterson et al. 2007; Berg et al. 2008).

Transcriptional dysregulation is not only caused directly by AML1/ETO but also by its effect on the expression and function of other hematopoietic transcription factors such as AML1 itself, PU.1 (Huang et al. 2008), C/EBPα (Pabst et al. 2001), E-box proteins (Zhang et al. 2004; Wei et al. 2007), and MEIS1 (Lasa et al. 2004).

The oncogenic properties of AML1/ETO are enhanced by the silencing of classical tumor suppressor genes like RARβ2 (Fazi et al. 2007a), a key protein in the retinoic acid signaling pathway, or neurofibromatosis-1 (NF-1) (Yang et al. 2005). Finally, AML1 and AML1/ETO also serve important roles in the transcriptional regulation of genes necessary for granulocyte functions, such as myeloperoxidase (MPO) (Nuchprayoon et al. 1994), neutrophil elastase (ELA2) (Lausen et al. 2006), and lysozyme (LZM) (Claus et al. 2006).

6.2.6 Epigenetic Modifications by AML1/ETO: Interaction with HDACs and DNMTs

Histone deacetylases (HDACs) are directly or indirectly recruited by AML1/ETO (Hug and Lazar 2004). HDAC1 indirectly interacts with ETO via SIN3A (Wang et al. 1998; Gelmetti et al. 1998), whereas HDAC2 and HDAC3 interact via the nuclear corepressors N-CoR and SMRT (Lutterbach et al. 1998; Amann et al. 2001). Thus, AML1/ETO recruits HDAC activity to promoters, modifying the acetylation status of histones around the transcriptional start site and, consequently, repressing the expression of its target genes (Wang et al. 1998; Amann et al. 2001; Hildebrand et al. 2001). As shown for the c-FMS promoter, the presence of AML1/ETO correlates with a decrease of histone acetylation and increase of histone H3 lysine 9 (H3K9me) methylation, a histone mark associated with transcriptional silencing (Follows et al. 2003). Very recently, two pivotal papers demonstrated that both induction of an AML1/ETO transgene and depletion of this oncofusion gene in AML1/ETO-positive blasts result in genome-wide changes in chromatin structure, confirming on a large scale that AML1/ETO acts as a reversible silencer at its genomic targets. Specifically, the histone modification studied by the two groups included acetylation at H3K9, which was induced with depletion of AML1/ETO, as well as the induction of silencing marks H3K9 trimethylation, and H4 acetylation at lysines 5, 8, 12, and 16. Interestingly, one of these studies showed that AML1/ETO acts not only by binding at its target genes via AML1 binding motifs but also via Sp1 binding motifs in the absence of an AML1 consensus binding site (Ptasinska et al. 2012; Maiques-Diaz et al. 2012).

Liu et al. (2005) were the first to describe that AML1/ETO recruits DNMT1 and DNMT3a to the *IL3*-promoter. This finding was corroborated by Fazi et al. (2007a, b), who described the association of AML1/ETO with DNMT3a and DNMT3b on the *RARβ2* promoter and with DNMT1 and DNMT3a on the *pre-miR-223*. Although a direct interaction between AML1/ETO and DNMTs has not been shown, this association may be mediated by the methyl-binding protein MeCP2 or HDAC1 (Jones et al. 1998; Nan et al. 1998; Fuks et al. 2000). Global DNA methylation analysis shows that AML1/ETO influences the DNA methylation patterns of leukemic cells (Figueroa et al. 2010; Wilop et al. 2011; Alvarez et al. 2010). However, these DNA methylation changes could not be corroborated in CD34+ hematopoietic progenitor cells transduced with AML1/ETO, suggesting that AML1/ETO may need secondary hits or longer exposure times to induce DNA methylation changes (Alvarez et al. 2010).

AML1/ETO may also act as a transcriptional activator, e.g., of BCL2 (Klampfer et al. 1996) and p21^{waf1} (Berg et al. 2008). AML1/ETO interacts via its NHR2 domain with the histone acetyltransferase p300, which acetylates lysine residues of histones in its target genes, thus activating gene transcription (Wang et al. 2011b). Recently, it has been shown that MLL interacts with AML1 and induces the activating H3K4me3 mark at the PU.1 promoter. This finding links the function of these two key hematopoietic transcription factors, at least, on the key AML1 target gene PU.1 (Huang et al. 2011).

In summary, through its interaction and recruitment of positive (HATs, E-box proteins, and MLL) and negative (HDACs and DNMTs) regulators, AML1/ETO dysregulates physiological gene transcription. AML1 has an important function during the differentiation of myeloid and lymphoid cells, and AML1/ETO contributes to the development of AML by blocking differentiation of myeloid progenitors through transcriptional dysregulation.

6.2.7 AML1/ETO and microRNAs

The roles of AML1/ETO and AML1 as transcriptional regulators extend to genes that encode microRNAs. For instance, *miR-223*, which regulates human granulopoiesis (Fazi et al. 2005), is transcriptionally downregulated by AML1/ETO (Fazi et al. 2007b). AML1 downregulates the expression of three miRNAs *(miR-17-5p, miR-20a,* and *miR-106a*), which in turn downregulate the expression of *AML1* and, consequently, expression of the AML1 target gene *M-CSF-R* (Fontana et al. 2007). This mutual negative feedback loop between a transcription factor and microRNAs illustrates the importance of microRNA regulation in normal and aberrant hematopoiesis.

6.2.8 Posttranslational Modifications of AML1 and AML1/ETO by Chromatin-Modifying Enzymes

Chromatin-modifying enzymes regulate gene transcription by posttranslational modifications of histones and also of transcription factors including AML1 and AML1/ETO. AML1 transcriptional activity is regulated by the histone arginine methyltransferase PRMT1. Methylation of two arginine residues in AML1 abrogates its interaction with the corepressor protein SIN3A, thus enhancing the transcriptional activity of AML1. AML1/ETO lacks these two arginine sites and, in addition, ETO interacts directly with SIN3A, which confers more stable repressor properties to AML1/ETO (Zhao et al. 2008). Nevertheless, AML1/ETO is also targeted by posttranslational modifications, such as lysine acetylation. The transcriptional coactivator p300 acetylates AML1/ETO at a specific lysine which is essential for transcriptional activation and its leukemogenic potential (Wang et al. 2011b). These data demonstrate that epigenetic gene regulation is mediated not only through modifications on histone tails but also on transcription factors responsible for the initiation, maintenance, or repression of transcription.

6.2.9 The Susceptibility of AML1/ETO Leukemias to HDAC and DNMT Inhibitors

The phenotypic features and epigenetic changes caused by AML1/ETO in myeloid cells may be reversed by HDAC and DNMT inhibitors. Several HDAC inhibitors enhance the acetylation of histones at AML1 and AML1/ETO target promoters (Göttlicher et al. 2001; Klisovic et al. 2003; Gozzini et al. 2003; Claus et al. 2006), reexpress genes silenced by AML1/ETO (Liu et al. 2005; Fazi et al. 2007a; Duque-Afonso et al. 2011b), and promote cell growth arrest, apoptosis, and differentiation of AML1/ETO-positive cells (Wang et al. 1999; Gozzini and Santini 2005; Liu et al. 2007; Barbetti et al. 2008). Target promoters with CpG islands can be demethylated by the DNMT inhibitors 5-azacytidine (Fazi et al. 2007a) and decitabine (Claus et al. 2006; Berg et al. 2007). Furthermore, HDAC inhibitors and DNMT inhibitors cooperate to induce histone acetylation and cell differentiation (Gozzini and Santini 2005). When these agents are combined with an inducer of differentiation such as all-*trans* retinoic acid (ATRA), AML1/ETO-positive cells differentiate synergistically into the granulocytic lineage. The enhanced susceptibility to differentiation by ATRA after treatment with a demethylating agent is, at least in part, due to demethylation of the RARβ2 promoter (Fazi et al. 2007a).

Genes repressed in core binding factor (CBF) leukemias are reexpressed after treatment with DNMT and HDAC inhibitors (Serrano et al. 2008). Other effects besides epigenetics may explain the biological activity of DNMT and HDAC inhibitors, such as degradation of AML1/ETO (Yang et al. 2007) and acetylation of non-histone substrates such as p53 (Luo et al. 2000).

In conclusion, HDAC and DNMT inhibitors show clinical and biological effects in AML1/ETO-positive cells, and their combination with other biological modifiers, such as ATRA, should be tested within clinical trials in patients not eligible for induction chemotherapy or allogeneic stem cell transplantation.

6.3 The Oncogenic MLL Fusion Proteins

6.3.1 Clinical Characteristics of MLL Leukemias

The mixed lineage leukemia gene (*MLL*, also known as *HRX*, *TRX1*, and *ALL1*) on human chromosome 11q23 is fused in frame with more than 50 partner genes in both acute lymphoblastic leukemia (ALL) and AML (Meyer et al. 2006). *MLL* fusion genes are highly diverse, but several of them share a common molecular pathomechanism (Slany 2009).

MLL fusions are present in approximately 10 % of adult leukemias but are much more prevalent in infant leukemias (>70 %) and therapy-related secondary leukemias, particularly those arising in the setting of previous topoisomerase II inhibitor treatment, e.g., etoposide (Super et al. 1993). Leukemias in adults bearing MLL translocations are mostly AMLs, whereas in children they are mostly ALLs. The most common MLL fusion partners are AF9 and ENL in adult leukemias and AF4 and ENL in children. Overall, translocations involving 11q23 are found in 5 % of ALL, 5–10 % of AML, and almost all biphenotypic (or mixed lineage) leukemia cases (Huret et al. 2001). A common characteristic is a poor prognosis with worse disease-free and overall survival, as compared with patients without MLL rearrangement (Secker-Walker et al. 1998; Döhner et al. 2010).

6.3.2 The MLL Protein

The MLL protein is a homolog of *Drosophila melanogaster gene trithorax* (Tkachuk et al. 1992), which was originally identified for its role in HOX gene regulation. It is essential for both fetal (Hess et al. 1997; Yagi et al. 1998) and adult hematopoiesis (Jude et al. 2007; McMahon et al. 2007). *Mll* knockout mice die at E10.5 with multiple developmental defects (Yu et al. 1995). Notably, expression of *HOX* genes is initiated normally at early stages, but does not persist (Yu et al. 1998), demonstrating that MLL has a function in the maintenance of *HOX* gene expression during embryonic development.

MLL is a large protein (430 kD) that undergoes extensive posttranslational processing including proteolytic cleavage into two functional portions (MLL-N and MLL-C) by the protease Taspase 1 (Hsieh et al. 2003; see Fig. 6.3). MLL-N contains several domains involved in chromatin localization, including AT hooks that mediate specific binding to AT-rich DNA (Tkachuk et al. 1992; Zeleznik-Le et al. 1994); two subnuclear localization motifs SNL1 and SNL2 (Yano et al. 1997); the zinc-finger motif CXXC homologous to DNMT1 and methyl-binding protein 1 (MBD1) (Cross et al. 1997); and the plant homology domains (PHD) 1-3, whose PHD3 domain binds the H3K4me3 mark necessary for transcriptional activity/maintenance (Chang et al. 2010; Milne et al. 2010) and interacts with the cyclophilin CYP33 (Wang et al. 2010). MLL-C, which associates with MLL-N to form a stable complex, contains a transcriptional activation domain (TA) that recruits CBP and histone acetyltransferases (Ernst et al. 2001) and a SET domain (Su(var)3-9 enhancer of zeste, trithorax), which possesses histone methyltransferase activity that creates the H3K4me3 mark (Milne et al. 2002).

MLL is part of a large nuclear chromatin-remodeling complex that regulates gene expression. MLL-N interacts with MENIN, the product of the tumor suppressor gene *MEN1*. MENIN acts as an adaptor to link MLL with the chromatin-associated protein LEDGF, thus facilitating physical association of the MLL/MENIN complex with chromatin (Yokoyama and Cleary 2008). Both MENIN and

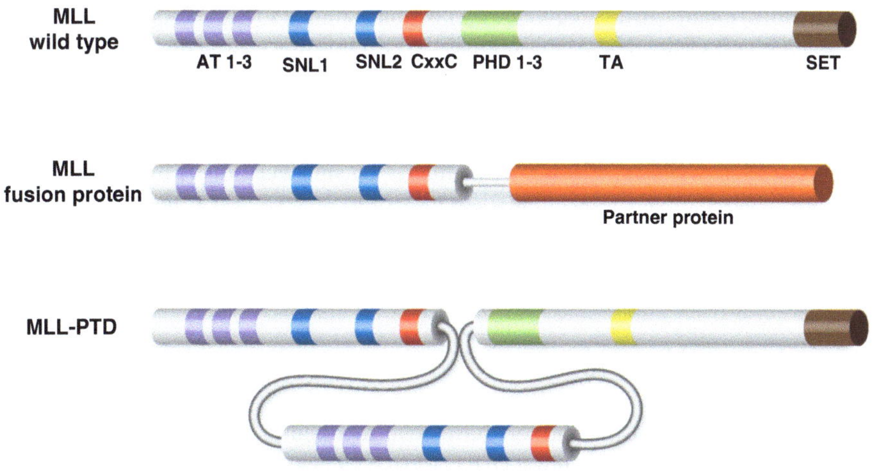

Fig. 6.3 Schematic representations of wild-type and mutant MLL proteins. Representative functional domains are shown as colored boxes. *Abbreviations*: *AT* AT hook DNA-binding motif, *SNL* speckled nuclear localization signals, *CXXC* cysteine-rich motif homologous to DNA methyltransferases and MBD1, *PHD* plant homology domain zinc-finger motifs, *TA* transactivation domain, *SET* Su(var)3-9 enhancer of zeste, trithorax domain, *PTD* partial tandem duplication (adapted from Ayton and Cleary (2003))

LEDGF are required for the transcriptional and oncogenic activities of MLL fusion proteins (Yokoyama et al. 2005, 2008). The DNA-binding CXXC motif, which is retained in all MLL fusion proteins, recognizes unmethylated CpG dinucleotides in pre-activated promoters (Birke et al. 2002) and preserves them from DNA methylation (Erfurth et al. 2008; Cierpicki et al. 2010). Point mutations in the CXXC motif abolish transformation of bone marrow myeloid progenitors *in vitro* (Ayton et al. 2004) and leukemogenic transformation *in vivo* by MLL fusion proteins (Cierpicki et al. 2010). The CXXC motif interacts with corepressor proteins such as HDAC1, the polycomb group protein BMI-1 (Xia et al. 2003), and the polymerase-associated factor complex (PAFc). PAFc stimulates the ubiquitination of histone H2B necessary for H3K4 trimethylation by the SET domain and associates with RNA polymerase II (Milne et al. 2010; Muntean et al. 2010).

The SET domain of MLL interacts with at least 4 proteins that are necessary for its chromatin-modifying activity: RBBP5 and ASH2L are essential for the methyltransferase activity of the SET domain (Dou et al. 2006; Southall et al. 2009); WDR5 is required to bind the methylated H3K4 introduced by MLL (Wysocka et al. 2005); and the histone acetyltransferase MOF acetylates the specific histone mark H4K16 (Dou et al. 2005). Although MLL interacts with corepressor proteins such as HDAC1, BMI-1 (Xia et al. 2003), and the cyclophilin CYP33 (Wang et al. 2010), accumulated evidence suggests that MLL functions as a positive regulator of gene expression through its own capacity to induce trimethylation of H3K4 and its interaction with HATs.

The function of MLL is regulated by posttranslational modifications, particularly within the cell cycle. The S-phase kinase ATR phosphorylates MLL at serine 516 after DNA damage, preventing the interaction and degradation of MLL by the SCF^{Skp2} E3 ligase. The accumulation of phosphorylated MLL leads to increased H3K4 methylation on chromatin. MLL fusion proteins lack serine 516 and consequently are not regulated by ATR-mediated phosphorylation (Liu et al. 2010). Further research on posttranslational modifications of MLL, MLL fusions, and their interaction partners will elucidate the complex functions of these proteins and might reveal pharmacological targets.

6.3.3 MLL Fusion Proteins

More than 50 MLL fusion partners have been reported in human leukemias. Most of them are rare but a small subset (AF4, AF6, AF9, and ENL) accounts for 80 % of MLL fusion proteins in leukemias (Krivtsov and Armstrong 2007). Although MLL partner proteins are heterogeneous, they comprise two general categories: nuclear proteins implicated in transcriptional regulation (e.g., AF4, AF9, AF10, ENL, and ELL) and cytoplasmic proteins involved in cell signaling (e.g., GAS7, EEN, AF6, and AFX) (Ayton and Cleary 2001; Krivtsov and Armstrong 2007). Several of the latter have been shown to mediate oligomeric self-association of their respective MLL fusion proteins (So et al. 2003; Liu et al. 2004; Liedtke et al. 2010). Other rare fusion partners include the histone acetyltransferases CBP (Taki et al. 1997) and p300 (Ida et al. 1997) and members of the septin protein family (SEPT2, SEPT5, SEPT6, SEPT9, and SEPT11) (Hall and Russell 2004).

A special case of MLL-induced leukemogenesis is the MLL-partial tandem duplication (PTD), in which selected exons (between exons 5 and 12) are duplicated and inserted between exons 11 and 12, showing that aberrations of MLL itself also might induce leukemia (see Fig. 6.3) (Schichman et al. 1994).

6.3.4 Chromatin Modifications by MLL Fusion Proteins

Several MLL fusion partners appear to have a common mechanism for transformation and are thought to aberrantly activate the transcriptional elongation of MLL target genes through epigenetic mechanisms (see Fig. 6.4). The PHD, TA, and SET domains of MLL are deleted in all fusion proteins, indicating that MLL loses its own transcriptional activation capacity. MLL is fused in 80 % of cases with one of the members of the ENL-associated protein (EAP) complex (ENL, AF9, AF4, AF5). The members of EAP complex interact physically with each other (Bitoun et al. 2007; Mueller et al. 2007) and with the positive transcription elongation factor b (P-TEFb), constituted by the cyclin-dependent kinase CDK9 and cyclin T1 (or T2) (Yokoyama et al. 2010). P-TEFb interacts with the MLL fusion partner ELL and together with EAP forms the super elongation complex (SEC). SEC phosphorylates RNA polymerase II, responsible for efficient transcriptional elongation, and requires the MLL fusion partner AF5 for stabilization and function (Lin et al. 2010). ENL,

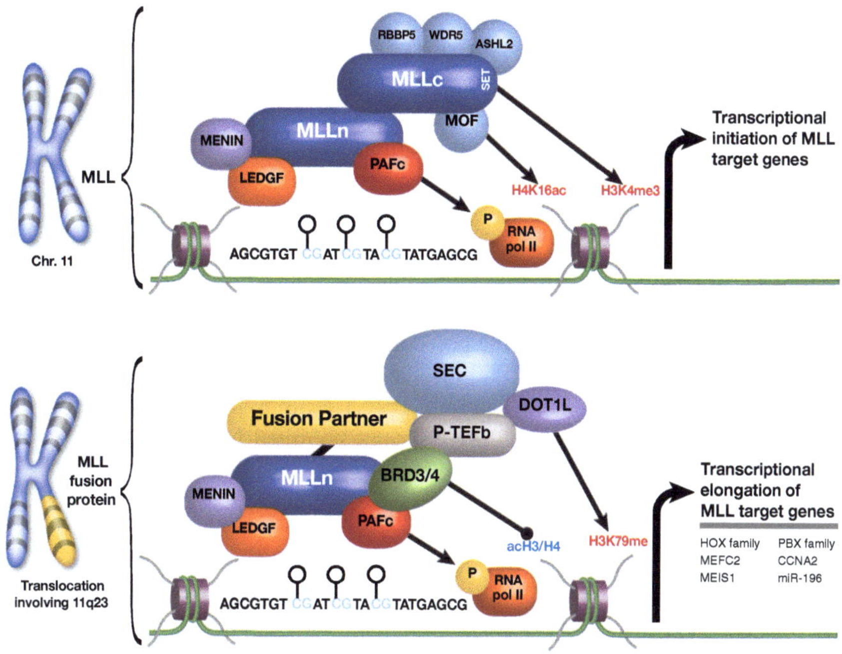

Fig. 6.4 Functional representations and protein interactions of MLL wild type and fusion proteins. The *MLL* gene is located on chromosome 11 band q23. The N-terminal part (MLL-N) of MLL interacts with MENIN and chromatin-associated protein LEDGF, permitting a physical interaction between MLL and chromatin. The CXXC motif binds unmethylated CpG dinucleotides of target promoters. The C-terminus (MLL-C) contains the SET domain, which induces methylation of histone H3 lysine 4 (H3K4) through its interaction with RBBP5, ASHL2, and WDR5. The histone acetyltransferase MOF interacts with MLL-C and acetylates the specific residue histone H4 lysine 16 (H4K16). The polymerase-associated factor complex (PAFc) interacts with MLL-N and phosphorylates RNA polymerase II (RNA pol II) activating the transcriptional initiation and elongation of MLL target genes such as *HOXA9, MEIS1, miR-196, CCNA2*, and *BCL2*. MLL fusion proteins contain the N-terminal part of MLL, which interacts with MENIN, LEDGF, and PAFc. The fusion partner protein interacts with other components of the ENL-associated protein (EAP) complex, including AF4, AF5, ENL, and AF9. The EAP complex recruits the positive elongation transcription factor b (P-TEFb) and the elongation factor ELL. The ENL protein family members recruit the histone H3 lysine 79 (H3K79) methyltransferase DOT1L, which aberrantly methylates the histones around target promoters and throughout gene bodies. The bromodomain and extraterminal (BET) family members BRD3 and BRD4 are recruited by P-TEFb and PAFc and bind to acetylated histones, regulating gene transcription. Through several epigenetic mechanisms, the transcriptional initiation and elongation of MLL target genes are aberrantly activated by MLL fusion proteins

AF9, and AF10 interact and recruit DOT1L to the MLL fusion complex. DOT1L is the unique known histone H3 lysine 79 (H3K79) methyltransferase in human cells and is essential to initiate and maintain aberrant transcription elongation of MLL target genes (Okada et al. 2005; Mueller et al. 2007; Bitoun et al. 2007). Recently, it was shown that the BET (bromodomain and extra terminal) chromatin regulators BRD3 and BRD4 are associated with the PAFc and P-TEFb complexes and may play a crucial role in MLL-induced leukemia binding to acetylated histones at activated target promoters (Dawson et al. 2011).

In addition to the aberrant H3K79 methylation activity and the activation of transcriptional elongation induced by several MLL fusion proteins, the co-expression of wild-type MLL is required for transformation. Wild-type MLL might activate the transcriptional initiation of target genes, but MLL fusion proteins link aberrant transcriptional initiation and elongation (Thiel et al. 2010; Milne et al. 2010).

Additional epigenetic mechanisms are also implicated in the molecular pathogenesis of specific MLL fusion proteins. For example, MLL-EEN recruits the histone arginine methyltransferase (PRMT1) to MLL target genes (Cheung et al. 2007), MLL-AF9 interacts with the polycomb group protein chromobox 8 (CBX8) and histone acetyltransferase TIP60 (Tan et al. 2011), and ENL interacts with the SWI/SNF chromatin-remodeling protein BRG1 (Nie et al. 2003), supporting the complexity of chromatin-remodeling enzymes recruited by MLL fusion proteins and the aberrant epigenetic reprogramming of gene transcription.

6.3.5 MLL and MLL Fusion Protein Target Genes

MLL target genes include *HOX* genes (especially *HOXA9*) (Ayton and Cleary 2003; Milne et al. 2005; Faber et al. 2009), *MEF2C* (Krivtsov et al. 2006), *PBX* genes (including *PBX2* and *PBX3*), and *MEIS1* (Wong et al. 2007; Kumar et al. 2009), which have been implicated in the transformation of leukemic cells. The proteins encoded by these MLL target genes activate the transcription of other genes, suggesting a hierarchy in gene expression with MLL oncoproteins at the apex (Kroon et al. 1998; Zeisig et al. 2004). Most of the aforementioned MLL target genes are oncogenes themselves involved in the regulation of cycling activity, self-renewal, and differentiation block (Wong et al. 2007; Kumar et al. 2009), demonstrating the importance of the aberrant transcriptional program activated by MLL fusion proteins.

Wild type MLL has been shown by ChIP-on-chip studies to bind more than 5000 human promoters, suggesting that MLL serves a general role in gene regulation. MLL exclusively co-localizes with RNA polymerase II and H3K4me3 at the 5′-end of actively transcribed genes (Guenther et al. 2005), whereas MLL fusion proteins aberrantly mislocalize along with H3K4me3 and H3K79me2 epigenetic marks throughout the length of target genes (Krivtsov et al. 2008; Guenther et al. 2008).

MLL fusion proteins deregulate global expression of microRNAs (Li et al. 2008; Stumpel et al. 2011; Arnold et al. 2011) with specific effects on *miR-196b* (Schotte et al. 2009) and *miR-17-92* (Li et al. 2008; Arnold et al. 2011). The *miR-196b* is located in a highly evolutionarily conserved region between *HOXA9* and *HOXA10* (Yekta et al. 2004) and might contribute to leukemic transformation by increasing proliferative capacity and blocking the differentiation of MLL-transformed cells (Popovic et al. 2009). The *miR-17-92* cluster, which acts as an oncogene in B-cell lymphoma (He et al. 2005), regulates MLL leukemia stem cell potential in part through repressing the expression of the cyclin-dependent kinase inhibitor p21 (Wong et al. 2010).

6.3.6 MLL Fusion Proteins Influence Global DNA Methylation

Epigenetic silencing by promoter methylation of tumor suppressor genes is implicated in the origin and maintenance of several cancers, including leukemia (Esteller 2008). Although an interaction between MLL fusion proteins and DNMTs has not been described, global and gene-specific changes in DNA methylation have been associated with MLL oncogenesis. Many genes have been identified to be silenced by promoter hypermethylation in MLL leukemias, such as DAPK1 (Gutierrez et al. 2003) and FHIT (Stam et al. 2006). Interestingly, AML samples with MLL-PTD exhibited an increased global methylation and, specifically, at the tumor suppressor gene SLC5A8 (Whitman et al. 2008).

Bone marrow samples of infants with ALL bearing MLL translocations show enhanced global DNA methylation compared to normal cells and non-MLL ALL (Schafer et al. 2010). The degree of promoter methylation is associated with adverse clinical outcomes in MLL-rearranged ALL (Stumpel et al. 2009, 2011).

6.3.7 Epigenetic Targeting of MLL Leukemias

The histone H3K79 methyltransferase DOT1L is recruited either directly or indirectly by several MLL fusion proteins to aberrantly maintain the transcription of MLL target genes (Okada et al. 2005; Mueller et al. 2007). Aberrant H3K79 methylation profiles distinguish MLL-rearranged leukemia and seem to be a common characteristic of most MLL fusion proteins (Krivtsov et al. 2008). Epigenetic profiling of hematopoietic progenitors versus leukemia stem cells revealed an aberrant H3K79 methylation profile in MLL-AF9 target genes, which correlated with gene expression. Furthermore, MLL-AF9-transformed cells are dependent on DOT1L for proliferation *in vitro* and *in vivo* (Bernt et al. 2011).

A potent and highly selective small-molecule inhibitor (EPZ0047777) of DOT1L displays biological activity and selectively kills MLL leukemia cells *in vitro*. *In vivo* administration of EPZ0047777 modestly extends overall survival in a xenograft model of MLL leukemia. This compound showed a low toxicity profile with no major hematopoietic defects at the plasma concentrations reached *in vivo* (Daigle et al. 2011). These data indicate that DOT1L is a crucial enzyme in sustaining MLL-transformed leukemia and is a candidate target for epigenetic therapy. HMT inhibitors with improved pharmacokinetic profiles will facilitate future clinical studies.

A novel class of epigenetic therapy compound targets chromatin "readers" that selectively bind specific histone marks, in contrast to the enzymes (HATs, HMTs) that "write" the histone code. Small molecules that specifically inhibit the acetyl-histone-binding bromodomains within the BET family members BRD3 and BRD4 that associate with MLL fusion proteins appear particularly promising (Rahman et al. 2011). BET inhibitors such as JQ1 and I-BET151 display potent efficacy against MLL-transformed cells *in vitro* and *in vivo*, at least in part due to the downregulation of key genes *BCL2*, *MYB*, *MYC*, and *CDK6*, and decreased recruitment of the transcription elongation complex (Zuber et al. 2011; Dawson et al. 2011). In addition to

AMLs, BET inhibitors appear promising in multiple myeloma (Delmore et al. 2011), squamous cell carcinomas with BRD4-NUT fusion proteins (Filippakopoulos et al. 2010), and in suppressing inflammatory responses (Nicodeme et al. 2010).

The interactions between MLL and its partner proteins provide novel therapeutic targets as shown by small-molecule inhibitors that block MLL-MENIN binding (Grembecka et al. 2012). Recently, the histone demethylase LSD1 (KDM1A) has been implicated in leukemogenesis induced by MLL fusion proteins, and pharmacological targeting of LSD1 leads to differentiation and apoptosis of MLL leukemia cells (Harris et al. 2012).

Conclusions

AML1/ETO aberrantly represses the transcription of its target genes through epigenetic modifications induced by the recruitment of HDACs and DNMTs. Conversely, MLL fusion proteins aberrantly maintain expression of their target genes by recruitment of various readers and writers of the histone code including transcriptional elongation factors, histone methyltransferases, or the chromatin-associated proteins BRD3/4. In leukemias bearing AML1/ETO or MLL fusion proteins, epigenetic therapies present as possible alternative treatments to target selectively these chimeric oncoproteins through their accessory factors at the molecular level, alone or in combination with standard chemotherapy.

Acknowledgments We would like to thank Heiko Becker and Leticia Solari for reviewing the manuscript and Norm Cyr for graphic design. J. Duque-Afonso was funded by a grant from LaCaixa-DAAD (ref. 314, A/05/29785), the Fellowship Program of the Department of Hematology/Oncology of the University of Freiburg, and is currently funded by the German Research Foundation (DFG, ref. DU 1287/2-1). M. Lübbert is supported by the DFG (SPP 1463 ref. LU 429/7-1 and CRC 992-C04 LU429/9-1). M. Cleary is supported by grants from the National Cancer Institute and Leukemia and Lymphoma Society. The authors have no conflicting financial interests.

References

Alcalay M, Meani N, Gelmetti V, Fantozzi A, Fagioli M, Orleth A, Riganelli D, Sebastiani C, Cappelli E, Casciari C, Sciurpi MT, Mariano AR, Minardi SP, Luzi L, Muller H, Di Fiore PP, Frosina G, Pelicci PG (2003) Acute myeloid leukemia fusion proteins deregulate genes involved in stem cell maintenance and DNA repair. J Clin Invest 112(11):1751–1761

Alvarez S, Suela J, Valencia A, Fernández A, Wunderlich M, Agirre X, Prósper F, Martín-Subero JI, Maiques A, Acquadro F, Rodriguez Perales S, Calasanz MJ, Roman-Gómez J, Siebert R, Mulloy JC, Cervera J, Sanz MA, Esteller M, Cigudosa JC (2010) DNA methylation profiles and their relationship with cytogenetic status in adult acute myeloid leukemia. PLoS One 5(8):e12197

Amann JM, Nip J, Strom DK, Lutterbach B, Harada H, Lenny N, Downing JR, Meyers S, Hiebert SW (2001) ETO, a target of t(8;21) in acute leukemia, makes distinct contacts with multiple histone deacetylases and binds mSin3A through its oligomerization domain. Mol Cell Biol 21(19):6470–6483

Arnold CP, Tan R, Zhou B, Yue SB, Schaffert S, Biggs JR, Doyonnas R, Lo MC, Perry JM, Renault VM, Sacco A, Somervaille T, Viatour P, Brunet A, Cleary ML, Li L, Sage J, Zhang DE, Blau

HM, Chen C, Chen CZ (2011) MicroRNA programs in normal and aberrant stem and progenitor cells. Genome Res 21(5):798–810

Ayton PM, Cleary ML (2001) Molecular mechanisms of leukemogenesis mediated by MLL fusion proteins. Oncogene 20(40):5695–5707

Ayton PM, Cleary ML (2003) Transformation of myeloid progenitors by MLL oncoproteins is dependent on Hoxa7 and Hoxa9. Genes Dev 17(18):2298–2307

Ayton PM, Chen EH, Cleary ML (2004) Binding to nonmethylated CpG DNA is essential for target recognition, transactivation, and myeloid transformation by an MLL oncoprotein. Mol Cell Biol 24(23):10470–10478

Barbetti V, Gozzini A, Rovida E, Morandi A, Spinelli E, Fossati G, Mascagni P, Lübbert M, Dello Sbarba P, Santini V (2008) Selective anti-leukaemic activity of low-dose histone deacetylase inhibitor ITF2357 on AML1/ETO-positive cells. Oncogene 27(12):1767–1778

Becker H, Pfeifer D, Afonso JD, Nimer SD, Veelken H, Schwabe M, Lübbert M (2008) Two cell lines of t(8;21) acute myeloid leukemia with activating c-KIT exon 17 mutation: models for the "second hit" hypothesis. Leukemia 22(9):1792–1794

Berg T, Guo Y, Abdelkarim M, Fliegauf M, Lübbert M (2007) Reversal of p15/INK4b hypermethylation in AML1/ETO-positive and -negative myeloid leukemia cell lines. Leuk Res 31(4): 497–506

Berg T, Fliegauf M, Burger J, Staege MS, Liu S, Martinez N, Heidenreich O, Burdach S, Haferlach T, Werner MH, Lübbert M (2008) Transcriptional upregulation of p21/WAF/Cip1 in myeloid leukemic blasts expressing AML1-ETO. Haematologica 93(11):1728–1733

Bernt KM, Zhu N, Sinha AU, Vempati S, Faber J, Krivtsov AV, Feng Z, Punt N, Daigle A, Bullinger L, Pollock RM, Richon VM, Kung AL, Armstrong SA (2011) MLL-rearranged leukemia is dependent on aberrant H3K79 methylztion by DOT1L. Cancer Cell 20(1):66–78

Birke M, Schreiner S, García-Cuéllar MP, Mahr K, Titgemeyer F, Slany RK (2002) The MT domain of the proto-oncoprotein MLL binds to CpG-containing DNA and discriminates against methylation. Nucleic Acids Res 30(4):958–965

Bitoun E, Oliver PL, Davies KE (2007) The mixed-lineage leukemia fusion partner AF4 stimulates RNA polymerase II transcriptional elongation and mediates coordinated chromatin remodeling. Hum Mol Genet 16(1):92–106

Bristow CA, Shore P (2003) Transcriptional regulation of the human MIP-1alpha promoter by RUNX1 and MOZ. Nucleic Acids Res 31(11):2735–2744

Calabi F, Pannell R, Pavloska G (2001) Gene targeting reveals a crucial role for MTG8 in the gut. Mol Cell Biol 21(16):5658–5666

Cameron S, Taylor DS, TePas EC, Speck NA, Mathey-Prevot B (1994) Identification of a critical regulatory site in the human interleukin-3 promoter by in vivo footprinting. Blood 83(10):2851–2859

Chang PY, Hom RA, Musselman CA, Zhu L, Kuo A, Gozani O, Kutateladze TG, Cleary ML (2010) Binding of the MLL PHD3 finger to histone H3K4me3 is required for MLL-dependent gene transcription. J Mol Biol 400(2):137–144

Cheung N, Chan LC, Thompson A, Cleary ML, So CW (2007) Protein arginine-methyltransferase-dependent oncogenesis. Nat Cell Biol 9(10):1208–1215

Chevalier N, Solari ML, Becker H, Pantic M, Gärtner F, Maul-Pavicic A, Hübner J, Wäsch R, Schmitt-Gräff A, Lübbert M (2010) Robust in vivo differentiation of t(8;21)-positive acute myeloid leukemia blasts to neutrophilic granulocytes induced by treatment with dasatinib. Leukemia 24(10):1779–1781

Cierpicki T, Risner LE, Grembecka J, Lukasik SM, Popovic R, Omonkowska M, Shultis DD, Zeleznik-Le NJ, Bushweller JH (2010) Structure of the MLL CXXC domain-DNA complex and its functional role in MLL-AF9 leukemia. Nat Struct Mol Biol 17(1):62–68

Claus R, Fliegauf M, Stock M, Duque AJ, Kolanczyc M, Lübbert M (2006) Inhibitors of DNA methylation and histone deacetylation independently relieve AML1/ETO-mediated lysozyme repression. J Leukoc Biol 80(6):1462–1472

Cleary ML (1991) Oncogenic conversion of transcription factors by chromosomal translocations. Cell 66(4):619–622

Cross SH, Meehan RR, Nan X, Bird A (1997) A component of the transcriptional repressor MeCP1 shares a motif with DNA methyltransferase and HRX proteins. Nat Genet 16(3):256–259

Daigle SR, Olhava EJ, Therkelsen CA, Majer CR, Sneeringer CJ, Song J, Johnston LD, Scott MP, Smith JJ, Xiao Y, Jin L, Kuntz KW, Chesworth R, Moyer MP, Bernt KM, Tseng JC, Kung AL, Armstrong SA, Copeland RA, Richon VM, Pollock RM (2011) Selective killing of mixed lineage leukemia cells by a potent small-molecule DOT1L inhibitor. Cancer Cell 20(1):53–65

Dawson MA, Prinjha RK, Dittmann A, Giotopoulos G, Bantscheff M, Chan WI, Robson SC, Chung CW, Hopf C, Savitski MM, Huthmacher C, Gudgin E, Lugo D, Beinke S, Chapman TD, Roberts EJ, Soden PE, Auger KR, Mirguet O, Doehner K, Delwel R, Burnett AK, Jeffrey P, Drewes G, Lee K, Huntly BJ, Kouzarides T (2011) Inhibition of BET recruitment to chromatin as an effective treatment for MLL-fusion leukaemia. Nature 478(7370):529–533

Delmore JE, Issa GC, Lemieux ME, Rahl PB, Shi J, Jacobs HM, Kastritis E, Gilpatrick T, Paranal RM, Qi J, Chesi M, Schinzel AC, McKeown MR, Heffernan TP, Vakoc CR, Bergsagel PL, Ghobrial IM, Richardson PG, Young RA, Hahn WC, Anderson KC, Kung AL, Bradner JE, Mitsiades CS (2011) BET bromodomain inhibition as a therapeutic strategy to target c-Myc. Cell 146(6):904–917

Dhanda RS, Lindberg SR, Olsson I (2008) The human SIN3B corepressor forms a nucleolar complex with leukemia-associated ETO homologues. BMC Mol Biol 9:8

Döhner H, Estey EH, Amadori S, Appelbaum FR, Büchner T, Burnett AK, Dombret H, Fenaux P, Grimwade D, Larson RA, Lo-Coco F, Naoe T, Niederwieser D, Ossenkoppele GJ, Sanz MA, Sierra J, Tallman MS, Löwenberg B, Bloomfield CD (2010) Diagnosis and management of acute myeloid leukemia in adults: recommendations from an international expert panel, on behalf of the European LeukemiaNet. Blood 115(3):453–474

Dou Y, Milne TA, Tackett AJ, Smith ER, Fukuda A, Wysocka J, Allis CD, Chait BT, Hess JL, Roeder RG (2005) Physical association and coordinate function of the H3 K4 methyltransferase MLL1 and the H4 K16 acetyltransferase MOF. Cell 121(6):873–885

Dou Y, Milne TA, Ruthenburg AJ, Lee S, Lee JW, Verdine GL, Allis CD, Roeder RG (2006) Regulation of MLL1 H3K4 methyltransferase activity by its core components. Nat Struct Mol Biol 13(8):713–719

Duque-Afonso J, Solari L, Essig A, Berg T, Pahl HL, Lübbert M (2011a) Regulation of the adaptor molecule LAT2, an in vivo target gene of RUNX1/RUNX1T1, during myeloid differentiation. Br J Haematol 153(5):612–622

Duque-Afonso J, Yalcin A, Berg T, Abdelkarim M, Heidenreich O, Lübbert M (2011b) The HDAC class I-specific inhibitor Entinostat (MS-275) effectively relieves epigenetic silencing of the LAT2 gene mediated by AML1/ETO. Oncogene 30(27):3062–3072

Erfurth FE, Popovic R, Grembecka J, Cierpicki T, Theisler C, Xia ZB, Stuart T, Diaz MO, Bushweller JH, Zeleznik-Le NJ (2008) MLL protects CpG clusters from methylation within the Hoxa9 gene, maintaining transcript expression. Proc Natl Acad Sci U S A 105(21):7517–7522

Erickson P, Gao J, Chang KS, Look T, Whisenant E, Raimondi S, Lasher R, Trujillo J, Rowley J, Drabkin H (1992) Identification of breakpoints in t(8;21) acute myelogenous leukemia and isolation of a fusion transcript, AML1/ETO, with similarity to Drosophila segmentation gene, runt. Blood 80:1825–1831

Ernst P, Wang J, Huang M, Goodman RH, Korsmeyer SJ (2001) MLL and CREB bind cooperatively to the nuclear coactivator CREB-binding protein. Mol Cell Biol 21(7):2249–2258

Esteller M (2008) Epigenetics in cancer. N Engl J Med 358(11):1148–1159

Faber J, Krivtsov AV, Stubbs MC, Wright R, Davis TN, van den Heuvel-Eibrink M, Zwaan CM, Kung AL, Armstrong SA (2009) HOXA9 is required for survival in human MLL-rearranged acute leukemias. Blood 113(11):2375–2385

Fazi F, Rosa A, Fatica A, Gelmetti V, De Marchis ML, Nervi C, Bozzoni I (2005) A minicircuitry comprised of microRNA-223 and transcription factors NFI-A and C/EBPalpha regulates human granulopoiesis. Cell 123(5):819–831

Fazi F, Zardo G, Gelmetti V, Travaglini L, Ciolfi A, Di Croce L, Rosa A, Bozzoni I, Grignani F, Lo-Coco F, Pelicci PG, Nervi C (2007a) Heterochromatic gene repression of the retinoic acid pathway in acute myeloid leukemia. Blood 109(10):4432–4440

Fazi F, Racanicchi S, Zardo G, Starnes LM, Mancini M, Travaglini L, Diverio D, Ammatuna E, Cimino G, Lo-Coco F, Grignani F, Nervi C (2007b) Epigenetic silencing of the myelopoiesis regulator microRNA-223 by the AML1/ETO oncoprotein. Cancer Cell 12(5):457–466

Figueroa ME, Lugthart S, Li Y, Erpelinck-Verschueren C, Deng X, Christos PJ, Schifano E, Booth J, van Putten W, Skrabanek L, Campagne F, Mazumdar M, Greally JM, Valk PJ, Löwenberg B, Delwel R, Melnick A (2010) DNA methylation signatures identify biologically distinct subtypes in acute myeloid leukemia. Cancer Cell 17(1):13–27

Filippakopoulos P, Qi J, Picaud S, Shen Y, Smith WB, Fedorov O, Morse EM, Keates T, Hickman TT, Felletar I, Philpott M, Munro S, McKeown MR, Wang Y, Christie AL, West N, Cameron MJ, Schwartz B, Heightman TD, La Thangue N, French CA, Wiest O, Kung AL, Knapp S, Bradner JE (2010) Selective inhibition of BET bromodomains. Nature 468(7327):1067–1073

Fliegauf M, Stock M, Berg T, Lübbert M (2004) Williams-Beuren syndrome critical region-5/non-T-cell activation linker: a novel target gene of AML1/ETO. Oncogene 23(56):9070–9081

Follows GA, Tagoh H, Lefevre P, Hodge D, Morgan GJ, Bonifer C (2003) Epigenetic consequences of AML1-ETO action at the human c-FMS locus. EMBO J 22(11):2798–2809

Fontana L, Pelosi E, Greco P, Racanicchi S, Testa U, Liuzzi F, Croce CM, Brunetti E, Grignani F, Peschle C (2007) MicroRNAs 17-5p-20a-106a control monocytopoiesis through AML1 targeting and M-CSF receptor upregulation. Nat Cell Biol 9(7):775–787

Frank R, Zhang J, Uchida H, Meyers S, Hiebert SW, Nimer SD (1995) The AML1/ETO fusion protein blocks transactivation of the GM-CSF promoter by AML1B. Oncogene 11(12):2667–2674

Fuks F, Burgers WA, Brehm A, Hughes-Davies L, Kouzarides T (2000) DNA methyltransferase Dnmt1 associates with histone deacetylase activity. Nat Genet 24(1):88–91

Gelmetti V, Zhang J, Fanelli M, Minucci S, Pelicci PG, Lazar MA (1998) Aberrant recruitment of the nuclear receptor corepressor-histone deacetylase complex by the acute myeloid leukemia fusion partner ETO. Mol Cell Biol 18(12):7185–7191

Göttlicher M, Minucci S, Zhu P, Krämer OH, Schimpf A, Giavara S, Sleeman JP, Lo Coco F, Nervi C, Pelicci PG, Heinzel T (2001) Valproic acid defines a novel class of HDAC inhibitors inducing differentiation of transformed cells. EMBO J 20(24):6969–6978

Gozzini A, Santini V (2005) Butyrates and decitabine cooperate to induce histone acetylation and granulocytic maturation of t(8;21) acute myeloid leukemia blasts. Ann Hematol 84(Suppl 1):54–60

Gozzini A, Rovida E, Dello Sbarba P, Galimberti S, Santini V (2003) Butyrates, as a single drug, induce histone acetylation and granulocytic maturation: possible selectivity on core binding factor-acute myeloid leukemia blasts. Cancer Res 63(24):8955–8961

Grembecka J, He S, Shi A, Purohit T, Muntean AG, Sorenson RJ, Showalter HD, Murai MJ, Belcher AM, Hartley T, Hess JL, Cierpicki T (2012) Menin-MLL inhibitors reverse oncogenic activity of MLL fusion proteins in leukemia. Nat Chem Biol 8(3):277–284

Guenther MG, Jenner RG, Chevalier B, Nakamura T, Croce CM, Canaani E, Young RA (2005) Global and Hox-specific roles for the MLL1 methyltransferase. Proc Natl Acad Sci U S A 102(24):8603–8608

Guenther MG, Lawton LN, Rozovskaia T, Frampton GM, Levine SS, Volkert TL, Croce CM, Nakamura T, Canaani E, Young RA (2008) Aberrant chromatin at genes encoding stem cell regulators in human mixed-lineage leukemia. Genes Dev 22(24):3403–3408

Gutierrez MI, Siraj AK, Bhargava M, Ozbek U, Banavali S, Chaudhary MA, El Solh H, Bhatia K (2003) Concurrent methylation of multiple genes in childhood ALL: Correlation with phenotype and molecular subgroup. Leukemia 17(9):1845–1850

Hall PA, Russell SE (2004) The pathobiology of the septin gene family. J Pathol 204(4):489–505

Harris WJ, Huang X, Lynch JT, Spencer GJ, Hitchin JR, Li Y, Ciceri F, Blaser JG, Greystoke BF, Jordan AM, Miller CJ, Ogilvie DJ, Somervaille TC (2012) The histone demethylase KDM1A sustains the oncogenic potential of MLL-AF9 leukemia stem cells. Cancer Cell 21(4):473–487

He L, Thomson JM, Hemann MT, Hernando-Monge E, Mu D, Goodson S, Powers S, Cordon-Cardo C, Lowe SW, Hannon GJ, Hammond SM (2005) A microRNA polycistron as a potential human oncogene. Nature 435(7043):828–833

Hess JL, Yu BD, Li B, Hanson R, Korsmeyer SJ (1997) Defects in yolk sac hematopoiesis in Mll-null embryos. Blood 90(5):1799–1806

Hildebrand D, Tiefenbach J, Heinzel T, Grez M, Maurer AB (2001) Multiple regions of ETO cooperate in transcriptional repression. J Biol Chem 276(13):9889–9895

Hsieh JJ, Ernst P, Erdjument-Bromage H, Tempst P, Korsmeyer SJ (2003) Proteolytic cleavage of MLL generates a complex of N- and C-terminal fragments that confers protein stability and subnuclear localization. Mol Cell Biol 23(1):186–194

Huang G, Shigesada K, Ito K, Wee HJ, Yokomizo T, Ito Y (2001) Dimerization with PEBP2beta protects RUNX1/AML1 from ubiquitin-proteasome-mediated degradation. EMBO J 20(4):723–733

Huang G, Zhang P, Hirai H, Elf S, Yan X, Chen Z, Koschmieder S, Okuno Y, Dayaram T, Growney JD, Shivdasani RA, Gilliland DG, Speck NA, Nimer SD, Tenen DG (2008) PU.1 is a major downstream target of AML1 (RUNX1) in adult mouse hematopoiesis. Nat Genet 40(1):51–60

Huang G, Zhao X, Wang L, Elf S, Xu H, Zhao X, Sashida G, Zhang Y, Liu Y, Lee J, Menendez S, Yang Y, Yan X, Zhang P, Tenen DG, Osato M, Hsieh JJ, Nimer SD (2011) The ability of MLL to bind RUNX1 and methylate H3K4 at PU.1 regulatory regions is impaired by MDS/AML-associated RUNX1/AML1 mutations. Blood 118(25):6544–6552

Hug BA, Lazar MA (2004) ETO interacting proteins. Oncogene 23(24):4270–4274

Huret JL, Dessen P, Bernheim A (2001) An atlas of chromosomes in hematological malignancies. Example: 11q23 and MLL partners. Leukemia 15(6):987–989

Ida K, Kitabayashi I, Taki T, Taniwaki M, Noro K, Yamamoto M, Ohki M, Hayashi Y (1997) Adenoviral E1A-associated protein p300 is involved in acute myeloid leukemia with t(11;22)(q23;q13). Blood 90(12):4699–4704

Jones PL, Veenstra GJ, Wade PA, Vermaak D, Kass SU, Landsberger N, Strouboulis J, Wolffe AP (1998) Methylated DNA and MeCP2 recruit histone deacetylase to repress transcription. Nat Genet 19(2):187–191

Jude CD, Climer L, Xu D, Artinger E, Fisher JK, Ernst P (2007) Unique and independent roles for MLL in adult hematopoietic stem cells and progenitors. Cell Stem Cell 1(3):324–337

Kelly LM, Gilliland DG (2002) Genetics of myeloid leukemias. Annu Rev Genomics Hum Genet 3:179–198

Kitabayashi I, Yokoyama A, Shimizu K, Ohki M (1998) Interaction and functional cooperation of the leukemia-associated factors AML1 and p300 in myeloid cell differentiation. EMBO J 17(11):2994–3004

Klampfer L, Zhang J, Zelenetz AO, Uchida H, Nimer SD (1996) The AML1/ETO fusion protein activates transcription of BCL-2. Proc Natl Acad Sci U S A 93(24):14059–14064

Klisovic MI, Maghraby EA, Parthun MR, Guimond M, Sklenar AR, Whitman SP, Chan KK, Murphy T, Anon J, Archer KJ, Rush LJ, Plass C, Grever MR, Byrd JC, Marcucci G (2003) Depsipeptide (FR 901228) promotes histone acetylation, gene transcription, apoptosis and its activity is enhanced by DNA methyltransferase inhibitors in AML1/ETO-positive leukemic cells. Leukemia 17:350–358

Krivtsov AV, Armstrong SA (2007) MLL translocations, histone modifications and leukaemia stem-cell development. Nat Rev Cancer 7(11):823–833

Krivtsov AV, Twomey D, Feng Z, Stubbs MC, Wang Y, Faber J, Levine JE, Wang J, Hahn WC, Gilliland DG, Golub TR, Armstrong SA (2006) Transformation from committed progenitor to leukaemia stem cell initiated by MLL-AF9. Nature 442(7104):818–822

Krivtsov AV, Feng Z, Lemieux ME, Faber J, Vempati S, Sinha AU, Xia X, Jesneck J, Bracken AP, Silverman LB, Kutok JL, Kung AL, Armstrong SA (2008) H3K79 methylation profiles define murine and human MLL-AF4 leukemias. Cancer Cell 14(5):355–368

Kroon E, Krosl J, Thorsteinsdottir U, Baban S, Buchberg AM, Sauvageau G (1998) Hoxa9 transforms primary bone marrow cells through specific collaboration with Meis1a but not Pbx1b. EMBO J 17(13):3714–3725

Kumar AR, Li Q, Hudson WA, Chen W, Sam T, Yao Q, Lund EA, Wu B, Kowal BJ, Kersey JH (2009) A role for MEIS1 in MLL-fusion gene leukemia. Blood 113(8):1756–1758

Lasa A, Carnicer MJ, Aventin A, Estivill C, Brunet S, Sierra J, Nomdedéu JF (2004) MEIS 1 expression is downregulated through promoter hypermethylation in AML1-ETO acute myeloid leukemias. Leukemia 18:1231–1237

Lausen J, Liu S, Fliegauf M, Lübbert M, Werner MH (2006) ELA2 is regulated by hematopoietic transcription factors, but not repressed by AML1-ETO. Oncogene 25(9):1349–1357

Li Z, Lu J, Sun M, Mi S, Zhang H, Luo RT, Chen P, Wang Y, Yan M, Qian Z, Neilly MB, Jin J, Zhang Y, Bohlander SK, Zhang DE, Larson RA, Le Beau MM, Thirman MJ, Golub TR, Rowley JD, Chen J (2008) Distinct microRNA expression profiles in acute myeloid leukemia with common translocations. Proc Natl Acad Sci U S A 105(40):15535–15540

Liedtke M, Ayton PM, Somervaille TC, Smith KS, Cleary ML (2010) Self-association mediated by the Ras association 1 domain of AF6 activates the oncogenic potential of MLL-AF6. Blood 116(1):63–70

Lin C, Smith ER, Takahashi H, Lai KC, Martin-Brown S, Florens L, Washburn MP, Conaway JW, Conaway RC, Shilatifard A (2010) AFF4, a component of the ELL/P-TEFb elongation complex and a shared subunit of MLL chimeras, can link transcription elongation to leukemia. Mol Cell 37(3):429–437

Linggi B, Müller-Tidow C, van de Locht L, Hu M, Nip J, Serve H, Berdel WE, van der Reijden B, Quelle DE, Rowley JD, Cleveland J, Jansen JH, Pandolfi PP, Hiebert SW (2002) The t(8;21) fusion protein, AML1 ETO, specifically represses the transcription of the p14(ARF) tumor suppressor in acute myeloid leukemia. Nat Med 8(7):743–750

Liu H, Chen B, Xiong H, Huang QH, Zhang QH, Wang ZG, Li BL, Chen Z, Chen SJ (2004) Functional contribution of EEN to leukemogenic transformation by MLL-EEN fusion protein. Oncogene 23(19):3385–3394

Liu S, Shen T, Huynh L, Klisovic MI, Rush LJ, Ford JL, Yu J, Becknell B, Li Y, Liu C, Vukosavljevic T, Whitman SP, Chang KS, Byrd JC, Perrotti D, Plass C, Marcucci G (2005) Interplay of RUNX1/MTG8 and DNA methyltransferase 1 in acute myeloid leukemia. Cancer Res 65(4):1277–1284

Liu Y, Cheney MD, Gaudet JJ, Chruszcz M, Lukasik SM, Sugiyama D, Lary J, Cole J, Dauter Z, Minor W, Speck NA, Bushweller JH (2006) The tetramer structure of the Nervy homology two domain, NHR2, is critical for AML1/ETO's activity. Cancer Cell 9(4):249–260

Liu S, Klisovic RB, Vukosavljevic T, Yu J, Paschka P, Huynh L, Pang J, Neviani P, Liu Z, Blum W, Chan KK, Perrotti D, Marcucci G (2007) Targeting AML1/ETO-histone deacetylase repressor complex: a novel mechanism for valproic acid-mediated gene expression and cellular differentiation in AML1/ETO-positive acute myeloid leukemia cells. J Pharmacol Exp Ther 321(3):953–960

Liu H, Takeda S, Kumar R, Westergard TD, Brown EJ, Pandita TK, Cheng EH, Hsieh JJ (2010) Phosphorylation of MLL by ATR is required for execution of mammalian S-phase checkpoint. Nature 467(7313):343–346

Löwenberg B, Downing JR, Burnett A (1999) Acute myeloid leukemia. N Engl J Med 341(14):1051–1062

Luo J, Su F, Chen D, Shiloh A, Gu W (2000) Deacetylation of p53 modulates its effect on cell growth and apoptosis. Nature 408(6810):377–381

Lütterbach B, Westendorf JJ, Linggi B, Patten A, Moniwa M, Davie JR, Huynh KD, Bardwell VJ, Lavinsky RM, Rosenfeld MG, Glass C, Seto E, Hiebert SW (1998) ETO, a target of t(8;21) in acute leukemia, interacts with the N-CoR and mSin3 corepressors. Mol Cell Biol 18(10):7176–7184

Maiques-Diaz A, Chou FS, Wunderlich M, Gómez-López G, Jacinto FV, Rodriguez-Perales S, Larrayoz MJ, Calasanz MJ, Mulloy JC, Cigudosa JC, Alvarez S (2012) Chromatin modifications induced by the AML1-ETO fusion protein reversibly silence its genomic targets through AML1 and Sp1 binding motifs. Leukemia 26(6):1329–1337

Marcucci G, Mrózek K, Ruppert AS, Maharry K, Kolitz JE, Moore JO, Mayer RJ, Pettenati MJ, Powell BL, Edwards CG, Sterling LJ, Vardiman JW, Schiffer CA, Carroll AJ, Larson RA, Bloomfield CD (2005) Prognostic factors and outcome of core binding factor acute myeloid leukemia patients with t(8;21) differ from those of patients with inv(16): a Cancer and Leukemia Group B study. J Clin Oncol 23(24):5705–5717

McMahon KA, Hiew SY, Hadjur S, Veiga-Fernandes H, Menzel U, Price AJ, Kioussis D, Williams O, Brady HJ (2007) Mll has a critical role in fetal and adult hematopoietic stem cell self-renewal. Cell Stem Cell 1(3):338–345

Meyer C, Schneider B, Jakob S, Strehl S, Attarbaschi A, Schnittger S, Schoch C, Jansen MW, van Dongen JJ, den Boer ML, Pieters R, Ennas MG, Angelucci E, Koehl U, Greil J, Griesinger F, Zur Stadt U, Eckert C, Szczepański T, Niggli FK, Schäfer BW, Kempski H, Brady HJ, Zuna J, Trka J, Nigro LL, Biondi A, Delabesse E, Macintyre E, Stanulla M, Schrappe M, Haas OA, Burmeister T, Dingermann T, Klingebiel T, Marschalek R (2006) The MLL recombinome of acute leukemias. Leukemia 20(5):777–784

Meyers S, Downing JR, Hiebert SW (1993) Identification of AML-1 and the (8;21) translocation protein (AML-1/ETO) as sequence-specific DNA-binding proteins: the runt homology domain is required for DNA binding and protein-protein interactions. Mol Cell Biol 13(10):6336–6345

Milne TA, Briggs SD, Brock HW, Martin ME, Gibbs D, Allis CD (2002) Hess JL MLL targets SET domain methyltransferase activity to Hox gene promoters. Mol Cell 10(5):1107–1117

Milne TA, Martin ME, Brock HW, Slany RK, Hess JL (2005) Leukemogenic MLL fusion proteins bind across a broad region of the Hox a9 locus, promoting transcription and multiple histone modifications. Cancer Res 65(24):11367–11374

Milne TA, Kim J, Wang GG, Stadler SC, Basrur V, Whitcomb SJ, Wang Z, Ruthenburg AJ, Elenitoba-Johnson KS, Roeder RG, Allis CD (2010) Multiple interactions recruit MLL1 and MLL1 fusion proteins to the HOXA9 locus in leukemogenesis. Mol Cell 38(6):853–863

Miyoshi H, Shimizu K, Kozu T, Maseki N, Kaneko Y, Ohki M (1991) t(8;21) breakpoints on chromosome 21 in acute myeloid leukemia are clustered within a limited region of a single gene, AML1. Proc Natl Acad Sci U S A 88(23):10431–10434

Mueller D, Bach C, Zeisig D, Garcia-Cuellar MP, Monroe S, Sreekumar A, Zhou R, Nesvizhskii A, Chinnaiyan A, Hess JL, Slany RK (2007) A role for the MLL fusion partner ENL in transcriptional elongation and chromatin modification. Blood 110(13):4445–4454

Müller AM, Duque-Afonso J, Shizuru JA, Lübbert M (2008) Complementing mutations in Core Binding Factor (CBF) leukemias: mechanisms und therapeutical implications. Oncogene 27(44):5759–5773

Muntean AG, Tan J, Sitwala K, Huang Y, Bronstein J, Connelly JA, Basrur V, Elenitoba-Johnson KS, Hess JL (2010) The PAF complex synergizes with MLL fusion proteins at HOX loci to promote leukemogenesis. Cancer Cell 17(6):609–621

Nan X, Ng HH, Johnson CA, Laherty CD, Turner BM, Eisenman RN, Bird A (1998) Transcriptional repression by the methyl-CpG-binding protein MeCP2 involves a histone deacetylase complex. Nature 393(6683):386–389

Nicodeme E, Jeffrey KL, Schaefer U, Beinke S, Dewell S, Chung CW, Chandwani R, Marazzi I, Wilson P, Coste H, White J, Kirilovsky J, Rice CM, Lora JM, Prinjha RK, Lee K, Tarakhovsky A (2010) Suppression of inflammation by a synthetic histone mimic. Nature 468(7327):1119–1123

Nie Z, Yan Z, Chen EH, Sechi S, Ling C, Zhou S, Xue Y, Yang D, Murray D, Kanakubo E, Cleary ML, Wang W (2003) Novel SWI/SNF chromatin-remodeling complexes contain a mixed-lineage leukemia chromosomal translocation partner. Mol Cell Biol 23(8):2942–2952

Nuchprayoon I, Meyers S, Scott LM, Suzow J, Hiebert S, Friedman AD (1994) PEBP2/CBF, the murine homolog of the human myeloid AML1 and PEBP2 beta/CBF beta proto-oncoproteins, regulates the murine myeloperoxidase and neutrophil elastase genes in immature myeloid cells. Mol Cell Biol 14(8):5558–5568

Ogawa E, Maruyama M, Kagoshima H, Inuzuka M, Lu J, Satake M, Shigesada K, Ito Y (1993) PEBP2/PEA2 represents a family of transcription factors homologous to the products of the Drosophila runt gene and the human AML1 gene. Proc Natl Acad Sci U S A 90(14):6859–6863

Okada Y, Feng Q, Lin Y, Jiang Q, Li Y, Coffield VM, Su L, Xu G, Zhang Y (2005) hDOT1L links histone methylation to leukemogenesis. Cell 121(2):167–178

Okuda T, van Deursen J, Hiebert SW, Grosveld G, Downing JR (1996) AML1, the target of multiple chromosomal translocations in human leukemia, is essential for normal fetal liver hematopoiesis. Cell 84(2):321–330

Otto F, Lübbert M, Stock M (2003) Upstream and downstream targets of RUNX proteins. J Cell Biochem 89:9–18

Pabst T, Mueller BU, Harakawa N, Schoch C, Haferlach T, Behre G, Hiddemann W, Zhang DE, Tenen DG (2001) AML1-ETO downregulates the granulocytic differentiation factor C/EBPalpha in t(8;21) myeloid leukemia. Nat Med 7(4):444–451

Peterson LF, Yan M, Zhang DE (2007) The p21/Waf1 pathway is involved in blocking leukemogenesis by the t(8;21) fusion protein AML1-ETO. Blood 109(10):4392–4398

Popovic R, Riesbeck LE, Velu CS, Chaubey A, Zhang J, Achille NJ, Erfurth FE, Eaton K, Lu J, Grimes HL, Chen J, Rowley JD, Zeleznik-Le NJ (2009) Regulation of mir-196b by MLL and its overexpression by MLL fusions contributes to immortalization. Blood 113(14):3314–3322

Ptasinska A, Assi SA, Mannari D, James SR, Williamson D, Dunne J, Hoogenkamp M, Wu M, Care M, McNeill H, Cauchy P, Cullen M, Tooze RM, Tenen DG, Young BD, Cockerill PN, Westhead DR, Heidenreich O, Bonifer C (2012) Depletion of RUNX1/ETO in t(8;21) AML cells leads to genome-wide changes in chromatin structure and transcription factor binding. Leukemia 26(8):1829–1841

Rahman S, Sowa ME, Ottinger M, Smith JA, Shi Y, Harper JW, Howley PM (2011) The Brd4 extraterminal domain confers transcription activation independent of pTEFb by recruiting multiple proteins, including NSD3. Mol Cell Biol 31(13):2641–2652

Schafer E, Irizarry R, Negi S, McIntyre E, Small D, Figueroa ME, Melnick A, Brown P (2010) Promoter hypermethylation in MLL-r infant acute lymphoblastic leukemia: biology and therapeutic targeting. Blood 115(23):4798–4809

Schichman SA, Caligiuri MA, Gu Y, Strout MP, Canaani E, Bloomfield CD, Croce CM (1994) ALL-1 partial duplication in acute leukemia. Proc Natl Acad Sci U S A 91(13):6236–6239

Schlenk RF, Benner A, Krauter J, Büchner T, Sauerland C, Ehninger G, Schaich M, Mohr B, Niederwieser D, Krahl R, Pasold R, Döhner K, Ganser A, Döhner H, Heil G (2004) Individual patient data-based meta-analysis of patients aged 16 to 60 years with core binding factor acute myeloid leukemia: a survey of the German Acute Myeloid Leukemia Intergroup. J Clin Oncol 22(18):3741–3750

Schotte D, Chau JC, Sylvester G, Liu G, Chen C, van der Velden VH, Broekhuis MJ, Peters TC, Pieters R, den Boer ML (2009) Identification of new microRNA genes and aberrant microRNA profiles in childhood acute lymphoblastic leukemia. Leukemia 23(2):313–322

Secker-Walker LM, Moorman AV, Bain BJ, Mehta AB (1998) Secondary acute leukemia and myelodysplastic syndrome with 11q23 abnormalities. EU Concerted Action 11q23 Workshop. Leukemia 12(5):840–844

Serrano E, Carnicer MJ, Lasa A, Orantes V, Pena J, Brunet S, Aventín A, Sierra J, Nomdedéu JF (2008) Epigenetic-based treatments emphasize the biologic differences of core-binding factor acute myeloid leukemias. Leuk Res 32(6):944–953

Shimizu K, Kitabayashi I, Kamada N, Abe T, Maseki N, Suzukawa K, Ohki M (2000) AML1-MTG8 leukemic protein induces the expression of granulocyte colony-stimulating factor (G-CSF) receptor through the up-regulation of CCAAT/enhancer binding protein epsilon. Blood 96(1):288–296

Slany RK (2009) The molecular biology of mixed lineage leukemia. Haematologica 94(7):984–993

So CW, Lin M, Ayton PM, Chen EH, Cleary ML (2003) Dimerization contributes to oncogenic activation of MLL chimeras in acute leukemias. Cancer Cell 4(2):99–110

Southall SM, Wong PS, Odho Z, Roe SM, Wilson JR (2009) Structural basis for the requirement of additional factors for MLL1 SET domain activity and recognition of epigenetic marks. Mol Cell 33(2):181–191

Stam RW, den Boer ML, Passier MM, Janka-Schaub GE, Sallan SE, Armstrong SA, Pieters R (2006) Silencing of the tumor suppressor gene FHIT is highly characteristic for MLL gene rearranged infant acute lymphoblastic leukemia. Leukemia 20(2):264–271

Stumpel DJ, Schneider P, van Roon EH, Boer JM, de Lorenzo P, Valsecchi MG, de Menezes RX, Pieters R, Stam RW (2009) Specific promoter methylation identifies different subgroups of MLL-rearranged infant acute lymphoblastic leukemia, influences clinical outcome, and provides therapeutic options. Blood 114(27):5490–5498

Stumpel DJ, Schotte D, Lange-Turenhout EA, Schneider P, Seslija L, de Menezes RX, Marquez VE, Pieters R, den Boer ML, Stam RW (2011) Hypermethylation of specific microRNA genes in MLL-rearranged infant acute lymphoblastic leukemia: major matters at a micro scale. Leukemia 25(3):429–439

Super HJ, McCabe NR, Thirman MJ, Larson RA, Le Beau MM, Pedersen-Bjergaard J, Philip P, Diaz MO, Rowley JD (1993) Rearrangements of the MLL gene in therapy-related acute myeloid leukemia in patients previously treated with agents targeting DNA-topoisomerase II. Blood 82(12):3705–3711

Tahirov TH, Inoue-Bungo T, Morii H, Fujikawa A, Sasaki M, Kimura K, Shiina M, Sato K, Kumasaka T, Yamamoto M, Ishii S, Ogata K (2001) Structural analyses of DNA recognition by the AML1/Runx-1 Runt domain and its allosteric control by CBFbeta. Cell 104(5):755–767

Taki T, Sako M, Tsuchida M, Hayashi Y (1997) The t(11;16)(q23;p13) translocation in myelodysplastic syndrome fuses the MLL gene to the CBP gene. Blood 89(11):3945–3950

Tan J, Jones M, Koseki H, Nakayama M, Muntean AG, Maillard I, Hess JL (2011) CBX8, a Polycomb Group Protein, Is Essential for MLL-AF9-Induced Leukemogenesis. Cancer Cell 20(5):563–575

Thiel AT, Blessington P, Zou T, Feather D, Wu X, Yan J, Zhang H, Liu Z, Ernst P, Koretzky GA, Hua X (2010) MLL-AF9-induced leukemogenesis requires coexpression of the wild-type Mll allele. Cancer Cell 17(2):148–159

Tkachuk DC, Kohler S, Cleary ML (1992) Involvement of a homolog of Drosophila trithorax by 11q23 chromosomal translocations in acute leukemias. Cell 71(4):691–700

Uchida H, Zhang J, Nimer SD (1997) AML1A and AML1B can transactivate the human IL-3 promoter. J Immunol 158(5):2251–2258

Walker H, Smith FJ, Betts DR (1994) Cytogenetics in acute myeloid leukaemia. Blood Rev 8(1):30–36

Wang Q, Stacy T, Miller JD, Lewis AF, Gu TL, Huang X, Bushweller JH, Bories JC, Alt FW, Ryan G, Liu PP, Wynshaw-Boris A, Binder M, Marín-Padilla M, Sharpe AH, Speck NA (1996) The CBFbeta subunit is essential for CBFalpha2 (AML1) function in vivo. Cell 87(4):697–708

Wang J, Hoshino T, Redner RL, Kajigaya S, Liu JM (1998) ETO, fusion partner in t(8;21) acute myeloid leukemia, represses transcription by interaction with the human N-CoR/mSin3/HDAC1 complex. Proc Natl Acad Sci U S A 95(18):10860–10865

Wang J, Saunthararajah Y, Redner RL, Liu JM (1999) Inhibitors of histone deacetylase relieve ETO-mediated repression and induce differentiation of AML1-ETO leukemia cells. Cancer Res 59(12):2766–2769

Wang Z, Song J, Milne TA, Wang GG, Li H, Allis CD, Patel DJ (2010) Pro isomerization in MLL1 PHD3-bromo cassette connects H3K4me readout to CyP33 and HDAC-mediated repression. Cell 141(7):1183–1194

Wang L, Gural A, Sun XJ, Zhao X, Perna F, Huang G, Hatlen MA, Vu L, Liu F, Xu H, Asai T, Xu H, Deblasio T, Menendez S, Voza F, Jiang Y, Cole PA, Zhang J, Melnick A, Roeder RG, Nimer SD (2011a) The leukemogenicity of AML1-ETO is dependent on site-specific lysine acetylation. Science 333(6043):765–769

Wang YY, Zhao LJ, Wu CF, Liu P, Shi L, Liang Y, Xiong SM, Mi JQ, Chen Z, Ren R, Chen SJ (2011b) C-KIT mutation cooperates with full-length AML1-ETO to induce acute myeloid leukemia in mice. Proc Natl Acad Sci USA 108(6):2450–2455

Wei Y, Liu S, Lausen J, Woodrell C, Cho S, Biris N, Kobayashi N, Wei Y, Yokoyama S, Werner MH (2007) A TAF4-homology domain from the corepressor ETO is a docking platform for positive and negative regulators of transcription. Nat Struct Mol Biol 14(7):653–661

Whitman SP, Hackanson B, Liyanarachchi S, Liu S, Rush LJ, Maharry K, Margeson D, Davuluri R, Wen J, Witte T, Yu L, Liu C, Bloomfield CD, Marcucci G, Plass C, Caligiuri MA (2008)

DNA hypermethylation and epigenetic silencing of the tumor suppressor gene, SLC5A8, in acute myeloid leukemia with the MLL partial tandem duplication. Blood 112(5):2013–2016

Wilop S, Fernandez AF, Jost E, Herman JG, Brümmendorf TH, Esteller M, Galm O (2011) Array-based DNA methylation profiling in acute myeloid leukaemia. Br J Haematol 155(1):65–72

Wong P, Iwasaki M, Somervaille TC, So CW, Cleary ML (2007) Meis1 is an essential and rate-limiting regulator of MLL leukemia stem cell potential. Genes Dev 21(21):2762–2774

Wong P, Iwasaki M, Somervaille TC, Ficara F, Carico C, Arnold C, Chen CZ, Cleary ML (2010) The miR-17-92 microRNA polycistron regulates MLL leukemia stem cell potential by modulating p21 expression. Cancer Res 70(9):3833–3842

Wysocka J, Swigut T, Milne TA, Dou Y, Zhang X, Burlingame AL, Roeder RG, Brivanlou AH, Allis CD (2005) WDR5 associates with histone H3 methylated at K4 and is essential for H3 K4 methylation and vertebrate development. Cell 121(6):859–872

Xia ZB, Anderson M, Diaz MO, Zeleznik-Le NJ (2003) MLL repression domain interacts with histone deacetylases, the polycomb group proteins HPC2 and BMI-1, and the corepressor C-terminal-binding protein. Proc Natl Acad Sci U S A 100(14):8342–8347

Yagi H, Deguchi K, Aono A, Tani Y, Kishimoto T, Komori T (1998) Growth disturbance in fetal liver hematopoiesis of Mll-mutant mice. Blood 92(1):108–117

Yan M, Kanbe E, Peterson LF, Boyapati A, Miao Y, Wang Y, Chen IM, Chen Z, Rowley JD, Willman CL, Zhang DE (2006) A previously unidentified alternatively spliced isoform of t(8;21) transcript promotes leukemogenesis. Nat Med 12(8):945–949

Yang G, Khalaf W, van de Locht L et al (2005) Transcriptional repression of the Neurofibromatosis-1 tumor suppressor by the t(8;21) fusion protein. Mol Cell Biol 25(14):5869–5879

Yang G, Thompson MA, Brandt SJ, Hiebert SW (2007) Histone deacetylase inhibitors induce the degradation of the t(8;21) fusion oncoprotein. Oncogene 26(1):91–101

Yano T, Nakamura T, Blechman J, Sorio C, Dang CV, Geiger B, Canaani E (1997) Nuclear punctate distribution of ALL-1 is conferred by distinct elements at the N terminus of the protein. Proc Natl Acad Sci U S A 94(14):7286–7291

Yekta S, Shih IH, Bartel DP (2004) MicroRNA-directed cleavage of HOXB8 mRNA. Science 304(5670):594–596

Yokoyama A, Cleary ML (2008) Menin critically links MLL proteins with LEDGF on cancer-associated target genes. Cancer Cell 14(1):36–46

Yokoyama A, Somervaille TC, Smith KS, Rozenblatt-Rosen O, Meyerson M, Cleary ML (2005) The menin tumor suppressor protein is an essential oncogenic cofactor for MLL-associated leukemogenesis. Cell 123(2):207–218

Yokoyama A, Lin M, Naresh A, Kitabayashi I, Cleary ML (2010) A higher-order complex containing AF4 and ENL family proteins with P-TEFb facilitates oncogenic and physiologic MLL-dependent transcription. Cancer Cell 17(2):198–212

Yu BD, Hess JL, Horning SE, Brown GA, Korsmeyer SJ (1995) Altered Hox expression and segmental identity in Mll-mutant mice. Nature 378(6556):505–508

Yu BD, Hanson RD, Hess JL, Horning SE, Korsmeyer SJ (1998) MLL, a mammalian trithorax-group gene, functions as a transcriptional maintenance factor in morphogenesis. Proc Natl Acad Sci U S A 95(18):10632–10636

Zeisig BB, Milne T, García-Cuéllar MP, Schreiner S, Martin ME, Fuchs U, Borkhardt A, Chanda SK, Walker J, Soden R, Hess JL, Slany RK (2004) Hoxa9 and Meis1 are key targets for MLL-ENL-mediated cellular immortalization. Mol Cell Biol 24(2):617–628

Zeleznik-Le NJ, Harden AM, Rowley JD (1994) 11q23 translocations split the "AT-hook" cruciform DNA-binding region and the transcriptional repression domain from the activation domain of the mixed-lineage leukemia (MLL) gene. Proc Natl Acad Sci U S A 91(22):10610–10614

Zhang DE, Fujioka K, Hetherington CJ, Shapiro LH, Chen HM, Look AT, Tenen DG (1994) Identification of a region which directs the monocytic activity of the colony-stimulating factor 1 (macrophage colony-stimulating factor) receptor promoter and binds PEBP2/CBF (AML1). Mol Cell Biol 14(12):8085–8095

Zhang J, Kalkum M, Yamamura S, Chait BT, Roeder RG (2004) E protein silencing by the leukemogenic AML1-ETO fusion protein. Science 305(5688):1286–1289

Zhao X, Jankovic V, Gural A, Huang G, Pardanani A, Menendez S, Zhang J, Dunne R, Xiao A, Erdjument-Bromage H, Allis CD, Tempst P, Nimer SD (2008) Methylation of RUNX1 by PRMT1 abrogates SIN3A binding and potentiates its transcriptional activity. Genes Dev 22(5):640–653

Zuber J, Shi J, Wang E, Rappaport AR, Herrmann H, Sison EA, Magoon D, Qi J, Blatt K, Wunderlich M, Taylor MJ, Johns C, Chicas A, Mulloy JC, Kogan SC, Brown P, Valent P, Bradner JE, Lowe SW, Vakoc CR (2011) RNAi screen identifies Brd4 as a therapeutic target in acute myeloid leukaemia. Nature 478(7370):524–528

Treatment of Hematologic Malignancies with DNA Hypomethylating Agents

7

Michael Daskalakis, Tina E. Joeckel, Michael Lübbert, and A. Kuendgen

7.1 5-Azacytidine (5-Aza)

7.1.1 Clinical Studies of 5-Azacytidine Before the Discovery of Its Hypomethylating Activity

5-Azacytidine (5-aza) and 5-aza-2′-deoxycytidine (decitabine, DAC) were both synthesized in 1964 and were developed in parallel as antileukemic agents. Early clinical studies in the 1970s focused on their application as intensive induction chemotherapy in acute leukemias as well as solid tumor treatment. These early clinical data on 5-aza were reviewed by von Hoff et al.: a total of 58 protocols and reviews received by the National Institutes of Health were analyzed, which included 821 patients who had been treated with 5-aza, 207 of them within phase I studies. 5-Aza revealed consistent antitumor activity in patients with AML, with an overall response rate of 36 % (20 % CR, 16 % PR) in 200 patients with AML refractory to previous treatment. The median duration of remission

M. Daskalakis (✉)
Department of Haematology and Central Haematology Laboratory, Inselspital, Bern, Switzerland
e-mail: michael.daskalakis@insel.ch

T.E. Joeckel, MD
Cancer Research, Peter MacCallum Cancer Centre, St Andrews Place, East Melbourne VIC 3002, Australia

M. Lübbert, MD, PhD (✉)
Department of Hematology/Oncology, University Medical Center Freiburg, University of Freiburg, Hugstetterstr. 55, Freiburg D-79106, Germany
e-mail: michael.luebbert@uniklinik-freiburg.de

A. Kuendgen
Department of Hematology, Oncology and Clinical Immunology, Heinrich-Heine-University, Düsseldorf, Germany
kuendgen@med.uni-duesseldorf.de

M. Lübbert, P.A. Jones (eds.), *Epigenetic Therapy of Cancer*,
DOI 10.1007/978-3-642-38404-2_7,

was between 15 and 19 weeks (von Hoff et al. 1976). Despite this activity of 5-aza as a single agent in AML, it never advanced through the US FDA review process as a leukemia therapy.

7.1.2 Clinical Studies of Low-Dose 5-Azacytidine in MDS

7.1.2.1 Development of 5-Azacytidine to First Approved MDS Therapy: CALGB Studies, AZA001 Trial

When the demethylating activity of 5-aza and DAC was observed at much lower dosages than administered before, myelodysplastic syndromes (MDS) appeared to be an ideal candidate disease to test this hypothesis, since MDS patients have a high probability to evolve to AML, hypermethylation of tumor suppressor genes seems to play a role in disease pathogenesis and progression (Uchida et al. 1997), and many patients are not candidates for intensive treatment approaches. 5-Aza was the first drug approved by the FDA for the treatment of MDS (2004). This decision was based on the results of 2 phase II (protocols 8421 and 8921) and one phase III trial (protocol 9221) conducted by the Cancer and Leukemia Group B (CALGB). All three studies administered the same dosage of 5-aza (75 mg/m^2/day for 7 days every 28 days) either by continuous IV infusion (CALGB 8421) or by subcutaneous administration (CALGB 8921 and 9221) (Silverman et al. 1994, 2002).

After initial promising results in the two aforementioned phase II trials, the phase III study including 191 patients with MDS according to FAB classification was initiated. The main study population consisted of higher-risk MDS, but lower-risk groups could be included if they had additional signs of significant marrow dysfunction. Patients were randomized between 5-aza at the abovementioned dose and supportive care only, with the possibility of a crossover to the treatment arm in case of disease progression. Responses occurred in 60 % of patients on the 5-aza arm (7 % CR, 16 % PR, 37 % HI) compared with 5 % (HI) receiving supportive care [$p<0.001$]. A significant prolongation of median time to leukemic transformation or death was observed in the 5-aza arm (21 months versus 13 months [$p = 0.007$]), while the difference in OS was not statistically significant for the whole group of patients. When a landmark analysis after 6 months was performed to eliminate the confounding effect of early crossover to 5-aza, a borderline difference in median survival of 18 months compared to 11 months [$p=0.03$] could be demonstrated. A recently published reanalysis of the 3 CALGB trials applying the WHO classification (Vardiman et al. 2002) for disease categorization as well as IWG criteria for response assessment (Cheson et al. 2000) showed a CR rate of 10–17 % for 5-aza treated patients; partial remissions were rare; 23–36 % of patients had hematologic improvement (HI). The median number of cycles to first response was 3, and 90 % of responses were seen by cycle 6 (Silverman et al. 2006).

To achieve approval for 5-aza in Europe as well, the worldwide confirmatory Aza001 trial has been performed (Fenaux et al. 2009). In this trial 5-aza at the standard dosage was compared to three different conventional care regimens, including supportive care, low-dose ara-C, and intensive chemotherapy, without an option to crossover. 358 patients have been included, 179 were randomized to 5-aza and 179 to conventional care (105 supportive care, 49 low-dose ara-C, 25 standard chemotherapy). With a median of 9 cycles, 5-aza was administered much longer compared to previous trials. 51 (28.5 %) patients achieved CR or PR. Altogether 49 % of patients showed hematologic improvement. After a median follow-up of 21.1 months, median overall survival (OS) was 24.5 months for the azacytidine group versus 15.0 months for the conventional care group [$p = 0.0001$]. At 2 years, 50.8 % of patients in the azacytidine group were alive compared with 26.2 % in the conventional care group [$p < 0.0001$]. The most common grade 3–4 adverse events were peripheral cytopenias. Differences in overall survival were seen consistently between 5-aza and the three different conventional care regimens: 9.6 (best supportive care, BSC), 9.2 (low-dose ara-C, LDAC), and 9.4 months (standard intensive chemotherapy, IC), respectively. Still, this difference achieved only statistical significance in the two larger subgroups of patients, due to the small number of patients in the intensive chemotherapy group [$p = 0.0045$, 0.0006, and 0.51, respectively]. Independent of patient characteristics like age, gender, FAB and WHO subtype, LDH, and karyotype, advantages for 5-aza were seen in all subgroups analyzed. Interestingly, data by Raj et al. indicate that patients with chromosome 7 anomalies, who generally have a poor prognosis, seem to achieve high response rates with 5-aza treatment (Raj et al. 2007). Mufti et al. have performed a subgroup analysis from the Aza001 study (Mufti et al. 2009) looking at the influence of karyotype for response to 5-aza. Karyotype groups with a significant benefit from 5-aza treatment were del 7/7q- (noncomplex), trisomy 8 (complex and noncomplex), del5/5q- without del7/7q- (noncomplex), and normal karyotype. The worse cytogenetic categories del 7/7q- and del 5/5q- with complex karyotype were associated with the poorest overall survival regardless of treatment. However, patient subgroups in this analysis were small and heterogeneous and only the four most frequent cytogenetic abnormalities could be evaluated. Further subgroup analyses from the Aza001 trial deal with elderly patients and AML according to WHO (RAEB-T). Of 113 elderly patients with a marrow blast count between 20 and 30 %, 55 received 5-aza and 58 conventional care regimens (CCR; 47 % BSC, 34 % LDAC, 19 % IC). At a median follow-up of 20.1 months, median OS for azacytidine-treated patients was 24.5 months compared with 16.0 months for CCR-treated patients [$p = 0.005$], and 2 years OS rates were 50 and 16 %, respectively [$p = 0.001$] (Fenaux et al. 2009). The other analysis compared 5-aza to CCR in the subset of 87 elderly (≥75 years) patients with higher-risk MDS (FAB (RAEB, RAEB-t, CMML) and IPSS (intermediate-2 or high)) from the Aza001 trial. In this subgroup as well, Aza significantly improved OS versus CCR [$p = 0.0193$] and 2-year OS rates were 55 % versus 15 % [$p < 0.001$], respectively.

Induction mortality with 5-aza is low, and side effects include mainly myelosuppression and associated effects, especially during the first cycles. Other side effects, including nausea and vomiting, are generally easily manageable. One side effect occurring in patients receiving 5-aza subcutaneously is skin reactions. Platzbecker et al. (2009) have shown that in some patients evening primrose oil might alleviate inflammatory skin reactions successfully. 5-Aza was approved by the FDA for SC administration based on the CALGB 9221 study. Since the earlier phase II studies with IV azacytidine indicated this to be a safe and efficacious way of drug administration, the FDA recently also approved the use of 5-aza for IV administration. However, no randomized trials show equivalency of the two routes of administration to date, and pharmacokinetics differ.

7.1.2.2 Alternative 5-Azacytidine Schedules and Formulation

An open question regarding the use of 5-aza is the optimal schedule. Most studies used the initially chosen 7-day schedule, but this is inconvenient for patients and doctors due to the necessity of weekend administrations and is clearly not the most frequent schedule chosen in clinical practice. Results of a US trial evaluating three different dosing schedules including 5, 7, or 10 days of 5-aza without weekend injections and including 151 patients show, independently of the alternative dosing regimen, a consistent response for HI, RBC transfusion independence, and safety profile across all subtypes of MDS (Lyons et al. 2009). Regrettably this study did not require pretreatment cytogenetics, did not examine marrow responses, and did not include the conventional 7-day schedule as control arm. Furthermore, most patients treated were lower-risk MDS. Thus, the optimal route of administration and the optimal treatment schedule for 5-aza currently are not clear. Data from named patient programs in Spain and Italy seem at least to point to an inferior effectiveness of reduced dosages like a 5-day schedule (75 mg/m^2) or 100 mg fixed dose versus 75 mg/m^2 (Musto et al. 2010; García et al. 2010). Independent from the optimal dosage, the good results from the confirmatory trial underline the importance of prolonged treatment.

In addition to the approved application in high-risk MDS, 5-aza is increasingly used off-label in lower-risk MDS as well as in AML patients. For both indications no phase III trials have yet demonstrated a survival benefit, except for the RAEB-T subgroup as AML with a low marrow blast count (Fenaux et al. 2010), but phase II trials or retrospective analyses from named patient programs have shown promising response rates (Musto et al. 2010; Thépot et al. 2009; Al-Ali et al. 2012). However given the expected survival time of patients with lower-risk MDS, the need for continuous treatment in case of response should be discussed with the patient in this subgroup with a special emphasis, and there is clearly a need for phase III safety data, regarding the risk for AML evolution.

An oral formulation of the drug has been developed and is currently in phase I trials. Preliminary data were presented at ASH 2009 and ASH 2010 (Garcia-Manero et al. 2011). These data demonstrated safety and a sufficient although variable bioavailability, but the number of patients published is too low to date, to assess efficacy compared to the standard SC administration, and phase III trials are needed.

Further new possibilities for 5-aza include its use as maintenance treatment and the combination with curative treatment approaches like allogeneic stem cell transplantation. As maintenance 5-aza was evaluated after intensive chemotherapy (Grövdal et al. 2010) and allogeneic stem cell transplantation (de Lima et al. 2010). 5-Aza treatment, at a dose of 60 mg/m^2 subsequent to chemotherapy and 32 mg/m^2 in patients after stem cell transplantation, was well tolerated. In both cases 5-aza treatment appeared safe and feasible and may be of benefit in a subset of patients, but again phase III trials are needed to sufficiently evaluate the role of 5-aza in the setting of maintenance therapy. 5-Aza has been used successfully as a bridge to transplantation or at the time of relapse (Czibere et al. 2010; Field et al. 2010); although the experience published to date is limited, this field of application appears very promising as well.

Table 7.1 depicts phase II and phase III studies of 5-aza in MDS patients.

Table 7.1 Clinical trials of 5-aza in MDS

Author	CALGB 8421 (*Ann Hematol*, 1994)	CALGB 8921 (*Ann Hematol*, 1994)	CALGB 9221 (*JCO*, 2002)	Fabre et al. (*ASH*, 2006)	Fenaux et al. (*Lancet Oncol*, 2009)	Lyons et al. (*JCO*, 2009)
Schedule	75 mg/m²/day civ × 7 days every 28 days	75 mg/m²/day SC × 7 days every 28 days	75 mg/m²/day SC × 7 days every 28 days	75 mg/m²/day SC × 7 days every 28 days	75 mg/m²/day SC × 7 days every 28 days	AZA 5-2-2 (75 mg/m²/day × 5 days, 2 days no Tx, 75 mg/m²/day × 2 days); AZA 5-2-5 (50 mg/m²/day × 5 days, 2 days no Tx, 50 mg/m²/day × 5 days); AZA 5 (75 mg/m²/day × 5 days)
Phase	II	II	III	Compassionate use	III	II
Patient number	*n* = 48	*n* = 70	*n* = 99	*n* = 61	*n* = 179	*n* = 139
Response	7 CR (15 %), 1 PR (2 %), 13 HI (27 %), 21 ORR (44 %)	12 CR (17 %), 0 PR (0 %), 16 HI (23 %), 28 ORR (40 %)	10 CR (10 %), 1 PR (1 %), 36 HI (36 %), 47 ORR (47 %)	10 CR (16 %), 15 PR (25 %), 13 HI (21 %), 38 ORR (62 %)	51 (28.5 %) CR and PR	AZA 5-2-2: 20 HI (44 %), AZA 5-2-5 : 23 HI (52 %), AZA 5: 28 HI (57 %)
Toxicity			Myelosuppression, nausea, vomiting	Myelosuppression, local reaction, grade 1–2 gastrointestinal	Myelosuppression, local reactions, nausea, vomiting, diarrhea, fatigue	Myelosuppression

Abbreviations: *civ* continuous intravenous, *SC* subcutaneous, *AZA* 5-azacytidine, *Tx* treatment, *CR* complete remission, *PR* partial remission, *HI* hematologic improvement, *ORR* overall response rate

7.1.3 Combination Treatment of 5-Azacytidine with Histone Deacetylase Inhibitors and Other Drugs

To improve response rate as well as duration, the future of epigenetic therapy probably lies in combination treatments. In this regard one promising approach appears to be the combination with inhibitors of histone deacetylase (HDAC). DNA methylation and modification of histone tails cooperate in the control of gene expression. Several preclinical studies support the view that pharmacologic targeting of both DNMTs and HDACs may result in synergistic anticancer activity (Cameron et al. 1999; Yang et al. 2005). Recently several phase I/II studies have reported encouraging results (Garcia-Manero et al. 2012; Soriano et al. 2007; Blum et al. 2007; Gore et al. 2006; Maslak et al. 2006).

Several phase II trials with 5-aza and valproic acid (VPA) have been performed to date, most of them combining 5-aza with VPA and ATRA, but some added theophylline as well. Phase II trials are often difficult to compare, due to varying patient and response characteristics, which are given in Table 7.2. In a trial conducted by our group with 5-aza (100 mg/m^2 for 5 days) and VPA (continuously, serum trough level of 80–110 μg/ml), 37 % of 24 patients with MDS or AML and 57 % of untreated patients responded. Especially encouraging was the high CR rate of 29 % overall and 55 % for untreated MDS patients (Kuendgen et al. 2011).

Soriano et al. (2007) employed a high-dose intermittent schedule of VPA (50 mg/kg for 7 days) combined with the approved 5-aza dosage and ATRA given at 45 mg/m^2 for 5 days. The study included 49 patients with AML and only 4 MDS patients. Overall response rate was 42 % (52 % in previously untreated patients). CR rate was 27 % (22 % CR and 5 % CRp), and 13 % of patients had only marrow responses. In contrast to the previous study, Voso and co-workers administered VPA at a relatively low dosage (600–1,500 mg) (Voso et al. 2009). ATRA was added in case of nonresponse. Sixty-two patients were enrolled, all with high-risk MDS, but only 26 patients completed 8 cycles and were evaluated for response. 30.7 % of these had CR or PR, and 15.4 % showed hematological improvement. The data from all three studies suggested, independent of the three different dosing regimens administered, that VPA serum levels, but not VPA dosage, had an influence on treatment response. Voso and colleagues postulated pharmacogenomic differences between patients to explain that discrepancy.

Craddock et al. (2013) used a shortened 5-aza schedule (75 mg/m^2 for 5 days) plus VPA, ATRA, and theophylline in 45 patients with AML or MDS. Responses were observed in 15 patients (33 %), after a median of 2 cycles. Finally, a trial by the French study group (Raffoux et al. 2010) combined Aza (75 mg/m^2 for 7 days) with VPA (35–50 mg/kg 7 days) and ATRA (45 mg/m^2 day 8–day 28). Fifty-one patients with high-risk AML or MDS were evaluable, of whom 31 % responded.

Other HDAC inhibitors evaluated in combination with 5-aza include phenylbutyrate (PB) (Gore et al. 2001, 2002), vorinostat (Garcia-Manero et al. 2006), and entinostat. In a phase II trial combining 5-aza with vorinostat at the time of an interim analysis, 17 patients were evaluable for response: 3 (17 %) achieved CR and 4 (23 %) complete marrow CRs (blasts less than 5 %) for an overall response rate 41 %.

Two further studies were conducted with PB plus 5-aza. In a pilot trial, 10 patients (8 AML, 2 MDS) were treated with 5-aza (75 mg/m^2, 7 days) followed by 5 days of

Table 7.2 Comparison of different combination studies with VPA and AZA

Author	Kuendgen et al. (2011)	Soriano et al. (2007)	Voso et al. (2009)	Craddock et al. (2008)	Raffoux et al. (2010)
Drugs	VPA, Aza	VPA, Aza, ATRA	VPA, Aza, ATRA[c]	VPA, Aza, ATRA, theophylline	VPA, Aza, ATRA
Dosage VPA	Median dosage 25 mg/kg continuously	50–75 mg/kg 7 days	600–1,500 mg continuously	ng	35–50 mg/kg 7 days
Dosage AZA	100 mg/m² 5 days	75 mg/m² 7 days	75 mg/m² 7 days	75 mg/m² 5 days	75 mg/m² 7 days
No. of pts.	$n=25$, evaluable 24	$n=53$	$n=62$, 26 evaluable[d]	$n=45$	$n=65$
Median age	73 years	69 years	70 years	66 years	72 years
No. AML/MDS	75 %/25 %[a]	92 %/8 %	31 %/69 %[e]	80 %/20 %	85 %/15 %
Pretreatment	$n=10$ (42 %)	$n=20$ (38 %)	ng	$n=30$ (67 %)	$n=13$ (20 %)
ORR	37 %	27 %[b]	31 %	33 %	26 %
CR/PR/HI/marrow response	7/2/0/4	27/0/0/7	3/5/4/ng	7/8/ng/ng	14/3/ng[g]/ng
Median cycles to response	2 (1–9)	2 (1–3)	5 (2–10) months[f]	2 (1–6)	ng
OS	9 months (23 in responders)	6.5 months (14+ in responders)	14.4 months	ng	12.4 months (19.5 in responders)

Abbreviations: *VPA* valproic acid, *Aza* 5-azacytidine, *ATRA* all-trans retinoic acid, *ORR* overall response rate, *CR* complete response, *PR* partial response, *HI* hematologic improvement, *OS* overall survival, *ng* not given

[a]46 %/54 % according to FAB
[b]42 % including marrow response
[c]Only in nonresponders
[d]At least 8 cycles to be evaluable
[e]100 % according to FAB
[f]Time to CR
[g]12.5 % of nonresponders had HI-erythroid

sodium PB (200 mg/kg) (Maslak et al. 2006). Five patients achieved a clinical response (PR or SD), and one patient received subsequent allogeneic stem cell transplantation. Another study by Gore et al. investigated the optimal dosing schedule for 5-aza in this combination (Gore et al. 2006). The overall response rate was 38 % (11/29), but it was 56 % (5/9) and 50 % (3/6) in the dose cohorts receiving prolonged 5-aza schedules (50 mg/m²/day for 10 days and 25 mg/m² for 14 days, respectively).

A randomized study comparing 5-aza to 5-aza plus entinostat (given simultaneously) could unfortunately not find a benefit for the combination arm but observed a relatively high response rate in general, possibly related to prolonged administration of 5-aza (50 mg/m² for 10 days) (Prebet et al. 2010). Simultaneous dosing may impact on the incorporation of the azanucleotide into DNA via G1 arrest induced by the HDAC inhibitor. Therefore presently a follow-up trial is testing this possibility by also studying the sequential dosing with 5-aza followed by entinostat.

5-Aza has not only been combined with HDAC inhibitors, but promising results from phase I/II studies exist for the combination with lenalidomide (Sekeres et al. 2010) and gemtuzumab ozogamicin (GO), as well. Nand et al. (2008) combined 5-aza with hydroxyurea (HU) and GO. Twenty patients with AML and MDS were treated, of which 14 (70 %) achieved a CR. The median duration of remission was 8 months after one induction and one consolidation cycle, and median survival was 10 months.

Sekeres and co-workers (2010) treated 18 patients with a combination of 5-aza and lenalidomide in a phase I setting. No dose-limiting toxicities occurred, and a maximum-tolerated dose was not reached. The overall response rate was 67 %: 8 patients (44 %) had a CR, 3 patients (17 %) had HI, and one patient (6 %) achieved a marrow CR.

Ongoing trials will furthermore look at the possibility of the combination with other chemotherapeutic agents and the inclusion in induction regimens.

7.2 5-Aza-2′-Deoxycytidine (Decitabine)

7.2.1 Clinical Studies of Decitabine

7.2.1.1 Studies in Previously Untreated MDS and Chronic Myelomonocytic Leukemia (CMML)

Decitabine was first used as a single agent at high doses in clinical trials for the treatment of children with acute leukemias, mostly ALL (Rivard et al. 1981; Momparler et al. 1985). The EORTC Leukemia Group also conducted trials with high-dose decitabine in AML (see below). However, the development of the drug at high doses was discontinued due to the high degree of hematologic and non-hematologic toxicities (reviewed by Lübbert 2000).

As with the 5-aza trials chaired by Prof. Silverman and conducted by the CALGB in the 1980s and 1990s, several clinical trials have been performed in Europe to investigate the effects of decitabine at low, well-tolerated doses in patients with MDS and AML.

First Pinto and co-workers from Aviano (Pinto et al. 1989) published their results of a phase I/II trial with low doses of decitabine in elderly AML/MDS patients, showing an overall response rate (ORR) of 45 % (15 % CR, 30 % PR). Since the early 1990s, Wijermans and co-workers conducted several large low-dose decitabine studies in elderly high-risk MDS patients. In two phase II trials with 29 and 66 patients, ORRs between 49 and 54 % were reached (Wijermans et al. 1997, 2000). CR was associated with cytogenetic remissions (Lübbert et al. 2001). Of note, after only 2 cycles of decitabine treatment, a remarkable improvement in thrombocytopenia was noted in 63 % of the MDS patients (van den Bosch et al. 2004).

In a randomized phase II study at the University of Texas M.D. Anderson Cancer Center (MDACC), dose intensity and subcutaneous route of administration were tested in three schedules of low-dose decitabine in patients with higher-risk MDS and CMML (Kantarjian et al. 2007a). They used total doses of 100 mg/m^2 decitabine given in three alternative schedules: 20 mg/m^2 intravenously (IV) daily for 5 days, 10 mg/m^2 IV daily for 10 days, or 20 mg/m^2 subcutaneously (SC) daily over 5 days.

By a Bayesian adaptive design, the 5-day intravenous schedule was selected as optimal. The arms scored as inferior contained only 14 and 17 patients, respectively. This study has been criticized for its overall statistical design, which may have underestimated the efficacy of the two arms it deemed inferior (Giagounidis 2007); also it did not recapitulate a preferential response of poor-risk cytogenetic patients which occurred with the continuous dosing of decitabine (Rüter et al. 2007). Kantarjian and his colleagues reported an update of this study with an ORR of 70 % (35 % CR) and a median survival of 22 months (Kantarjian et al. 2007b).

In a North American phase III trial of low-dose decitabine (Kantarjian et al. 2006), 170 MDS patients were randomized to receive either decitabine or best supportive care (BSC). The ORR in the study group was 30 % (9 % CR, 8 % PR, 13 % HI), with a median response duration of 10.3 months compared to 7 % HI in the BSC group. Notably, decitabine-treated patients had a prolonged median time to progression to AML or death compared to patients receiving BSC, but this was statistically significant only for IPSS high-risk patients (all patients, 12.1 months versus 7.8 months [$p=0.16$]; patients with IPSS intermediate-2/high-risk disease, 12.0 months versus 6.8 months [$p=0.03$]). Quality of life (QOL) measures were performed and demonstrated a statistically superior quality of life during decitabine treatment regarding global health status, fatigue and dyspnea, when compared to the control arm.

A large European phase III Intergroup trial (EORTC Leukemia Group, German MDS Study Group) randomized 233 patients (decitabine *versus* BSC) with almost exclusively intermediate-2 or high-risk MDS by IPSS (Lübbert et al. 2011). The ORR in the decitabine arm was 34 % (13 % CR, 6 % PR, 15 % HI) *versus* 2 % in the BSC group (2 % HI). Decitabine led to a significant ($p=0.004$) improvement of progression-free survival (0.55 years) as compared to the BSC arm (0.25 years). The median overall survival was not significantly different in both arms (0.84 years (decitabine) *versus* 0.71 years (BSC)). Again QOL was improved by decitabine.

Results of a phase II trial of decitabine in 39 patients with advanced CMML (Braun et al. 2011) revealed an ORR of 38 % (10 % CR, 21 % marrow responses, and 8 % SD with HI). In addition 46 % of all patients demonstrated SD without HI. The median overall survival was 18.2 months. Lee and colleagues reported on 101 patients with MDS and CMML who were treated with decitabine in a Korean observational study (Lee et al. 2011). The overall response rate was 55 % (13 % CR, 23 % marrow CR with or without HI, 1 % PR, 19 % HI). Furthermore 11 % of all patients showed SD. The median overall survival was 17.7 months.

7.2.1.2 Decitabine in the Outpatient Setting

The ADOPT (Alternative Dosing for Outpatient Treatment) trial, a multicenter, nonrandomized, and open-label North American trial, investigated the efficacy and safety of an outpatient regimen using decitabine in 99 MDS patients (Steensma et al. 2009). An ORR of 32 % (CR+mCR) and an overall improvement rate (CR+mCR+PR+HI) of 51 % were reached. In the subgroup of CMML patients, the improvement rate was 73 %. Cytogenetic responses were associated with higher rates of hematological responses, longer durations of transfusion independence, and doubling of projected survival, thus supporting early cytogenetic analysis to predict the hematological response (Goldberg and Steensma 2009).

An international, multicenter, nonrandomized, and open-label study from Argentina and South Korea treated 106 MDS and CMML patients using the same treatment schedule as the ADOPT trial (Iastrebner et al. 2010). The overall improvement rate of 99 assessable patients was 35 % (19 % CR+4 % mCR+4 % PR+8 % HI).

Taking into account the above studies, decitabine is feasible and effective in an outpatient setting. However, this treatment is associated with frequent grade 3–4 hematologic toxicity, requiring dose reduction and frequent dose delay. Cornelison and colleagues (2010) examined this topic further by analyzing data of 124 patients with MDS enrolled in phase II trials using decitabine in different schedules for frontline therapy. The main reasons for dose reduction or dose delay were myelosuppression and infection. There was no impact on clinical outcome (2-year OS, median OS, median TFS) if dose reduction or dose delay took place after achieving the best objective response. Therefore, prospective studies evaluating a treatment approach of decitabine using an induction loading dose for gaining the best objective response followed by a maintenance schedule should be considered.

7.2.1.3 Efficacy of Decitabine in Recurrent Disease

Lübbert, Wijermans, and co-workers addressed the question whether retreatment with decitabine is beneficial in patients with MDS and disease recurrence, given its low nonhematologic toxicity profile, which allows for repeated treatment courses. Twenty-two patients were retreated with low-dose decitabine after a median of 11 months (range: 3–27 months) from the last course of initial therapy. The ORR was 45 %, including one CR, two PR, and seven HI. The duration of this second response was 4 months, approximately 2.5 times shorter in duration than at the first response. The data also suggested superiority of prolonged initial treatment with low-dose decitabine (Rüter et al. 2006).

In MDS patients, even after failure of previous azacitidine treatment, decitabine can still induce responses. Borthakur and colleagues treated 14 patients with low-dose decitabine after failure of prior azacitidine therapy. The ORR was 28 % (21 % CR, 7 % HI), the median duration of remission was 5.3 months, and the median survival time was 6 months (Borthakur et al. 2008).

7.2.1.4 Decitabine in MDS and CMML: Prognostic Factors

Jabbour and colleagues (2013) searched for prognostic factors associated with progression of MDS to AML in patients treated with decitabine. In a combined analysis, 163 MDS patients, treated with two different schedules of decitabine, were stratified on the basis of AML progression or not. Prognostic factors associated with higher risk of transformation to AML were anemia (hemoglobin <10), thrombocytopenia (platelets <50,000/μl), and a cytogenetic risk profile that includes a del(5q) and/or chromosome 7 anomaly. The authors concluded that for this subgroup of patients, additional treatment options beside decitabine should be considered.

We investigated the duration of MDS prior to decitabine treatment as being a novel predictor of poor outcome in patients with high-risk MDS or sAML (Lübbert et al. 2011, 2012). Analysis of the 06011 EORTC-GMDSSG phase III trial (n=233) and the 00331 AML multicenter phase II decitabine trial (n=227, see below) revealed longer duration from MDS diagnosis to start of decitabine to be associated with better outcome. This was found for patients with intermediate-2 and high-risk

MDS. Also AML patients who had a longer MDS duration prior to developing secondary AML and consecutively starting with decitabine also had a better outcome.

The prognosis of patients with MDS or CMML after decitabine failure is usually poor. Jabbour and co-workers (2010) reviewed data from 87 patients with MDS ($n=67$) and CMML ($n=20$) after failure of decitabine treatment. After a median follow-up of 21 months from decitabine failure, 15 % of the patients remained alive. The median survival was 4.3 months and the estimated 12-month survival rate 28 %, with allografted patients having, as expected, the relatively still best outcome.

7.2.2 Clinical Studies of Decitabine in AML

7.2.2.1 Single-Agent Studies

The treatment of elderly patients with AML remains controversial due to the poor outcomes associated with intensive chemotherapy regimens. Hypomethylating agents have shown to improve quality of life and survival in subgroups of patients with AML. The EORTC Leukemia Cooperative Group investigated the efficacy of decitabine in combination with conventional chemotherapy already more than 20 years ago in a phase II study, demonstrating that decitabine has an antileukemic activity in relapsed AML (Willemze et al. 1997).

Evaluating several prolonged low-dose schedules of decitabine in relapsed and refractory leukemias, the dose of 15 mg/m^2 for 10 days appeared to induce the most responses (65 %) (Issa et al. 2004).

Recently, several phase II trials have been published, investigating the treatment with decitabine in older patients with previously untreated AML. The study of Blum and colleagues (2010b) with 53 patients showed an ORR of 64 %. In patients with complex karyotype ($n=16$), the CR rate was 50 % and in patients with normal karyotype 52 %, resulting in an overall CR rate of 47 %. Durations of median overall and disease-free survival were 55 and 46 weeks, respectively. The multicenter study reported by Cashen and co-workers (2010) assessed 55 patients who were treated with decitabine. The ORR was 25 % (24 % CR) and the SD rate was 29 %. The response rate was consistent across subgroups, and the overall median survival was 7.7 months.

Very recently Kantarjian et al. (2012) reported data of a randomized phase III trial of 485 AML patients treated with decitabine *versus* low-dose cytarabine or BSC. Decitabine-treated patients showed higher response rates (CR/CRp 17.8 % in the decitabine arm versus 7.8 % in the cytarabine/BSC arm) and an overall survival advantage (statistically not significant) without relevant differences in safety.

Regarding the clinical activity as second- or third-line treatment, a recent report about decitabine-based salvage therapy in relapsed or refractory AML demonstrated efficacy with low treatment toxicity with a median survival rate of 209 days and a CR rate of 13 % (Ritchie et al. 2009). Therefore, this is an option with low non-hematologic treatment toxicity especially in elderly patients with comorbidities. Table 7.3 depicts clinical trials of decitabine in patients with MDS and CMML, and Table 7.4 summarizes clinical trials of decitabine in acute leukemia and chronic myelogenous leukemia (CML).

Table 7.3 Clinical trials of 5-aza-2′-deoxycytidine (decitabine) in patients with MDS and CMML

Reference	Phase	*N*	Age (range) years	Schedule	% Responses (% CR/PR/HI)	RD (months)	OS (months)
Zagonel et al. (1993)	II	10	68	DAC 45 mg/m^2/day × 3 (IV) (=15 mg/m^2/4 h tid) DAC 50 mg/m^2/day × 3 (civ)	50 (40/10/0)	11	NA
Wijermanset al. (1997)	II	29	72 (58–82)	DAC 40–75 mg/m^2/day × 3 (civ)	54 (28/18/7)	7.3	10.5
Wijermanset al. (2000)	II	66	68 (38–84)	DAC 45 mg/m^2/day × 3 (IV) (=15 mg/m^2/4 h tid)	49 (20/5/24)	7	15
Wijermans et al. (2005)	II	169	70 (38–89)	DAC 45–50 mg/m^2/day × 3 (IV) every 6 weeks	49	40 weeks	15
Rüter et al. (2006)	II (retreatment)	22	71 (51–81)	DAC 45 mg/m^2/day × 3 (IV) (=15 mg/m^2/4 h tid)	14 (4/9/32)	4	27.5[b]
Kantarjian et al (2007a)	II	95	66 (39–90)	20 mg/m^2/day IV q5d every 4 weeks; 20 mg/m^2/day SC q5d every 4 weeks; 10 mg/m^2/day IV q10d every 4 weeks	73 (34/1/28)	NA	19
Kantarjian et al. (2006)	III	89[a]	70 (65–76)	DAC 15 mg/m^2/3 h tid q3d every 6 weeks	17 (9/8/13)	10.3	14
Borthakur et al. (2008)	II	14	74.5 (58–85)	DAC 20 mg/m^2/day IV 1h q5d every 4 weeks	28 (21/0/7)	4	6
Lübbert et al. (2011)	III	233	70 (60–90)	DAC 45 mg/m^2/day × 3 (IV) (=15 mg/m^2/4 h tid)	34 (13/6/15)	8.6	10
Braun et al. (2011)	II	39	71 (54–88)	DAC 20 mg/m^2/day IV q5d every 4 weeks	38 (10/21/8)	NA	18.2
Lee et al. (2011)	IV	101	65 (23–80)	DAC 20 mg/m^2/day IV q5d every 4 weeks	55 (13/24/19)	13.2	17.7
Steensma et al. (2009)	II	99	72 (34–87)	DAC 20 mg/m^2/day IV 1 h q5d every 4 weeks	32 (17/0/18)	10	19.4
Iastrebner et al. (2010)	IV	99	64 (23–84)	DAC 20 mg/m^2/day IV 1 h q5d every 4 weeks	36 (19/8/8)	NA	71 % at 2 years

Table notes: *N* number of patients, *CR* complete response, *PR* partial response, *HI* hematologic improvement, *RD* median response duration, *OS* overall survival, *DAC* decitabine, *IV* intravenous infusion, *civ* continuous intravenous infusion, *q* for, *tid* three times daily, *NA* not available

[a]Patients randomized to receive decitabine;

[b]OS calculated from start of initial decitabine treatment

Table 7.4 Clinical trials of 5-aza-2′-deoxycytidine (decitabine) in acute leukemia and chronic myelogenous leukemia

Patients	*N*	Age (range) years	Drug schedule	% ORR (%CR)	Reference
AML, ALL (relapsed/refractory)	22 (7.15)	9 (2–15)	DAC 0.75–80 mg/kg (12–44 h civ)	14 (9)	Rivard et al. (1981)
AML, ALL (relapsed/refractory)	27 (6.21)	NA (1–20)	DAC 37–80 mg/kg (36–60 h civ)	37 (22)	Momparler et al. (1985)
AML, ALL (relapsed/refractory), CML (myeloid blast crisis)	26 (21.2, 3)	55 (24–74)	DAC 300–500 mg/m^2 (24–120 h civ)	26 (4)	Debusscher et al. (1990)
De novo AML, AML from MDS, CML (not previously treated)	22 (12.8, 2)	74 (62–83)	DAC 45–180 mg/m^2/day × 3 IV (=15–60 mg/m^2/4 h tid)	68 (11)	Zagonel et al. (1990)
AML (not previously treated)	12	64 (47–77)	DAC 270–360 mg/m^2/day × 3 IV (=90–120 mg/m^2/4 h tid)	40 (30)	Petti et al. (1993)
AML (relapsed/refractory)	11	51 (20–63)	DAC 125–250 mg/m^2 bid × 12, amsacrine 120 mg/m^2/day × 2	82 (73)	Richel et al. (1991)
AML (relapsed/refractory)	49	52 (18–65)	DAC 125–250 mg/m^2 bid × 12, amsacrine 120 mg/m^2/day × 2	41 (41)	Willemze et al. (1993, 1997)
AML (relapsed/refractory)	36	57 (NA)	DAC 125–250 mg/m^2 bid × 12, idarubicin 12 mg/m^2/day × 3	44(44)	Willemze et al. (1993, 1997)
De novo AML (not previously treated)	8	44 (30–59)	DAC 90 mg/m^2/day × 5, daunorubicin 50 mg/m^2/day × 3	100 (100)	Schwartsmann et al. (1997)
AML, MDS, CML, ALL (phase I)	48 (35, 7, 5, 1)	60 (2–84)	5, 10, 15, or 20 mg/m^2/day IV 1 h q5d for 2 consecutive weeks	32 (18)	Issa et al. (2004)
De novo AML, high-risk MDS	81 (37.44)	66 (37–85)	DAC 20 mg/m^2/day × 5 every 4 weeks or Aza 75 mg/m^2/day × 7 every 4 weeks	NA (41)	Ravandi et al. (2009)
De novo AML, AML from MDS (phase II)	55	74 (61–87)	DAC 20 mg/m^2/day × 5 IV	25 (24)	Cashen et al. (2010)
De novo AML, therapy-related AML (phase II)	53	74 (60–85)	DAC 20 mg/m^2/day ×10 IV; HU before/during cycle 1 possible	64 (47)	Blum et al. (2010b)

(continued)

Table 7.4 (continued)

Patients	*N*	Age (range) years	Drug schedule	% ORR (%CR)	Reference
AML	227	72 (56–86)	DAC 45 mg/m2/day × 3 IV; ATRA 45 mg/m2/day × 28	26 (13)	Lübbert et al. (2012)
De novo and secondary AML	485	73 (64–91)	DAC 20 mg/m²/day IV 1h q5d every 4 weeks	CR + CRp = 17.8 (15.7)	Kantarjian et al. (2012)
CML (myeloid blast crisis)	31	52 (23–78)	DAC 50–100 mg/m² bid × 10	84 (10)	Kantarjian et al. (1997a, b), Sacchi et al. (1999)
CML (accelerated phase)	17	NA	DAC 50–100 mg/m² bid × 10	53 (0)	Kantarjian et al. (1997a, b)
CML (Ph-positive) blastic phase (BP), accelerated phase (AP), chronic phase (CP)	123	55 (16–78)	DAC 50–100 mg/m² bid × 10	BP: 28 (10) AP: 55 (23) CP: 63 (13)	Kantarjian et al. (2003)

Table notes: *ALL* acute lymphoblastic leukemia, *AML* acute myeloid leukemia, *bid* twice daily, *civ* continuous intravenous infusion, *CML* chronic myeloid leukemia, *CR* complete remission, *DAC* decitabine, *HU* hydroxyurea, *IV* intravenous, *MDS* myelodysplastic syndrome, *NA* not available, *tid* three times daily

7.2.2.2 Clinical Studies of Decitabine in Combination Treatment Regimens in MDS and AML

In a multicenter phase II study (00331), 227 AML patients received decitabine, and patients not having achieved CR or PR but an antileukemic effect (ALE) or SD received an additional treatment of all-*trans* retinoic acid (ATRA) during the second course of decitabine (Lübbert et al. 2012). Best response rate was 52 % (13 % CR, 13 % PR, 26 % ALE). The median survival time was 5.5 months with comparable survival of patients receiving decitabine alone or in combination with ATRA.

Several preclinical studies support the view that pharmacologically targeting both DNA methyltransferase (DNMT) and histone deacetylase (HDAC) may result in synergistic anticancer activity (Cameron et al. 1999; Boivin et al. 2002; Garcia-Manero 2012; Garcia-Manero and Issa 2005).

As a single agent, valproic acid (VPA) has shown HDAC inhibitory activity in lower-risk MDS (Kuendgen et al. 2004). Recently, several phase I/II studies using decitabine or 5-azacytidine in combination with HDAC inhibitors have reported encouraging results (Garcia-Manero et al. 2006; Gore et al. 2006; Maslak et al. 2006; Soriano et al. 2007; Blum et al. 2007). Garcia-Manero and co-workers (2006) treated 54 patients (AML or high-risk MDS) with low-dose decitabine administered concomitantly with escalating doses of VPA. The ORR (CR and PR) was 22 % (19 % CR, 3 % CR but incomplete platelet recovery). It is notable that responses were already achieved after a median of one cycle of treatment, which is earlier than expected with decitabine monotherapy.

A smaller phase I study (Blum et al. 2007) of decitabine plus VPA in 25 AML patients could not verify this beneficial effect of VPA, although responses appeared to occur earlier with the combination treatment *versus* single-agent decitabine, as well. In assessable patients ($n=21$) the ORR was 52 %, but additional VPA led to frequent toxicity in this elderly patient population and revealed no further benefit in respect of clinical responses.

Presently a prospective, randomized, four-armed multicenter phase II study (DECIDER trial) of the German-Austrian Acute Myeloid Leukemia Study Group (AMLSG) is investigating the efficacy of low-dose decitabine alone or in combination with VPA and/or ATRA in patients >60 years with AML who are ineligible for induction chemotherapy (00332/AMLSG14-09; NCT00867672).

Kirschbaum and co-workers (2009) presented their data on a phase I dose-escalation study of the HDAC inhibitor vorinostat (suberoylanilide hydroxamic acid, SAHA) in combination with decitabine for relapsed or newly diagnosed AML or MDS patients ($n=72$). Overall, CR or CRi was achieved by 18 % of the patients with MDS, by 8 % with relapsed/refractory AML and by 36 % with untreated AML. The authors conclude that even with their preliminary data, the combination of vorinostat with decitabine, either concurrently or sequentially, is feasible without significant toxicity.

Panobinostat (LBH589) is a pan-deacetylase inhibitor of both histones and nonhistone proteins and has demonstrated activity in a broad range of hematologic malignancies including AML with in vitro studies demonstrating synergistic mechanism of action with a number of agents including DNA hypomethylating agents. Uy and colleagues (2010) have conducted a phase I study of panobinostat plus decitabine as first-line therapy in elderly patients with advanced MDS ($n=7$) and AML ($n=21$). Of 27 evaluable patients, 7 patients (22 %) achieved a CR and 2 patients a CRi. Response rates were more frequently observed at higher doses of panobinostat (>30 mg/day). Based on this phase I data, a phase II cohort using an increased dose of panobinostat is currently being enrolled (NCT00691938).

Recently, several studies investigated the combination of decitabine with gemtuzumab ozogamicin (GO) in high-risk MDS and AML. Treatment of AML cells with the hypomethylating agent 5-azacytidine increased expression of Ski, a tumor suppressor in AML cells, which interacts with the intracellular part of the CD33 antigen. Untreated AML patients showed high remission rates (70 %) with combined treatment of 5-azacytidine, GO, and hydroxyurea in a phase II study (Nand et al. 2008). Therefore, Borthakur and co-workers (2009) investigated the efficacy and safety of GO with decitabine in previously untreated patients with high-risk MDS ($n=10$) and AML ($n=23$): 24 % of the patients achieved CR, 15 % had clearance of marrow blasts, and one patient had a HI.

In addition, Chowdhury et al. treated a small group of 12 patients with relapsed or refractory AML with a combination of decitabine and GO: 42 % of the patients achieved a CR and subsequently underwent hematopoietic stem cell transplantation (Chowdhury et al. 2009).

Based on these first data, further clinical studies exploring decitabine in combination treatment regimens are needed to achieve higher antitumor efficacy, find optimal dose schedules, and overcome acquired drug resistance due to DNA methylation and gene silencing.

7.2.3 Decitabine Treatment in Other Hematologic Malignancies

7.2.3.1 Decitabine in Patients with Acute Lymphocytic Leukemia (ALL)

The prognosis of refractory acute lymphoblastic leukemia (ALL) after allogeneic hematopoietic stem cell transplantation is very poor, and novel therapeutic agents are warranted to change this situation. Hypermethylation of multiple promoter-associated CpG islands has been frequently identified in ALL patients (Garcia-Manero et al. 2002a, b, 2003; Roman-Gomez et al. 2004, 2007a; Hoshino et al. 2007). Moreover, aberrant methylation is associated with poor prognosis in childhood and adult acute lymphocytic leukemia (Shen et al. 2003; Roman-Gomez et al. 2007b; Kuang et al. 2008; Garcia-Manero et al. 2009a).

Residual DNA methylation at the time of morphologic remission of ALL might predict for worse prognosis. Having this hypothesis, Yang and colleagues (2009) analyzed the methylation levels of p73, p15, and p57 (KIP2) at the time of initial remission in 199 patients with ALL (Philadelphia chromosome (Ph)-negative and MLL-negative). In 123 patients, pretreatment samples were available and compared with remission ones. The presence of residual p73 methylation was associated with a significant lower disease-free survival and overall survival.

Treatment of ALL-derived cell lines with decitabine results in hypomethylation and reexpression of putative tumor suppressor genes (Yang et al. 2005). Garcia-Manero and co-workers designed a phase I study of different dose levels of decitabine in patients with relapsed or refractory ALL (Garcia-Manero 2009c). The ORR was 23 % (one CRp and five complete marrow responses). For patients with relapsed or refractory ALL who do not respond or progress after single-agent decitabine, a parallel study of decitabine combined with hyperCVAD is ongoing. Garcia-Manero and colleagues (2010a) reported the results of the combined treatment schedule at the ASH meeting in 2010. Of 25 patients 52 % achieved a response (16 % CR, 8 % CRp, and 28 % complete marrow responses). No significant toxicity related to the combination was observed.

In summary, these two recent studies indicate decitabine as a single agent and in combination with hyperCVAD to be feasible and safe in patients with relapsed or refractory ALL. Based on these data, further results of additional phase I and II trials investigating the activity of decitabine alone or in combination with conventional intensive chemotherapy in patients with recurrent or refractory ALL are pending.

7.2.3.2 Decitabine in Patients with CML

Prognosis is very poor once CML accelerates and progresses from the chronic phase to blast crisis. If myeloid blast crisis develops, however, remission rates with standard AML-induction chemotherapy regimens are below 20 % (Kantarjian et al. 1993). From 1986 to 1997, high-dose decitabine was used at the MDACC in the treatment of 31 patients with CML in myeloid blast crisis (Sacchi et al. 1999) and 17 patients with CML in accelerated phase (Kantarjian et al. 1997a, b). Objective responses were observed in 26 % of patients in blast crisis, with a median survival of 29 weeks. One of the patients with a complete response had suppression of the Philadelphia (Ph)-positive clone to 25 % of metaphases. Of 17 patients with accelerated phase of CML, 53 % responded to decitabine, with 6 patients achieving a second chronic phase of CML and 2 showing Ph suppression. Prolonged myelosuppression was the major side effect, but no severe non-hematological toxicity was observed. During the same period, a total of 162 adult patients with the diagnosis of CML in nonlymphoid blastic phase were treated at the MDACC either with intensive chemotherapy ($n=90$), with other single agents ($n=41$), or with decitabine ($n=31$), as described above. Decitabine showed similar objective response rates compared to intensive chemotherapy (26 % versus 28 %), whereas other single agents showed objective response rates of 7 %. The median survival times were 29 weeks with decitabine, 21 weeks with intensive chemotherapy, and 22 weeks with other agents. In elderly patients, survival was significantly better with decitabine compared to the other treatment options ($p<0.01$) (Sacchi et al. 1999).

Another study investigated the activity, toxicity, and different dose levels of decitabine in all phases of CML (Kantarjian et al. 2003) in 123 patients with Ph-positive CML (64 blastic, 51 accelerated, 8 chronic) and 7 patients with Ph-negative CML. Objective response rates were 28 % in patients with blastic phase (six complete hematologic responses (CHR), two partial hematologic responses

(PHR), seven HI, and three patients returned to a second chronic phase (CP)), 55 % in patients with accelerated phase (12 CHR, 10 PHR, 3 HI, and 3 second CP), and 63 % in the chronic phase patients. Four of seven patients with Ph-negative CML had objective responses (57 %). The estimated 3-year survival rate was less than 5 % for patients with blastic phase and 27 % for patients in accelerated phase.

In a phase II study, 35 patients with imatinib-resistant CML (12 patients in chronic phase, 17 patients in accelerated phase, and 6 patients in blastic phase) received low-dose decitabine treatment for a total of ten doses (Issa et al. 2005). A CHR was achieved by 34 % of the patients and 20 % of the patients achieved a PHR, resulting in an ORR of 54 %. Complete cytogenetic responses were seen in 6 patients.

In another phase II trial, the combination of low-dose decitabine and imatinib was investigated in 28 patients with CML (25 of whom had already imatinib resistance) (Oki et al. 2007): 32 % of the patients achieved CHR, 4 % PHR, and 7 % showed HI. In addition 18 % achieved major cytogenetic responses and 11 % minor cytogenetic responses.

Decitabine appears to have significant activity in all CML phases; additional studies should evaluate decitabine dose schedules in tyrosine kinase inhibitor (TKI)-resistant CML as well as combinations of decitabine and TKIs in different CML phases.

7.2.3.3 Decitabine in Patients with Idiopathic Myelofibrosis (IMF)

Several investigators have shown that epigenetic changes are implicated in the pathogenesis of idiopathic myelofibrosis (IMF) (Wang et al. 2002; Jones et al. 2004; Bogani et al. 2008).

In a small phase II study, Odenike and co-workers (2006) could demonstrate activity of decitabine given SC in seven patients with myelofibrosis. One patient achieved a CHR; a second patient showed a HI in platelet counts and a decrease in peripheral circulating blasts.

To report on response rates of the combination of decitabine with GO in IMF, Al-Ameri and co-workers (2010) reviewed the records of patients with IMF. They found seven patients being treated with this combination before the FDA withdrew GO from the market due to side effects. Overall, four patients had stable disease, one patient had clearance of marrow blasts, and two patients had no response. The splenic size was decreased in three patients. Summarizing that this combination shows clinical activity in IMF, future investigations will be limited due to the lack of access to GO.

7.3 Conclusion and Future Perspectives

Epigenetic drugs represent a major improvement in our treatment modalities against hematologic malignancies. The most widely used demethylating single agents, 5-azacytidine and decitabine have shown significant activity in MDS and AML at lower dose schedules in many clinical trials. To improve this activity in MDS and

AML, further clinical studies investigating combination regimens with other agents such as HDAC inhibitors, growth factors, cytarabine, and other chemotherapeutic agents are needed. While DNMT inhibitors are already an integral part of treatment, especially in high-risk disease, HDAC inhibitors, particularly the newer substances, have until now mainly been tested in phase I and II trials.

Further investigation of decitabine in CML after treatment failure of tyrosine kinase inhibitors, as well as the use in ALL and other hematologic diseases, i.e., chronic lymphocytic leukemia and other non-Hodgkin lymphomas (Blum et al. 2010a), should be undertaken.

For all epigenetic drugs, the optimal treatment schedules still have to be determined in monotherapy and also in combination regimens. Further analysis is needed to determine which patients, e.g., cytogenetic subgroups, benefit most from the different approaches. Thus biomarkers that will identify those patients with a high or low probability of response are needed.

The development of new compounds with more potent hypomethylating activity is of clinical importance. And hopefully, these new compounds and drug combinations will translate into longer overall survival.

References

Al-Ali HK, Jaekel N, Junghanss C, Maschmeyer G, Krahl R, Cross M, Hoppe G, Niederwieser D (2012) Azacitidine in patients with acute myeloid leukemia medically unfit for or resistant to chemotherapy: a multicenter phase I/II study. Leuk Lymphoma 53:110–117

Al-Ameri AA, Kantarjian H, Malik A, Badoux X, Andreeff M, Quintas-Cardama A, Borthakur G (2010) Decitabine and gemtuzumab ozogamicin in patients with advanced myelofibrosis. Blood (ASH Annu Meet Abstr) 116:5061

Blum W, Klisovic RB, Hackanson B, Liu Z, Liu S, Devine H, Vukosavljevic T, Huynh L, Lozanski G, Kefauver C, Plass C, Devine SM, Heerema NA, Murgo A, Chan KK, Grever MR, Byrd JC, Marcucci G (2007) Phase I study of decitabine alone or in combination with valproic acid in acute myeloid leukemia. J Clin Oncol 25:3884–3891

Blum KA, Liu Z, Lucas DM, Chen P, Xie Z, Baiocchi R, Benson DM, Devine SM, Jones J, Andritsos L, Flynn J, Plass C, Marcucci G, Chan KK, Grever MR, Byrd JC (2010a) Phase I trial of low dose decitabine targeting DNA hypermethylation in patients with chronic lymphocytic leukaemia and non-Hodgkin lymphoma: dose-limiting myelosuppression without evidence of DNA hypomethylation. Br J Haematol 150:189–195

Blum W, Garzon R, Klisovic RB, Schwind S, Walker A, Geyer S, Liu S, Havelange V, Becker H, Schaaf L, Mickle J, Devine H, Kefauver C, Devine SM, Chan KK, Heerema NA, Bloomfield CD, Grever MR, Byrd JC, Villalona-Calero M, Croce CM, Marcucci G (2010b) Clinical response and miR-29b predictive significance in older AML patients treated with a 10-day schedule of decitabine. Proc Natl Acad Sci USA 107:7473–7478

Bogani C, Ponziani V, Guglielmelli P, Desterke C, Rosti V, Bosi A, Le Bousse-Kerdiles MC, Barosi G, Vannucchi AM (2008) Hypermethylation of CXCR4 promoter in CD34+ cells from patients with primary myelofibrosis. Stem Cells 26:1920–1930

Boivin AJ, Momparler LF, Hurtubise A, Momparler RL (2002) Antineoplastic action of 5-aza-2′-deoxycytidine and phenylbutyrate on human lung carcinoma cells. Anticancer Drugs 13:869–874

Borthakur G, Ahdab SE, Ravandi F, Faderl S, Ferrajoli A, Newman B, Issa JP, Katarjian H (2008) Activity of decitabine in patients with myelodysplastic syndrome previously treated with azacitidine. Leuk Lymphoma 49:690–695

Borthakur G, Garcia-Manero G, Estrov Z, Konopleva M, Burger JA, Thomas DA, Kadia T, Williams B, George S, Kantarjian H (2009) Phase 2 study of decitabine and gemtuzumab ozogamicin in acute myelogenous leukemia and high-risk myelodysplastic syndrome – outcome in previously untreated patients. Blood (ASH Annu Meet Abstr) 114:1053

Braun T, Itzykson R, Renneville A, de Renzis B, Dreyfus F, Laribi K, Bouabdallah K, Vey N, Toma A, Recher C, Royer B, Joly B, Vekhoff A, Lafon I, Sanhes L, Meurice G, Orear C, Preudhomme C, Gardin C, Ades L, Fontenay M, Fenaux P, Droin N, Solary E, on behalf of the Groupe Francophone des Myelodysplasies (2011) Molecular predictors of response to decitabine in advanced chronic myelomonocytic leukemia: a phase 2 trial. Blood 118:3824–3831

Cameron EE, Bachman KE, Myohanen S, Herman JG, Baylin SB (1999) Synergy of demethylation and histone deacetylase inhibition in the re-expression of genes silenced in cancer. Nat Genet 21:103–107

Cashen AF, Schiller GJ, O'Donnell MR, DiPersio JF (2010) Multicenter, phase II study of decitabine for the first-line treatment of older patients with acute myeloid leukemia. J Clin Oncol 28:556–561

Cheson BD, Bennett JM, Kantarjian H, Pinto A, Schiffer CA, Nimer SD, Löwenberg B, Beran M, de Witte TM, Stone RM, Mittelman M, Sanz GF, Wijermans PW, Gore S, Greenberg PL, World Health Organization (WHO) International Working Group (2000) Report of an international working group to standardize response criteria for myelodysplastic syndromes. Blood 96:3671–3674

Chowdhury S, Seropian S, Marks PW (2009) Decitabine combined with fractionated gemtuzumab ozogamicin therapy in patients with relapsed or refractory acute myeloid leukemia. Am J Hematol 84:599–600

Cornelison AM, Garcia Manero G, Kantarjian H, Ravandi F, Kadia T, Cortes J, O'Brien S, Borthakur G, Brandt M, Jabbour EJ (2010) Decitabine (DAC) can be safely reduced after achievement of best response in patients (pts) with myelodysplastic syndrome (MDS). Blood (ASH Annu Meet Abstr) 116:1858

Craddock C, Quek L, Goardon N, Freeman S, Siddique S, Raghavan M et al (2013) Azacitidine fails to eradicate leukemic stem/progenitor cell populations in patients with acute myeloid leukemia and myelodysplasia. Leukemia 27(5):1028–1036

Czibere A, Bruns I, Kröger N, Platzbecker U, Lind J, Zohren F, Fenk R, Germing U, Schröder T, Gräf T, Haas R, Kobbe G (2010) 5-Azacytidine for the treatment of patients with acute myeloid leukemia or myelodysplastic syndrome who relapse after allo-SCT: a retrospective analysis. Bone Marrow Transplant 45:872–876

de Lima M, Giralt S, Thall PF, de Padua Silva L, Jones RB, Komanduri K, Braun TM, Nguyen HQ, Champlin R, Garcia-Manero G (2010) Maintenance therapy with low-dose azacitidine after allogeneic hematopoietic stem cell transplantation for recurrent acute myelogenous leukemia or myelodysplastic syndrome: a dose and schedule finding study. Cancer 116:5420–5431

Debusscher L, Marie JP, Dodion P, Blanc GM, Arrigo C, Zittoun R, Stryckmans P (1990) Phase-I-II trial of 5-aza-2′-deoxycytidine in adult patients with acute leukemia. In: Momparler RL, de Vos D (eds) 5-Aza-2′-deoxycytidine: preclinical and clinical studies. PCH, Haarlem, pp 131–142

Fabre, Claire, Chermat, Fatsiha, Legros, Laurence, Park, Sophie, Dreyfus, Francois, Isnard, Francoise, Nowak, Florence, Marfaing, Anne, de Botton, Stephane, Noel, Marie-Pierre, Fruchart, Christophe, Prebet, Thomas, Vey, Norbert, Dartigeas, Caroline, Fenaux, Pierre (2006) Treatment of high risk MDS and AML Post-MDS with Azacytidine (AZA): preliminary results of the French ATU program. ASH Annual Meeting Abstracts 108:2664

Fenaux P, Mufti GJ, Hellstrom-Lindberg E, Santini V, Finelli C, Giagounidis A, Schoch R, Gattermann N, Sanz G, List A, Gore SD, Seymour JF, Bennett JM, Byrd J, Backstrom J, Zimmerman L, McKenzie D, Beach C, Silverman LR, International Vidaza High-Risk MDS Survival Study Group (2009) Efficacy of azacitidine compared with that of conventional care regimens in the treatment of higher-risk myelodysplastic syndromes: a randomized, open-label, phase III study. Lancet Oncol 10:223–232

Fenaux P, Mufti GJ, Hellström-Lindberg E, Santini V, Gattermann N, Germing U, Sanz G, List AF, Gore S, Seymour JF, Dombret H, Backstrom J, Zimmerman L, McKenzie D, Beach CL,

Silverman LR (2010) Azacitidine prolongs overall survival compared with conventional care regimens in elderly patients with low bone marrow blast count acute myeloid leukemia. J Clin Oncol 28:562–569

Field T, Perkins J, Huang Y, Kharfan-Dabaja MA, Alsina M, Ayala E, Fernandez HF, Janssen W, Lancet J, Perez L, Sullivan D, List A, Anasetti C (2010) 5-Azacitidine for myelodysplasia before allogeneic hematopoietic cell transplantation. Bone Marrow Transplant 45:255–260

García R, Arnar M, Luño E, Bargay J, Ma Mar Romero, Besalduch J, Amutio E, Garrido R, Carnicero F, Grupo Andaluz de Smd (2010) Efficacy and effectiveness of azacitidine in elderly patients with acute myeloid leukemia and blasts counts below 30%: experience of the Spanish registry. Blood (ASH Annu Meet Abstr) 116:4354

Garcia-Manero G, Issa JP (2005) Histone deacetylase inhibitors: a review of their clinical status as antineoplastic agents. Cancer Invest 23:635–642

Garcia-Manero G, Daniel J, Smith TL, Kornblau SM, Lee MS, Kantarjian HM, Issa JP (2002a) DNA methylation of multiple promoter-associated CpG islands in adult acute lymphocytic leukemia. Clin Cancer Res 8:2217–2224

Garcia-Manero G, Bueso-Ramos C, Daniel J, Williamson J, Kantarjian HM, Issa JP (2002b) DNA methylation patterns at relapse in adult acute lymphocytic leukemia. Clin Cancer Res 8:1897–1903

Garcia-Manero G, Jeha S, Daniel J, Williamson J, Albitar M, Kantarjian HM, Issa JP (2003) Aberrant DNA methylation in pediatric patients with acute lymphocytic leukemia. Cancer 3:695–702

Garcia-Manero G, Kantarjian HM, Sanchez-Gonzalez B, Yang H, Rosner G, Verstovsek S, Rytting M, Wierda WG, Ravandi F, Koller C, Xiao L, Faderl S, Estrov Z, Cortes J, O'brien S, Estey E, Bueso-Ramos C, Fiorentino J, Jabbour E, Issa JP (2006) Phase 1/2 study of the combination of 5-aza-2′-deoxycytidine with valproic acid in patients with leukemia. Blood 108:3271–3279

Garcia-Manero G, Couriel DR, Tambaro FP, Gabrail N, Nadeem A, Kadia T, Jabbour E, Borthakur G, Faderl S, Newsome W, Yang H, Chen K, Stein K, Kantarjian H (2009a) A phase II Randomized Bayesian Study of very low dose subcutaneous decitabine administered daily or weekly times three in patients with lower risk myelodysplastic syndrome (MDS). Blood (ASH Annu Meet Abstr) 114:119

Garcia-Manero G, Yang H, Kuang SQ, O'Brien S, Thomas D, Kantarjian H (2009b) Epigenetics of acute lymphocytic leukemia. Semin Hematol 46:24–32

Garcia-Manero G, Thomas D, Rytting M, Zweidler-McKay PA, Yang H, Fang Z, Kuang S, Dara S, O'Brien S, Kantarjian HM (2009c) A phase 1 study of dose-dense 5-Aza-2′-deoxycitidine (decitabine) in relapse refractory acute lymphocytic leukemia (ALL). Blood (ASH Annu Meet Abstr) 114:2030

Garcia-Manero G, Thomas DA, Rytting ME, O'Brien S, Franklin ARK, Borthakur G, Kwari M, Dara S, Yang H, Kantarjian H (2010) Final report of a phase I trial of decitabine with or without hyperCVAD in relapsed acute lymphocytic leukemia (ALL). Blood (ASH Annu Meet Abstr) 116:Abstract 867

Garcia-Manero G, Gore SD, Cogle C, Ward R, Shi T, Macbeth KJ, Laille E, Giordano H, Sakoian S, Jabbour E, Kantarjian H, Skikne B (2011) Phase I study of oral azacitidine in myelodysplastic syndromes, chronic myelomonocytic leukemia, and acute myeloid leukemia. J Clin Oncol 29(18):2521–2527

Garcia-Manero G, Tambaro FP, Bekele NB, Yang H, Ravandi F, Jabbour E, Borthakur G, Kadia TM, Konopleva MY, Faderl S, Cortes JE, Brandt M, Hu Y, McCue D, Newsome WM, Pierce SR, de Lima M, Kantarjian HM (2012) Phase II trial of vorinostat with idarubicin and cytarabine for patients with newly diagnosed acute myelogenous leukemia or myelodysplastic syndrome. J Clin Oncol 30(18):2204–2210

Giagounidis AA (2007) Decitabine dosage in myelodysplastic syndromes. Blood 110:1082–1083

Goldberg SL, Steensma DP (2009) Myelodysplastic syndrome patients obtaining a cytogenetic response to outpatient decitabine experience improved hematological responses and longer survival: additional analyses from the ADOPT trial. Blood (ASH Annu Meet Abstr) 114:3817

Gore SD, Weng LJ, Figg WD, Zhai S, Donehower RC, Dover G, Grever MR, Griffin C, Grochow LB, Hawkins A, Burks K, Zabelena Y, Miller CB (2001) Impact of the putative differentiating agent sodium phenylbutyrate on myelodysplastic syndromes and acute myeloid leukemia. Clin Cancer Res 7:2330–2339

Gore SD, Weng LJ, Zhai S, Figg WD, Donehower RC, Dover GJ, Grever M, Griffin CA, Grochow LB, Rowinsky EK, Zabalena Y, Hawkins AL, Burks K, Miller CB (2002) Impact of prolonged infusions of the putative differentiating agent sodium phenylbutyrate on myelodysplastic syndromes and acute myeloid leukemia. Clin Cancer Res 8:963–970

Gore SD, Baylin S, Sugar E, Carraway H, Miller CB, Carducci M, Grever M, Galm O, Dauses T, Karp JE, Rudek MA, Zhao M, Smith BD, Manning J, Jiemjit A, Dover G, Mays A, Zwiebel J, Murgo A, Weng LJ, Herman JG (2006) Combined DNA methyltransferase and histone deacetylase inhibition in the treatment of myeloid neoplasms. Cancer Res 66:6361–6369

Grövdal M, Karimi M, Khan R, Aggerholm A, Antunovic P, Astermark J, Bernell P, Engström LM, Kjeldsen L, Linder O, Nilsson L, Olsson A, Holm MS, Tangen JM, Wallvik J, Oberg G, Hokland P, Jacobsen SE, Porwit A, Hellström-Lindberg E (2010) Maintenance treatment with azacytidine for patients with high-risk myelodysplastic syndromes (MDS) or acute myeloid leukaemia following MDS in complete remission after induction chemotherapy. J Haematol 150:293–302

Hoshino K, Quintás-Cardama A, Yang H, Sanchez-Gonzalez B, Garcia-Manero G (2007) Aberrant DNA methylation of the Src kinase Hck, but not of Lyn, in Philadelphia chromosome negative acute lymphocytic leukemia. Leukemia 21:906–911

Iastrebner M, Jang JH, Nucifora E, Kim K, Sackmann F, Kim DH, Orlando S, Jung CW, Basquiera A, Klein G, Santini F, Bernard HI, Korin J, Taborda G (2010) Decitabine in myelodysplastic syndromes and chronic myelomonocytic leukemia: Argentinian/South Korean multi-institutional clinical experience. Leuk Lymphoma 12:2250–2257

Issa J-PJ, Garcia-Manero G, Giles FJ, Mannari R, Thomas D, Faderl S, et al (2004) Phase 1 study of low-dose prolonged exposure schedules of the hypomethylating agent 5-aza-2′-deoxycytidine (decitabine) in hematopoietic malignancies. Blood 103(5):1635–40

Issa JP, Gharibyan V, Cortes J, Jelinek J, Morris G, Verstovsek S, Talpaz M, Garcia-Manero G, Kantarjian HM (2005) Phase II study of low dose decitabine in patients with chronic myelogenous leukemia resistant to imatinib mesylate. J Clin Oncol 23:3948–3956

Jabbour E, Garcia-Manero G, Batty N, Shan J, O'Brien S, Cortes J, Ravandi F, Issa JP, Kantarjian H (2010) Outcome of patients with myelodysplastic syndrome after failure of decitabine therapy. Cancer 116:3830–3834

Jabbour E, Garcia-Manero G, Ravandi F, Faderl S, O'Brien S, Fullmer A, Cortes JE, Wierda W, Kantarjian H (2013) Prognostic factors associated with disease progression and overall survival in patients with myelodysplastic syndromes treated with decitabine. Clin Lymphoma Myeloma Leuk 13(2):131–138

Jones LC, Tefferi A, Idos GE, Kumagai T, Hofmann WK, Koeffler HP (2004) RARbeta2 is a candidate tumor suppressor gene in myelofibrosis with myeloid metaplasia. Oncogene 23:7846–7853

Kantarjian HM, Deisseroth A, Kurzrock R, Estrov Z, Talpaz M (1993) Chronic myelogenous leukemia: a concise update. Blood 82:691–703

Kantarjian HM, O'Brien SM, Estey E, Giralt S, Beran M, Rios MB, Keating M, De Vos D, Talpaz M (1997a) Decitabine studies in chronic and acute myelogenous leukemia. Leukemia 11(Suppl 1):35–36

Kantarjian HM, O'Brien SM, Keating M, Beran M, Estey E, Giralt S, Kornblau S, Rios MB, De Vos D, Talpaz M (1997b) Results of decitabine therapy in the accelerated and blastic phases of chronic myelogenous leukemia. Leukemia 11:1617–1620

Kantarjian HM, O'Brien S, Cortes J, Giles FJ, Faderl S, Issa JP, Garcia-Manero G, Rios MB, Shan J, Andreeff M, Keating M, Talpaz M (2003) Results of decitabine (5-aza-2′-deoxycytidine) therapy in 130 patients with chronic myelogenous leukemia. Cancer 98:522–528

Kantarjian HM, Issa JP, Rosenfeld CS, Bennett JM, Albitar M, DiPersio J, Klimek V, Slack J, de Castro C, Ravandi F, Helmer R 3rd, Shen L, Nimer SD, Leavitt R, Raza A, Saba H (2006) Decitabine improves patient outcomes in myelodysplastic syndromes: results of a phase III randomized study. Cancer 106:1794–1803

Kantarjian HM, Oki Y, Garcia-Manero G, Huang X, O'Brien S, Cortes J, Faderl S, Bueso-Ramos C, Ravandi F, Estrov Z, Ferrajoli A, Wierda W, Shan J, Davis J, Giles F, Saba HI, Issa JP

(2007a) Results of a randomized study of 3 schedules of low-dose decitabine in higher-risk myelodysplastic syndrome and chronic myelomonocytic leukemia. Blood 109:52–57

Kantarjian HM, O'Brien S, Shan J, Aribi A, Garcia-Manero G, Jabbour E, Ravandi F, Cortes J, Davisson J, Issa JP (2007b) Update of the decitabine experience in higher risk myelodysplastic syndrome and analysis of prognostic factors associated with outcome. Cancer 109(2):265–273

Kantarjian HM, Thomas XG, Dmoszynska A, Wierzbowska A, Mazur G, Mayer J, Gau J-P, Chou W-C, Buckstein R, Cermak J, Kuo C-Y, Oriol A, Ravandi F, Faderl S, Delaunay J, Lysák D, Minden M, Arthur C (2012) Multicenter, randomized, open-label, phase III trial of decitabine versus patient choice, with physician advice, of either supportive care or low-dose cytarabine for the treatment of older patients with newly diagnosed acute myeloid leukemia. J Clin Oncol 30:2670–2677

Kirschbaum M, Gojo I, Goldberg SL, Kujawski L, Atallah E, Marks P, Gravio D, Pyle L, Rizvi S, Issa JP (2009) Vorinostat in combination with decitabine for the treatment of relapsed or newly diagnosed acute myelogenous leukemia (AML) or myelodysplastic syndrome (MDS): a phase I, dose-escalation study. Blood (ASH Annu Meet Abstr) 114:2089

Kuang SQ, Tong WG, Yang H, Lin W, Lee MK, Fang ZH, Wei Y, Jelinek J, Issa JP, Garcia-Manero G (2008) Genome-wide identification of aberrantly methylated promoter associated CpG islands in acute lymphoblastic leukemia. Leukemia 8:1529–1538

Kuendgen A, Strupp C, Aivado M, Bernhardt A, Hildebrandt B, Haas R, Germing U, Gattermann N (2004) Treatment of myelodysplastic syndromes with valproic acid alone or in combination with all-trans retinoic acid. Blood 104:1266–1269

Kuendgen A, Bug G, Ottmann OG, Haase D, Schanz J, Hildebrandt B, Nachtkamp K, Neukirchen J, Dienst A, Haas R, Germing U, Gattermann N (2011) Treatment of poor-risk myelodysplastic syndromes and acute myeloid leukemia with a combination of 5-azacytidine and valproic acid. Clin Epigenetics 2(2):389–399

Lee J-H, Jang JH, Park J, Park S, Joo Y-D, Kim Y-K, Kim H-G, Choi CW, Kim S-H, Park SK, Park E, Min YH (2011) A prospective multicenter observational study of decitabine treatment in Korean patients with myelodysplastic syndrome. Haematologica 96:1441–1447

Lübbert M (2000) DNA methylation inhibitors in the treatment of leukemias, myelodysplastic syndromes and hemoglobinopathies: clinical results and possible mechanisms of action. Curr Top Microbiol Immunol 249:135–164

Lübbert M, Wijermans P, Kunzmann R, Verhoef G, Bosly A, Ravoet C, Andre M, Ferrant A (2001) Cytogenetic responses in high-risk myelodysplastic syndrome following low-dose treatment with DNA methylation inhibitor 5-aza-2′-deoxycytidine. Br J Haematol 114:349–357

Lübbert M, Suciu S, Baila L, Rüter BH, Platzbecker U, Giagounidis A, Selleslag D, Labar B, Germing U, Salih HR, Beeldens F, Muus P, Pflüger KH, Coens C, Hagemeijer A, Schaefer HE, Ganser A, Aul C, de Witte T, Wijermans PW (2011) Low-dose decitabine versus best supportive care in elderly patients with intermediate- or high-risk myelodysplastic syndrome (MDS) ineligible for intensive chemotherapy: final results of the randomized phase III study of the European Organization for Research and Treatment of Cancer Leukemia Group and the German MDS Study Group. J Clin Oncol 29:1987–1996

Lübbert M, Rüter BH, Claus R, Schmoor C, Schmid M, Germing U, et al (2012) A multicenter phase II trial of decitabine as first-line treatment for older patients with acute myeloid leukemia judged unfit for induction chemotherapy. Haematologica 97(3):393–401

Lyons RM, Cosgriff TM, Modi SS, Gersh RH, Hainsworth JD, Cohn AL, McIntyre HJ, Fernando IJ, Backstrom JT, Beach CL (2009) Hematologic response to three alternative dosing schedules of azacitidine in patients with myelodysplastic syndromes. J Clin Oncol 27:1850–1856

Maslak P, Chanel S, Camacho LH, Soignet S, Pandolfi PP, Guernah I, Warrell R, Nimer S (2006) Pilot study of combination transcriptional modulation therapy with sodium phenylbutyrate and 5-azacytidine in patients with acute myeloid leukemia or myelodysplastic syndrome. Leukemia 2:212–217

Momparler RL, Rivard GE, Gyger M (1985) Clinical trial on 5-aza-2′-deoxycytidine in patients with acute leukemia. Pharmacol Ther 30:277–286

Mufti GH, Gore SD, Santini V, Fenaux P, Silverman LR, Hagemeijer A, Skikne B, Hellstrom-Lindberg E, Seymour JF, Beach CL, Backstrom J, Fernando I (2009) Influence of karyotype on overall survival in patients with higher-risk myelodysplastic syndrome treated with azacitidine or a conventional care regimen. Blood (ASH Annu Meet Abstr) 114:1755

Musto P, Maurillo L, Spagnoli A, Gozzini A, Rivellini F, Lunghi M, Villani O, Aloe-Spiriti MA, Venditti A, Santini V, Ad Hoc Italian Cooperative Study Group on Azacitidine in Myelodysplastic Syndromes Acute Leukemias (2010) Azacitidine for the treatment of lower risk myelodysplastic syndromes: a retrospective study of 74 patients enrolled in an Italian named patient program. Cancer 116:1485–1494

Nand S, Godwin J, Smith S, Barton K, Michaelis L, Alkan S, Veerappan R, Rychlik K, Germano E, Stiff P (2008) Hydroxyurea, azacitidine and gemtuzumab ozogamicin therapy in patients with previously untreated non-M3 acute myeloid leukemia and high-risk myelodysplastic syndromes in the elderly: results from a pilot trial. Leuk Lymphoma 49:2141–2147

Odenike OM, Godwin JE, van Besien K, Huo D, Stiff PJ, Sher D, Klekowski N, Green M, Larson RA, Stock W (2006) Phase II study of decitabine in myelofibrosis with myeloid metaplasia. Blood (ASH Annu Meet Abstr) 108:4923

Oki Y, Kantarjian H, Gharibyan V, Jones D, O'brien S, Verstovsek S, Cortes J, Morris GM, Garcia-Manero G, Issa JP (2007) Phase II study of low-dose decitabine in combination with imatinib mesylate in patients with accelerated or myeloid blastic phase of chronic myelogenous leukemia. Cancer 109:899–906

Petti MC, Mandelli F, Zagonel V, De Gregoris C, Merola MC, Latagliata R, Gattei V, Fazi P, Monfardini S, Pino A (1993) Pilot study of 5-aza-2′-deoxycytidine (decitabine) in the treatment of poor prognosis acute myelogenous leukemia patients: preliminary results. Leukemia 7:36–41

Pinto A, Zagonel V, Attadia V, Bullian PL, Gattei V, Carbone A, Monfardini S, Colombatti A (1989) 5-aza-2′-deoxycytidine as a differentiation inducer in acute myeloid leukaemias and myelodysplastic syndromes of the elderly. Bone Marrow Transplant 4(Suppl 3):28–32

Platzbecker U, Aul C, Ehninger G, Giagounidis A (2009) Reduction of 5-azacitidine induced skin reactions in MDS patients with evening primrose oil. Ann Hematol 89:427–428

Prebet T, Gore SD, Sun Z, Greenberg PL, Juckett M, Malick L, Smith MR, Paietta E, Czader M, Gabrilove J, Erba HP, Tallman MS (2010) Prolonged administration of azacitidine with or without entinostat increases rate of hematologic normalization for myelodysplastic syndrome and acute myeloid leukemia with myelodysplasia-related changes: results of the US Leukemia Intergroup Trial E1905. Blood (ASH Annu Meet Abstr) 116:601

Raffoux E, Cras A, Recher C, Boëlle PY, de Labarthe A, Turlure P, Marolleau JP, Reman O, Gardin C, Victor M, Maury S, Rousselot P, Malfuson JV, Maarek O, Daniel MT, Fenaux P, Degos L, Chomienne C, Chevret S, Dombret H (2010) Phase 2 clinical trial of 5-azacitidine, valproic acid, and all-trans retinoic acid in patients with high-risk acute myeloid leukemia or myelodysplastic syndrome. Oncotarget 1:34–42

Raj K, John A, Ho A, Chronis C, Khan S, Samuel J, Pomplun S, Thomas NS, Mufti GJ (2007) CDKN2B methylation status and isolated chromosome 7 abnormalities predict responses to treatment with 5-azacytidine. Leukemia 21:1937–1944

Ravandi F, Issa JP, Garcia-Manero G, O'Brien S, Pierce S, Shan J, Borthakur G, Verstovsek S, Faderl S, Cortes J, Kantarjian H (2009) Superior outcome with hypomethylating therapy in patients with acute myeloid leukemia and high-risk myelodysplastic syndrome and chromosome 5 and 7 abnormalities. Cancer 115:5746–5751

Richel DJ, Colly LP, Kluin-Nelemans JC, Willemze R (1991) The antileukemic activity of 5-aza-2′-deoxycytidine (Aza-dC) in patients with relapsed and resistant leukemia. Br J Cancer 64:144–148

Ritchie EK, Arnason J, Feldman EJ, Gergis US, Mayer SA, Ippoliti C, Scandura JM, Roboz G (2009) Decitabine-based salvage therapy in adults with acute myeloid leukemia. Blood (ASH Annu Meet Abstr) 114:2063

Rivard GE, Momparler RL, Demers J, Benoit P, Raymond R, Lin K, Momparler LF (1981) Phase I study on 5-aza-2′-deoxycytidine in children with acute leukemia. Leuk Res 5:453–462

Roman-Gomez J, Jimenez-Velasco A, Castillejo JA, Agirre X, Barrios M, Navarro G, Molina FJ, Calasanz MJ, Prosper F, Heiniger A, Torres A (2004) Promoter hypermethylation of cancer-related genes: a strong independent prognostic factor in acute lymphoblastic leukemia. Blood 10:2492–2498

Roman-Gomez J, Cordeu L, Agirre X, Jimenez-Velasco A, San Jose-Eneriz E, Garate L, Calasanz MJ, Heiniger A, Torres A, Prosper F (2007a) Epigenetic regulation of Wnt-signaling pathway in acute lymphoblastic leukemia. Blood 8:3462–3469

Roman-Gomez J, Jimenez-Velasco A, Barrios M, Prosper F, Heiniger A, Torres A, Agirre X (2007b) Poor prognosis in acute lymphoblastic leukemia may relate to promoter hypermethylation of cancer-related genes. Leuk Lymphoma 48:1269–1282

Rüter B, Wijermans PW, Lübbert M (2006) Superiority of prolonged low-dose azanucleoside administration? Results of 5-aza-2′-deoxycytidine retreatment in high risk myelodysplasia patients. Cancer 106:1744–1750

Rüter B, Wijermans P, Claus R, Kunzmann R, Lübbert M (2007) Preferential cytogenetic response to continuous intravenous low-dose decitabine (DAC) administration in myelodysplastic syndrome with chromosome 7 abnormalities. Blood 110:1080–1082

Sacchi S, Kantarjian HM, O'Brien S, Cortes J, Rios MB, Giles FJ, Beran M, Koller CA, Keating MJ, Talpaz M (1999) Chronic myelogenous leukemia in nonlymphoid blastic phase: analysis of the results of first salvage therapy with three different treatment approaches for 162 patients. Cancer 86:2632–2641

Schwartsmann G, Fernandes MS, Schaan MD, Moschen M, Gerhardt LM, DiLeone L, Loitzembauer B, Kalakun L (1997) Decitabine (5-aza-2′-deoxycytidine; decitabine) plus daunorubicin as a first line treatment in patients with acute myeloid leukemia: preliminary observations. Leukemia 11(Suppl 1):28–31

Sekeres MA, List AF, Cuthbertson D, Paquette R, Ganetzky R, Latham D, Paulic K, Afable M, Saba HI, Loughran TP Jr, Maciejewski JP (2010) Phase I combination trial of lenalidomide and azacitidine in patients with higher-risk myelodysplastic syndromes. J Clin Oncol 28:2253–2258

Shen L, Toyota M, Kondo Y, Obata T, Daniel S, Pierce S, Imai K, Kantarjian HM, Issa JP, Garcia-Manero G (2003) Aberrant DNA methylation of p57KIP2 identifies a cell cycle regulatory pathway with prognostic impact in adult acute lymphocytic leukemia. Blood 101:4131–4136

Silverman LR, Holland JF, Demakos EP (1994) Azacitidine (aza C) in myelodysplastic syndromes (MDS), CALGB studies 8421 and 8921. Ann Hematol 68:A12

Silverman LR, Demakos EP, Peterson BL, Kornblith AB, Holland JC, Odchimar-Reissig R, Stone RM, Nelson D, Powell BL, DeCastro CM, Ellerton J, Larson RA, Schiffer CA, Holland JF (2002) Randomized controlled trial of azacitidine in patients with the myelodysplastic syndrome: a study of the cancer and leukemia group B. J Clin Oncol 20:2429–2440

Silverman LR, McKenzie DR, Peterson BL, Holland JF, Backstrom JT, Beach CL, Larson RA, Cancer and Leukemia Group B (2006) Further analysis of trials with azacitidine in patients with myelodysplastic syndrome: studies 8421, 8921, and 9221 by the Cancer and Leukemia Group B. J Clin Oncol 24:3895–3903

Soriano AO, Yang H, Faderl S, Estrov Z, Giles F, Ravandi F, Cortes J, Wierda WG, Ouzounian S, Quezada A, Pierce S, Estey EH, Issa JP, Kantarjian HM, Garcia-Manero G (2007) Safety and clinical activity of the combination of 5-azacytidine, valproic acid, and all-trans retinoic acid in acute myeloid leukemia and myelodysplastic syndrome. Blood 110:2302–2308

Steensma DP, Baer MR, Slack JL, Buckstein R, Godley LA, Garcia-Manero G, Albitar M, Larsen JS, Arora S, Cullen MT, Kantarjian H (2009) Multicenter study of decitabine administered daily for 5 days every 4 weeks to adults with myelodysplastic syndromes: the alternative dosing for outpatient treatment (ADOPT) trial. J Clin Oncol 27:3842–3848

Thépot S, Itzykson R, Seegers V, Recher C, Quesnel B, Delaunay J, Cluzeau T, Marfaing Koka A, Stamatoullas A, Chaury MP, Dartigeas C, Cheze S, Salanoubat C, Morel P, Plantier I, Taksin A, Marolleau JP, Pautas C, Wattel E, Isnard F, Sanhes L, Harel S, de Botton S, Chait Y, Uzunov M, Guerci A, Dahoun M, Vey N, Dombret H, Dreyfus F, Ades L, Fenaux P, Gardin C (2009) Azacytidine (AZA) as first line therapy in AML: results of the French ATU program. Blood (ASH Annu Meet Abstr) 114:843

Uchida T, Kinoshita T, Nagai H, Nakahara Y, Saito H, Hotta T, Murate T (1997) Hypermethylation of the p15INK4B gene in myelodysplastic syndromes. Blood 90:1403–1409

Uy GL, Abboud CN, Cashen AF, DiPersio JF, Stockerl-Goldstein KE, Vij R, Westervelt P (2010) Phase I study of panobinostat plus decitabine in elderly patients with advanced MDS or AML. Blood (ASH Annu Meet Abstr) 116:1060

van den Bosch J, Lübbert M, Verhoef G, Wijermans PW (2004) The effects of 5-aza-2′-deoxycytidine (decitabine) on the platelet count in patients with intermediate and high-risk myelodysplastic syndrome. Leuk Res 28:785–790

Vardiman JW, Harris NL, Brunning RD (2002) The World Health Organization (WHO) classification of the myeloid neoplasms. Blood 100:2292–2302

von Hoff DD, Slavik M, Muggia FM (1976) 5-azacytidine. A new anticancer drug with effectiveness in acute myelogenous leukemia. Ann Intern Med 85:237–245

Voso MT, Santini V, Finelli C, Musto P, Pogliani E, Angelucci E, Fioritoni G, Alimena G, Maurillo L, Cortelezzi A, Buccisano F, Gobbi M, Borin L, Di Tucci A, Zini G, Petti MC, Martinelli G, Fabiani E, Fazi P, Vignetti M, Piciocchi A, Liso V, Amadori S, Leone G (2009) Valproic acid at therapeutic plasma levels may increase 5-azacytidine efficacy in higher risk myelodysplastic syndromes. Clin Cancer Res 15:5002–5007

Wang JC, Chen W, Nallusamy S, Chen C, Novetsky AD (2002) Hypermethylation of the P15INK4b and P16INK4a in agnogenic myeloid metaplasia (AMM) and AMM in leukaemic transformation. Br J Haematol 116:582–586

Wijermans PW, Krulder JW, Huijgens PC, Neve P (1997) Continuous infusion of low-dose 5-aza-2′-deoxycytidine in elderly patients with high-risk myelodysplastic syndrome. Leukemia 11:19–23

Wijermans PW, Lübbert M, Verhoef G, Bosly A, Ravoet C, Andre M, Ferrant A (2000) Low-dose 5-aza-2′-deoxycytidine, a DNA hypomethylating agent, for the treatment of high-risk myelodysplastic syndrome: a multicenter phase II study in elderly patients. J Clin Oncol 18:956–962

Wijermans PW, Luebbert M, Verhoef G, Klimek V, Bosly A (2005) An epigenetic approach to the treatment of advanced MDS; the experience with the DNA demethylating agent 5-aza-2′-deoxycytidine (decitabine) in 177 patients. Ann Hematol 84(Suppl 1):9–17

Willemze R, Archimbaud E, Muus P (1993) Preliminary results with 5-aza-2′deoxycytidine (DAC)-containing chemotherapy in patients with relapsed or refractory acute leukemia. The EORTC Leukemia Cooperative Group. Leukemia 7(Suppl 1):49–50

Willemze R, Suciu S, Archimbaud E, Muus P, Stryckmans P, Louwagie EA, Berneman Z, Tjean M, Wijermans P, Döhner H, Jehn U, Labar B, Jaksic B, Dardenne M, Zittoun R (1997) A randomized phase-II study on the effects of 5-aza-2′-deoxycytidine combined with either amsacrine or idarubicin in patients with relapsed acute leukemia: an EORTC Leukemia Cooperative Group phase-II study. Leukemia 11(Suppl 1):24–27

Yang H, Hoshino K, Sanchez-Gonzalez B, Kantarjian H, Garcia-Manero G (2005) Antileukemia activity of the combination of 5-aza-2′-deoxycytidine with valproic acid. Leuk Res 29:739–748

Yang H, Kadia T, Xiao L, Bueso-Ramos CE, Hoshino K, Thomas DA, O'Brien S, Jabbour E, Pierce S, Rosner GL, Kantarjian HM, Garcia-Manero G (2009) Residual DNA methylation at remission is prognostic in adult Philadelphia chromosome-negative acute lymphocytic leukemia. Blood 113:1892–1898

Zagonel V, Pinto A, Bullian PL, Sorio R, Gattei V, Curri G, De Rosa L, Attadia V, Monfardini S (1990) 5-aza-2′-deoxycytidine as a differentiation inducer in human hemopoietic malignancies: preliminary clinical report. In: Momparler RL, de Vos D (eds) 5-aza-2′-deoxycytidine: preclinical and clinical studies. PCH, Haarlem

Zagonel V, Lo Re G, Marotta G, Barbare R, Sardeo R, Gattei V, De Angelis V, Montardinni S, Pinto A (1993) 5-aza-2′-deoxycytidine (decitabine) induces trilineage response in unfavorable myelodysplastic syndrome. Leukemia 7(Suppl 1):30–35

Pharmacodynamic Responses to DNA Methyltransferase Inhibition

8

Elizabeth Griffiths, Richard L. Momparler, and Adam R. Karpf

8.1 Introduction

The clinically relevant DNA methyltransferase inhibitors (DNMTi), 5-azacytidine (Vidaza, here abbreviated as Aza) and decitabine (Dacogen, here abbreviated as Dac), are nucleoside analogues first synthesized in 1964 and initially evaluated clinically as classical cytotoxics administered at high dose to multiply relapsed patients with refractory leukemias (Sorm and Vesely 1964; Pliml and Sorm 1964, McCredie 1973; Von Hoff 1976; Momparler et al. 1985; Rivard 1981). These agents, both azanucloside analogues of cytosine, substitute nitrogen for carbon in the C-5 position of the pyrimidine ring, making methyl substitution, as mediated in vivo by DNA methyltransferase inhibitors (DNMTi), impossible (Leone et al. 2003) (Fig. 8.1). In 1980, Peter Jones and Shirley Taylor demonstrated that in vitro treatment of mouse embryo cells with Aza and Dac resulted in both differentiation and demethylation (Jones and Taylor 1980). This observation, in concert with the recognition of methylation-induced silencing of tumor suppressor genes as a hallmark of malignancy (Holliday 1979; Makos et al. 1992), has led to the approval of these agents at low dose for the treatment of myelodysplasia and acute myeloid leukemia and to their development for the treatment of a variety of cancer subtypes (Piekarz

E. Griffiths, MD (✉)
Department of Medicine, Roswell Park Cancer Institute, CGP Building Room 5301B, Elm & Carlton Sts, Buffalo, NY 14263, USA
e-mail: elizabeth.griffiths@roswellpark.org

R.L. Momparler, PhD
CHU Sainte-Justine, Centre de recherche, 3175 Chemin de la Côte Sainte-Catherine, Montréal, QC H3T 1C5, Canada
e-mail: richard.l.momparler@umontreal.ca

A.R. Karpf, PhD
Eppley Institute for Research in Cancer, University of Nebraska Medical Center, DRC2, Room 4030, 985950 Nebraska Medical Center, Omaha, NE 68198-5950, USA
e-mail: adam.karpf@unmc.edu

M. Lübbert, P.A. Jones (eds.), *Epigenetic Therapy of Cancer*,
DOI 10.1007/978-3-642-38404-2_8,

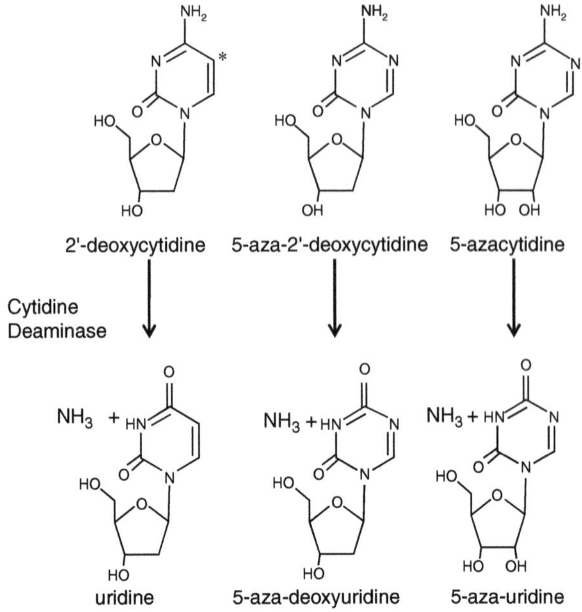

Fig. 8.1 Chemical structure of deoxycytidine, Dac and Aza. Breakdown of these compounds is mediated by cytidinedeaminase, present at high levels in human liver and other cell types, which removes nitrogen from the ring, rendering the compound inactive. The * indicates the carbon 5 position, substitution of which for nitrogen, as in Dac and Aza, blocks the action of DNMT enzymes

and Bates 2009). While the mechanism responsible for the activity of Aza and Dac in myeloid malignancy remains a matter of some controversy, there is little doubt that responses depend, at least in part, on incorporation into DNA, irreversible binding with and degradation of DNMTi, and resultant demethylation.

8.2 Preclinical Comparison of Antineoplastic Activity of Aza and Dac

It is important to evaluate carefully the preclinical data on Aza and Dac so as to assign a priority for clinical investigation on these analogues in patients with cancer. Which analogue has more potential in cancer chemotherapy? In brief, Aza and Dac are prodrugs that are activated by phosphorylation by deoxycytidine kinase and uridine/cytidine kinase, respectively. Leukemic cells lacking these enzymes are drug resistant to these analogues. About 80–90 % of Aza is incorporated into RNA and 10–20 % incorporated into DNA, after conversion to its deoxyribose form by ribonucleotidereductase (Li et al. 1970; Hollenbach et al. 2010). The incorporation of Aza and Dac into DNA is responsible for their inhibition of DNA methylation. The preclinical data suggest that the incorporation of Aza into RNA is also responsible for part of its antineoplastic action.

Initial reports showed that the incorporation of Aza into RNA reduced the function of tRNA in protein synthesis (Momparler et al. 1976) and its acceptor activity (reviewed by Cihak 1974). Reichman and Penman (1973) showed that Aza

Table 8.1 Comparison of in vitro and in vivo antineoplastic activity of 5-AZA-CdR and 5-azacytidine on murine L1210 leukemic cells

Parameter	Dac	Aza
Growth inhibition at 48 h	IC50 ~ 0.01 μM	IC50 ~ 0.02 μM
Loss of clonogenicity after 6 h exposure	LC50 ~ 0.1 μM	LC50 ~ 1.0 μM
Inhibit DNA methylation after 15 h exposure	51 % at 0.1 μM	<1 % at 0.1 μM
	69 % at 1.0 μM	63 % at 1.0 μM
Increase life span of mice with leukemia after 15 h infusion	384 % 10.1 mg/kg	63 % 11.7 mg/kg
	674 % 20.6 mg/kg	115 % 24.1 mg/kg
"Curative therapy" of mice with leukemia after 15 h infusion	60 % 20.6 mg/kg	0 % 24.1 mg/kg

Modified from Momparler et al. (1984a). IC50 = concentration 50 % growth inhibition LC50 = concentration 50 % loss of clonogenicity (colony assay). "Curative therapy" = ≥60 days survival after IV injection 10^4 L1210 leukemic cells. Control leukemic mice survival time = 6.1 ± 0.5 days

inhibited protein synthesis and proposed that this analogue interfered with the initiation of translation due to the formation of defective RNAs. Aza was shown to inhibit ribosomal maturation (Weiss and Pitot 1974). Recently, Aza, but not Dac, was shown to inhibit cytosine methylation in $tRNA^{asp}$ (Schaefer et al. 2009), which can also modify its function. The action of Aza on RNA function and protein synthesis was most likely responsible for its liver toxicity observed in both preclinical studies (Palm and Kensler 1971) and clinical studies (Von Hoff et al. 1976). These reports suggest that the antineoplastic action on cancer cells by Aza is due to both its incorporation into RNA and DNA. The complex action of Aza due to its dual action of RNA function and DNA methylation may be responsible for the major differences between this riboside analogue and Dac with respect to their action on global gene expression as shown by microarray array analysis (Flotho et al. 2009; Hollenbach et al. 2010).

It should be noted that the inhibition of protein synthesis by Aza has the potential to interfere with cell cycle transit, since progression of cells from G1 to S phase is dependent in part on protein synthesis (Vermeulen et al. 2003). This could explain the results of Tobey (1972) who reported that Aza inhibited the progression of cells from G1 into S phase. The inhibition of the progression of some neoplastic cells into S phase by Aza has the potential to make its antineoplastic action self-limiting. If G1 phase cells are blocked from entering S phase, Aza cannot inhibit DNA methylation, which can permit some cells to escape from its therapeutic action. In this regard, the action of Dac is not self-limiting since it does not inhibit the progression of G1 phase cells into S phase (Chabot and Momparler 1986; Momparler et al. 1984b).

The relative chemotherapeutic potential of Aza and Dac was evaluated in the murine model of L1210 leukemia (Table 8.1, Momparler et al. 1984a,). The in vitro experiments showed that Dac was about tenfold more potent than Aza with respect to the loss of clonogenicity as determined by a colony assay and with respect to the inhibition of DNA methylation. These results are in accord with the data on the metabolism of Aza, which showed that only 10–20 % of this analogue is incorporated into DNA. The in vivo chemotherapeutic potential of these analogues was evaluated in the mice with L1210 leukemia. L1210 murine leukemic cells are a prototype of leukemic stem cells since one cell will produce death from leukemia in 14 days (Momparler and Gonzales 1978). Data obtained from this L1210 leukemia mouse model were very predictive of the clinical activity of the related deoxycytidine analogue, cytosine arabinoside, in patients with acute myeloid leukemia (Skipper et al. 1967; Mayer et al. 1994). The mice were injected intravenously (IV) with 10^4 L1210 leukemic cells and 24 h later administered a 15 h IV infusion of Dac or Aza. Dac at a dose of 10.1 mg/kg and Aza at a dose of 11.7 mg/kg increased the life span of the leukemic mice by 384 and 63 %, respectively (Table 8.1). Remarkably, Dac at 20.6 mg/kg cured 60 % of the mice, whereas no cures were observed with Aza at 24.1 mg/kg. Even at higher doses, in the range of the maximal tolerated dose, treatment with Aza did not cure the leukemic mice (Momparler et al. 1984a). One explanation for the marked differences in chemotherapeutic activity between these analogues is that Aza blocked the progression of some leukemic cells into S phase, preventing its curative action.

In summary, the incorporation of Aza into RNA is responsible for part of its cytotoxic action on cells and may limit some of its antileukemic activity. The preclinical data indicate that Dac is a more potent antileukemic agent than Aza. Whether this difference in antineoplastic activity between these two cytosine nucleoside analogues will also be observed in the clinical treatment of hematological malignancies can only be determined by randomized clinical trials using the optimal dose schedule for each agent. It is interesting to note that some patients with MDS that lack response (resistance or intolerance) to Aza can respond to Dac (Borthakur et al. 2008).

8.3 Pharmacokinetics

Both Aza and Dac are relatively unstable in alkaline and acid solution and undergo spontaneous decomposition under such conditions resulting in a half-life between 3 and 4 h for both compounds (Notari and DeYoung 1975; Lin et al. 1981; Tomankova and Zyka 1980). By contrast, they are relatively stable in neutral aqueous solution at 37 °C with half-lives of 7 h for Aza and 12–20 h for Dac (Momparler 2005; Stresemann and Lyko 2008). As a result of their instability in an acid environment, and concerns about the risk of instability at room temperature, initial phase I trials with Dac in children with acute leukemia were undertaken using an IV continuous infusion. With this protocol, doses of 36–80 mg/kg over 36–44 h were demonstrated to be effective, while lower doses and shorter infusion times were not (Rivard et al. 1981). A later phase I study in adults with solid tumors chose a strategy of serial 1 h infusions given every 8 h (now the FDA-approved dosing strategy for MDS), and these authors identified myelosuppression as the predominant toxicity and suggested that the drug might also have been responsible for the development of transient renal insufficiency, with one renal biopsy demonstrating tubulointerstitial nephritis, in a small percentage of patients (van Groeningen et al. 1986). This study demonstrated that following IV infusion at the highest dose studied (100 mg/m^2), Dac reached a maximum concentration of 4 μM which was cleared to less than 0.1 μM within 1 h after infusion and was undetectable after 3 h. Using these data, the mean clearance rate was estimated to be ~126 ml/min/kg, with a volume of distribution of ~4.6 l/kg. Less than 1 % of drug was recovered in the urine. Later studies demonstrated that the alpha half-life, which occurred on the order of 5–7 min, resulted from rapid equilibration between the extra- and intracellular compartments mediated by nucleoside-specific transport by means of the transporters hENT1 and hENT2 (van Groeningen et al. 1986; Wiley et al. 1982). The secondary phase of elimination, or beta half-life, of 25–30 min was demonstrated to result from metabolism by cytidinedeaminase, an enzyme present at high levels in human liver and many other tissues (Rivard et al. 1981).

By contrast with the relatively mild toxicities associated with IV dosing of Dac, early studies with Aza were notable for excessive gastrointestinal toxicity, and a strategy of continuous infusion dosing, rather than IV bolus administration, was suggested (Karon et al. 1973; McCredie et al. 1973; Troetel et al. 1972). These studies calculated the pharmacokinetics of Aza using carbon-14 labeled drug, but results were complicated by an inability to distinguish active drug from its metabolites (Troetel et al. 1972; Israili et al. 1976). As a result of interest in the activity of Aza as a demethylating agent, Aza was reinvestigated at lower doses for the treatment of myelodysplastic syndrome (MDS). Phase II studies in MDS exploring a dose of 75 mg/m^2, one giving the drug IV and the other subcutaneously (SQ), were done, followed by a phase III study by the Cancer and Leukemia Group B (CALGB 9221) (Silverman et al. 1993, 1994, 2002). These studies demonstrated pronounced activity in MDS, but pharmacokinetics were not possible due to technical limitations. In 2005, with the recognition that Aza was active in MDS and following the development of an HPLC-based method for analysis of drug levels, Guido Marcucci and colleagues at the Ohio State University performed the first pharmacokinetic study to accurately measure levels of active drug given either IV or SQ (Zhao et al. 2004; Marcucci et al. 2005). This study demonstrated the time to peak plasma concentration following IV infusion to be between 5 and 11 min and that for SQ administration to be 30 min. The elimination half-life was significantly longer for SQ compared to IV administration (0.69 h ± 0.14 vs. 0.36 h ± 0.02), although clearance was similar when given by the two routes, and exceeded the glomerular filtration rate and total renal blood flow, demonstrating that metabolism by cytidinedeaminase and hydrolysis, as with Dac, are the most important mechanisms of drug elimination (Chabner et al. 1973; Chabot et al. 1983). SQ bioavailability was ~90 % of the IV dose.

Currently studies are under way to develop oral formulations of both drugs (Celgene Corp 2009, 2010). The first phase I study of oral Aza was published by Guillermo Garcia-Manero in 2011 and was designed to compare the pharmacokinetics of oral and SQ Aza (Garcia-Manero et al. 2011). This study design used intra-patient comparisons of pharmacokinetic behavior by giving the first cycle of Aza subcutaneously and subsequent cycles orally. In all patients, the first cycle was given at the standard dose of 75 mg/m^2/day for 7 days, and subsequently, patients were assigned to oral Aza at doses between 120 and 600 mg for each subsequent 7 days cycle. This study enrolled 41 patients with MDS, CMML, and AML and identified 480 mg as the maximally tolerated dose of oral Aza. Common side effects of the oral formulation were gastrointestinal disorders, headache, and edema. Dose-limiting diarrhea (grades 3 and 4) was observed at the 600 mg dose. Oral Aza demonstrated significant inter-patient variability in pharmacokinetic parameters with Cmax observed within 0.5 h (range 0.2–1.1) for SQ dosing and 1.0 h (range 0.3–3.6) for oral dosing. Oral bioavailability ranged from 6.3 to 20 % and at the MTD of 480 mg was 13 ± 9 %. The elimination half-life for the oral formulation was 0.62 ± 0.25 h and for the SQ dosing, 1.6 ± 0.7 h. Both SQ and oral dosing resulted in significant changes in methylation at multiple loci using the Infinium Human Methylation27 BeadArray system, although fewer genes were affected by oral than by SQ dosing. The overall response in the 15 MDS or CMML patients who were hypomethylating agent naive was 73 % (11/15) and in this group overall was 42 % (17/32); 8 patients with AML were treated on study and 2 had stable disease for 14 or 15 cycles. Overall these results were encouraging for the development of oral Aza, although some controversy arose regarding the relative contribution of the first cycle of SQ Aza in producing responses. Recently, and in order to quash the question of whether oral Aza could effect a response without SQ priming, Garcia-Manero's group presented results in abstract from second phase I trial of oral Aza in which a dose of 300 mg orally was examined in International Prognostic Scoring System Low or Int-1 MDS patients, but with extended dosing schedules of either 14, 21, or 28 days (Garcia-Manero et al. 2012). To date, 53 hypomethylating agent-naïve patients with lower-risk MDS have been enrolled; a median of 6 cycles have been given to patients on the 14 days arm and 4 on the 21 days arm. In the patients who received a minimum of four courses, the overall response rates (including CR, PR, or HI) were 47 % (9/19) in the 14 days arm and 50 % (7/14) in the 21 days arm. Adverse events were chiefly gastrointestinal. There is also an ongoing phase I study to examine the bioavailability of a single oral dose of Dac in patients with MDS, but results from this trial are not yet available (Eisai 2009). Overall the data from these phase I trials demonstrate that despite concerns about stability, the development of oral formulations of the hypomethylating drugs may be feasible with preserved efficacy, although it remains to be seen whether such oral formulations will be sufficient to supplant IV or SQ dosing entirely.

Issues of drug interaction and treatment of unusual populations, like those with liver or kidney dysfunction, are relatively limited. There is no evidence to demonstrate an interaction between either Aza or Dac and the cytochrome P450 enzymes; furthermore, the very high clearance rates for both drugs make renal elimination of marginal importance (Chen et al. 2010). Although there are no formal studies of either drug in patients on dialysis, theoretically treatment of these patients should be feasible. Patients with significant liver dysfunction should be treated with caution, however, given the possible importance of liver cytidinedeaminase for drug clearance. Figures 8.1 and 8.2 demonstrate schematic representations of the metabolism and activation of both Dac and Aza.

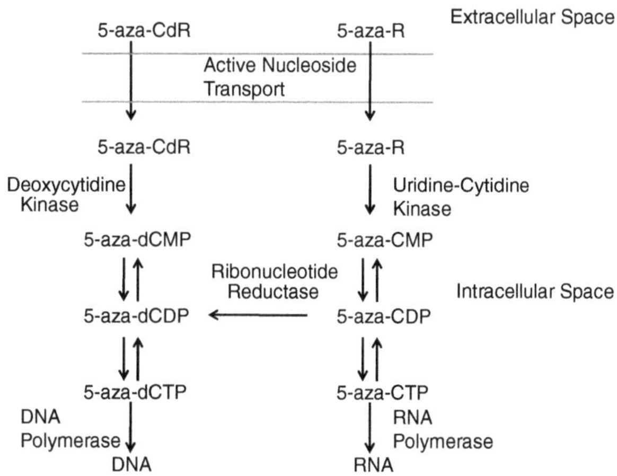

Fig. 8.2 Schematic detailing the cellular uptake and serial activation of azanucleotides which render these compounds active

8.4 Activation and Incorporation

The antineoplastic activity, with respect to demethylation and cytotoxicity, of both Aza and Dac requires incorporation into nucleic acid, and these drugs are thus S-phase specific. Several authors have demonstrated that in nondividing cells, the impact of both agents is blunted and DNMT levels are not diminished (Issa et al. 1993; Robertson et al. 2000). Neither drug is active in its parent form but requires activation by phosphorylation. As illustrated in Fig. 8.2, Dac is subject to phosphorylation by deoxycytidine kinase, while Aza is activated by uridine/cytidine kinase (Momparler and Derse 1979; Van Rompay et al. 2001). As might be expected from Fig. 8.2, alterations in deoxycytidine kinase expression have been shown to result in cross-resistance between cytarabine (AraC) and Dac, but not to impact sensitivity to Aza, due to the differential activation of the latter by uridine/cytidine kinase (Stegmann et al. 1995; Kong et al. 1991). Subsequently, the same enzymes act upon both compounds, adding successive phosphate groups until the active, triphosphate form has been achieved. Most (~80 %) of the activated triphosphate Aza (Aza-CTP) will be incorporated into RNA, but about 10–30 % will be converted to the same diphosphate intermediate as Dac (Dac-dCDP), by the activity of ribonucleotidereductase (Li et al. 1970; Hollenbach et al. 2010). All of the activate triphosphate Dac (Dac-dCTP) is available for DNA incorporation by DNA polymerase. As a result of this clean target profile, Dac has been favored for use in the laboratory as a typical DNMTi.

8.5 Therapeutic Targets

The recrudescence of interest in Dac and Aza stemmed from recognition of DNA methylation as a potentially reversible epigenetic mechanism regulating gene transcription by modification at cytosines in the context of cytosine phosphoguanine

(CpG) dinucleotides in CpG-dense regions surrounding gene promoters. Identification of this phenomenon as a cancer-specific event has further spurred both gene-specific and genome-wide analysis of methylation events as a readout for response to Aza and Dac in vivo. Although initially considered to be relatively similar compounds with near-identical mechanisms of action (demethylation of silenced tumor suppressor genes), the discrepancy in observed clinical response between the two agents has prompted additional investigation. Both agents clearly result in gene reexpression and reversal of methylation both in vitro and in patients. To date, however, studies examining reexpression of gene-specific targets have been unable to definitively demonstrate that response to therapy is a result of these events (Yang et al. 2006; Kantarjian et al. 2007; Fandy et al. 2009). Controversy remains as to the relative contribution of demethylation events, with subsequent gene reexpression and differentiation, and DNA damage events (due to double-strand breaks from DNMT-DNA adduct formation), both of which are certainly a result of treatment with both Aza and Dac. For Aza, the additional impact of incorporation into RNA and the effect of this event on RNA methylation (particularly of specific sites on tRNA which appear to be specific targets of DNMT2), processing, and protein translation to disease response remain a matter of considerable interest and investigation (Schaefer et al. 2009).

In vitro studies directly comparing both agents in AML cell lines have been performed by Hollenbach and colleagues (Hollenbach et al. 2010). These authors demonstrated that, in four different AML cell lines, at equimolar concentrations, Aza was more potent at inhibiting cell growth than Dac. Furthermore, they demonstrated a ratio of RNA to DNA incorporation for Aza into KG1a cells in the order of 65:35, slightly lower than the previously reported rate of 85:15 into L1210 leukemia cells; they did not replicate this experiment for Dac; however, presumably this agent is not incorporated into RNA (Li et al. 1970). The impact of Aza and Dac at a concentration of 2 μM, once daily (a level achievable only briefly in vivo immediately following IV injection for both agents) for 48 h on protein synthesis, was directly compared at using metabolically labeled ^{35}S-methionine and ^{35}S-cysteine. Protein synthesis was reduced by ~50 % by Aza, while no changes were observed following Dac treatment. Both Aza and Dac effectively depleted DNMT1 and induced DNA hypomethylation; this was achieved at a concentration of 1 μM for Aza and 0.3 μM for Dac, highlighting the relative potency for demethylation of the latter compound and confirming previously published reports of relative potency for this endpoint (Stresemann and Lyko 2008). Additionally DNA damage, as measured by phosph-H2AX induction as a measure of DNA double-strand breaks, was observed following in vitro treatment with both agents; interestingly this induction occurred at concentrations synonymous with those necessary for depletion of DNMT1 (Hollenbach et al. 2010). Effects of the two agents on cell cycle were somewhat different. At concentrations less than 1 μM, Aza had no impact upon the cell cycle of KG1a cells, while concentrations above 1 μM resulted in an increase in the sub-G1 fraction of cells; treatment with Dac also resulted in an increase in the sub-G1 fraction of cells but also increased the number of cells in the G2-M phase, most notably occurring at a concentration above 0.3 μM (Hollenbach et al. 2010). This differential effect on cell cycle was paralleled by an increase in markers of apoptosis which occurred above a dose of 1 μM for Aza and above 0.3 μM for Dac. At biologically equivalent doses (1 and 0.3 μM), respectively, the two agents appeared to induce approximately the same degree of apoptosis (Hollenbach et al. 2010). Finally, these authors reported alterations in gene expression profile following treatment with the two agents, demonstrating significant differences between the two agents in both number (596 vs. 87 following 24 h of treatment at 1 and 0.3 μM, respectively) and type of genes regulated; notably Aza treatment resulted in alterations in gene pathways important for metabolic processes, aminoacyl-tRNA ligase activity and mitochondria, as well as mitosis, cell cycle, and cell division, while Dac treatment resulted primarily in genes associated with cell differentiation (Hollenbach et al. 2010). This in vitro work highlights the differences between the two FDA-approved DNMTi and suggests that they may very well have distinct therapeutic effects and targets.

8.5.1 Epigenetic Targets

8.5.1.1 DNA Methylation

The importance of gene-specific DNA methylation events, most notably of recognized tumor suppressor genes (TSGs) as prognostic factor in MDS and AML, has been previously examined (reviewed in Issa 2010). Hypermethylation of several of these, including $p15^{INK4B}$, *HIC1*, *CDH1*, and *ERα*, has been described by a number of groups, and methylation of these genes, either alone (for $p15^{INK4B}$) or in combination (for the other genes), has been demonstrated to correlate with adverse prognosis in MDS (Christiansen et al. 2003; Aggerholm et al. 2006). While several authors have suggested that quantitative differences in methylation density may predict responsiveness to Aza therapy, with intermediate methylation density associated with a higher incidence of therapeutic efficacy (Daskalakis et al. 2002; Raj et al. 2007; Herman et al. 2009), other authors, using nonquantitative assays, have failed to establish this correlation. In contrast, clear evidence exists for the occurrence of demethylation events following therapy (Yang et al. 2006; Kantarjian et al. 2007; Fandy et al. 2009). Among the clinical trials responsible for the establishment of these agents for the therapy of MDS, none have definitively shown that methylation states at diagnosis, reversal of methylation of specific genes, or alterations in global methylation states correlate with therapeutic efficacy when evaluated at early time points following therapy. Several reports have demonstrated that patients who respond to therapy with these agents do demonstrate decreased levels of global methylation; notably, one large study reported that following Dac treatment, reduced methylation levels correlated with response (Shen et al. 2010). Since responses may result in loss of clonal dominance of the malignant clone, however, analyses of methylation changes at later time points, as frequently reported, may be a surrogate marker for replacement of marrow elements with more normal cells, rather than alterations to the underlying methylated population of cells, as suggested by Mund and colleagues (Shen et al. 2010; Mund et al. 2005). These results emphasize the

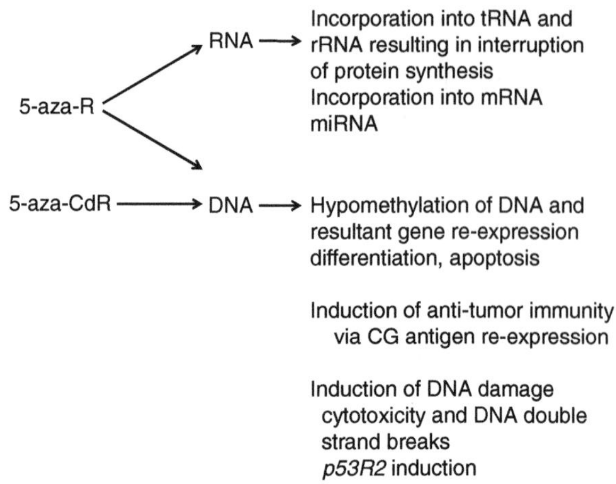

Fig. 8.3 Aza and Dac are incorporated into RNA and DNA; they have a variety of different effects on cellular processes, any one or combination of which may be responsible for their clinical efficacy

mixed observations in terms of response to therapy and methylation and demonstrate the continued need for investigation with more comprehensive microarray techniques and other more sensitive strategies to definitively address the contribution of TSG demethylation events to response (Fig. 8.3).

In addition to reexpression of silenced TSG, new evidence has come to light demonstrating that many micro-RNAs (miRs) are regulated epigenetically and that treatment of a variety of cancer cell lines with either Aza or Dac results in enhanced expression of these important RNAs (Tsai et al. 2009). The relative importance of this reexpression for disease response to demethylating therapy remains unclear, but certainly there is evidence to suggest that dysregulation of miR signaling is a common event in a variety of cancer subtypes and that epigenetic therapy with Aza or Dac may well be altering miR expression and signaling (Davalos and Esteller 2010).

In addition to the reexpression of TSG, several authors have suggested that activation of cancer testis antigens (also known as cancer germline or CG antigens) may be involved in responses to DNMTi (Sigalotti et al. 2003; Karpf 2006; Glazer et al. 2009; Loriot et al. 2009). These genes, which are expressed uniquely in immunologically privileged sites (germ cells of the testis and ovary), are frequently reexpressed in cancer cells treated with Aza or Dac and have variable baseline expression and frequent methylation in a variety of tumor subtypes (Akers et al. 2010). Reexpression of these genes using DNMTi has been suggested as a mechanism for the induction of host antitumor immunity. Clear evidence for this phenomenon in patients has not yet been proven, however trials in ovarian cancer are ongoing to address this question (Roswell Park Cancer Institute 2009).

During initial development of DNMTi for clinical use, considerable concern existed regarding the theoretical risk for induction of genomic instability in normal tissues or worsening the malignancy of the underlying therapeutic target as a result of hypomethylation of repetitive elements, or alternatively reexpression of silenced oncogenes within DNA (Toyota and Issa 2005). To date these concerns have not borne fruit. In fact, there has been no evidence to suggest that pretreatment with demethylating agents results in more resistant secondary AML or that secondary malignancies other the AML are a frequent event in those responders to Aza or Dac treated over the longer term (El-Osta 2003). Furthermore, there is evidence to suggest that cross-resistance to azanucleotides may not be significant, since gene expression profiles following treatment are relatively nonoverlapping and responses have been observed when patients are switched from one agent to another (Borthakur et al. 2008; Hollenbach et al. 2010).

Recently Hsing-Chen Tsai and colleagues published an intriguing paper suggesting that transient exposure to especially low doses of Aza (500 nM) and Dac (10–100 nM) might have long-term effects upon the repopulating capacity of cancer cell lines (leukemic and breast) and primary cancer cells (AML and breast cancer cells harvested from malignant pleural effusions) (Tsai et al. 2012). In this paper the authors expose cancer cell lines to very low doses of hypomethylating drugs and demonstrate relatively short-term effects upon DNA methylation (lasting up to 11 days) which appear to translate into longer-term effects on gene expression (lasting up to 14 days) which correlate with sustained impacts on cell repopulation capacity in vitro and serial xenografting in vivo. These authors suggest that the observed impact upon long-term repopulation capacity indicates that epigenetic drugs can induce a "memory" antitumor response which results from a resetting of the epigenetic state of the malignancy. Although these data have yet to be confirmed, they provide a tantalizing suggestion for the novel combination of these drugs in a variety of cancer types.

8.5.1.2 RNA Methylation

The incorporation of Aza-CTP into RNA has been demonstrated to have an impact on protein synthesis, but it may also result in demethylation of specific transfer RNAs (tRNAs), most notably $tRNA^{Asp}$, in which specific demethylation of cytosine 38 resulted following in vitro Aza treatment, possibly resulting from the irreversible binding and degradation of DNMT2 (Schaefer et al. 2009). Since tRNA methylation has been linked to the function of these molecules, this may suggest yet another alternative mechanism for the efficacy of Aza (Helm 2006). The impact of RNA demethylation remains the subject of investigation; however, in vitro treatment of AML cell lines with low-dose Aza (0.5 μM) was sufficient to result in tRNA demethylation at sites proposed to be specific DNMT2 targets and was correlated with reduced metabolic activity in cancer cell lines (Schaefer et al. 2009). Given these findings, Schaefer and colleagues suggest that tRNA methylation reversal may represent a possible biomarker for Aza responsiveness.

8.5.1.3 Effects on Histones

The interaction between histone-modifying enzymes and DNMTs is well established (Fuks et al. 2000; Rountree et al. 2000; Estève et al. 2006). Extensive literature exists on the synergistic reexpression of epigenetically silenced tumor suppressor genes following sequential application of Dac and an HDAC inhibitor first described by Elizabeth Cameron in 1999, but a direct effect for azanucleotides on histones was not universally appreciated (Cameron et al. 1999). In 2006, during a dose-finding study to evaluate synergy between Aza and an HDAC inhibitor, sodium phenylbutyrate, in patients with MDS or AML, a direct effect on histone acetylation by Aza alone, with induction of acetylated histones H3 and H4, was observed in the peripheral blood and bone marrow mononuclear cells of 11/23 enrolled patients (Gore et al. 2006). Given that in vivo, multi-protein complexes containing both DNMTs and histone-modifying enzymes exist, all of which influence the silencing of euchromatic genes, there has been some question as to whether these "off target" effects are modulating response to DNMTi (Cedar and Bergman 2009; Vire et al. 2006; Hernandez-Munoz et al. 2005; Li et al. 2006; Smallwood et al. 2007). In a recent study by Komashko and colleagues, the authors undertook an analysis of gene expression changes following in vitro treatment of HEK 293 embryonic kidney cells with Aza to assess whether genes associated with altered histone marks were overrepresented (Komashko and Farnham 2010). This study highlighted that the genes whose expression was most frequently altered by Aza treatment were neither primarily those with methylated promoters nor those with methylated histones and reiterated the findings generated by Hollenbach and colleagues demonstrating marked gene expression changes with Aza treatment, in excess of those demonstrated following treatment with Dac (Hollenbach et al. 2010). As described in AML cell lines by Hollenbach and colleagues, increased expression of categories of genes associated with C2H2 zinc finger transcription factors and decreases in expression of genes important for mitochondria and oxidoreductase activity were observed (Hollenbach et al. 2010). Surprisingly, they found that the overall levels of both H3K9me3 and H3K27me3 greatly increased in Aza-treated cells, while gene-specific H3K27me3 and H3K9me3 marks from the promoter regions of methylated genes decreased, suggesting that, as with DNA methylation, the impact of histone modifications with Aza treatment is complex. They conclude that most changes in gene expression due to Aza treatment are not due to relief of repression, although, as with all in vitro drug studies assessing time points after prolonged (>24–48 h) drug exposure, it is difficult to know which of the observed changes in gene expression represent direct response to treatment with the drugs and which reflect downstream alterations. Since epigenetic gene reexpression can occur relatively quickly following drug exposure (several hours, rather than days), it might be reasonable to assess earlier time points to determine which gene expression signatures occur first. Notably, in the study by Hollenbach and colleagues, only ~600 and 87 genes demonstrated altered expression following 24 h of exposure to biologically equivalent doses of Aza and Dac, respectively. Closer examination of these smaller groups of genes may disclose more insight into the fundamental biological processes that underlie response to therapy.

8.5.2 DNA Damage and Cytotoxicity

As mentioned previously, in vitro studies have clearly demonstrated that treatment with both Aza and Dac can result in DNA damage and cytotoxicity (Karpf et al. 2001; Jiemjit et al. 2008; Palii et al. 2008; Hollenbach et al. 2010). These events are felt to be mediated by the formation of DNA-DNMT adducts and subsequent double-strand DNA breaks. In vitro studies have demonstrated that in cancer cell lines, these double-strand breaks do not generally result in cell death but instead result in a G2 arrest during which the cancer cells undergo a program of DNA repair mediated by double-strand break and homologous recombination response pathways (Palii et al. 2008). Clinically this is manifested in some patients by prolonged cytopenias following treatment at even the "hypomethylation targeted" doses currently clinically in use and FDA-approved for MDS (Silverman et al. 2002; Steensma et al. 2009). Cytotoxicity is frequently evident even in 40–50 % of patients who do not ultimately respond to treatment, a phenomenon which generally requires repeated cycles of exposure (at least 4–6 cycles for Aza and at least 2–4 cycles for Dac) and is manifested by improved cytopenias as well as delayed transformation to AML (Fenaux et al. 2009; Kantarjian et al. 2006). Although studies examining induction of DNA damage in patients are limited, a combination study in MDS and AML patients treated with Aza and entinostat (MS-275), a histone deacetylase inhibitor, has clearly demonstrated that induction of γH2AX occurs in patient samples, as well as in vitro (Fandy et al. 2009).

One study has demonstrated a link between induction of DNA damage via p53 and response to therapy. Link and colleagues identified induction of *p53R2/RRMB2*, a p53 target gene important for the resolution of cellular damage which provides deoxynucleotides in cells undergoing cycle arrest following p53 activation, as a novel transcriptional target of Dac (Link et al. 2008). They demonstrated induction of the mRNA and protein of this gene, which they also demonstrated was not subject to methylation-induced silencing, in cell lines following Dac treatment at clinically relevant doses (0.5 μM), and further that this induction is due to direct transcriptional activation by p53. Loss of *p53R2* induction following Dac treatment, mediated by siRNA knockdown, was shown to significantly reduce G1 arrest. These authors further demonstrated that *p53R2* induction (both at the mRNA and protein level) occurs in primary patient samples following treatment with Dac, using the FDA-approved dosing strategy (15 mg/m^2 over 3 hours every 8 hours (45 mg/m^2/day) for 3 days every 6 weeks) in MDS ($n=10$), AML (n-4), and CMMoL ($n=1$), and correlated this with response to therapy (complete and partial responses in one patient each and stable disease in six patients). In this small sample, 7/8 (88 %) responders demonstrated induction of *p53R2* mRNA, while 0/5 (0) % nonresponders were induced ($p=0.0047$, Fisher's exact test). Similarly, p53R2 protein was induced in 4/5 (80 %) responders, while 2/4 nonresponders induced the protein ($p=0.5238$). Although small, in conjunction with prior in vitro data, these findings reiterate the importance of DNA damage response to the clinical efficacy of DNMTi.

Conclusions

The extent to which each of the mechanisms discussed above contribute to the observed clinical responses to DNMTi in patients with cancer remains the subject of debate and is clearly not a simple matter of DNA demethylation. Clearly, both Aza and Dac can reexpress genes silenced by methylation and induce DNA damage and cytotoxicity. In addition, the impact of Aza incorporation into RNA of various subtypes may also be important for the observed response to this agent. Despite the manifest differences between these two agents, their similarities remain marked in terms of both the degree of exposure (months) over which responses are observed as well as the patient populations in which they are most efficacious (myeloid malignancy). Given the complex transcriptional responses observed in cell lines treated with these agents, an understanding of the underlying mechanism responsible for this activity will likely depend on more than one of the pathways described above.

References

Aggerholm A, Holm MS, Guldberg P et al (2006) Promoter hypermethylation of p15INK4B, HIC1, CDH1, and ER is frequent in myelodysplastic syndrome and predicts poor prognosis in early-stage patients. Eur J Haematol 76:23–32

Akers SN, Odunsi K, Karpf AR (2010) Regulation of cancer germline antigen gene expression: implications for cancer immunotherapy. Future Oncol 6:717–732

Borthakur G, El Ahdab S, Ravandi F et al (2008) Activity of decitabine in patients with myelodysplastic syndrome previously treated with azacitidine. Leuk Lymphoma 49:690–695

Cameron EE, Bachman KE, Myöhänen S (1999) Synergy of demethylation and histone deacetylase inhibition in the re-expression of genes silenced in cancer. Nat Genet 21:103–107

Cedar H, Bergman Y (2009) Linking DNA methylation and histone modification: patterns and paradigms. Nat Rev Genet 10:295–304

Celgene Corp (2009) Safety, pharmacokinetics, and pharmacodynamics of oral azacitidine in subjects with myelodysplastic syndromes, chronic myelomonocytic leukemia and acute myelogenous leukemia (NCT00528983). http://clinicaltrials.gov

Celgene Corp (2010) Safety & pharmacokinetics study of azacitidine (SC and oral) in subjects with MDS, CMML, AML, lymphoma and multiple myeloma (NCT00761722). http://clinicaltrials.gov

Chabner BA, Drake JC, Johns DG (1973) Deamination of 5-azacytidine by a human leukemia cell cytidinedeaminase. Biochem Pharmacol 22:2763–2765

Chabot GG, Momparler RL (1986) Effects of 5-aza-2′-deoxycytidine on survival and cell cycle progression of L1210 leukemic cells. Leuk Res 10:533–537

Chabot GG, Rivard GE, Momparler RL (1983) Kinetics of deamination of 5-aza-2′-deoxycytidine and cytosine arabinoside by human liver cytidinedeaminase and its inhibition by 3-deazauriridine, thymidine or uracil arabinoside. Biochem Pharmacol 32:1327–1328

Chen Y, Liu L, Laille E et al (2010) In vitro assessment of cytochrome P450 inhibition and induction potential of azacitidine. Cancer Chemother Pharmacol 65:995–1000

Christiansen DH, Andersen MK, Pedersen-Bjergaard J (2003) Methylation of p15INK4B is common, is associated with deletion of genes on chromosome arm 7q and predicts a poor prognosis in therapy-related myelodysplasia and acute myeloid leukemia. Leukemia 17: 1813–1819

Cihak A (1974) Biological effects of 5-azacytidine in eukaryotes. Oncol 30:405–422

Daskalakis M, Nguyen TT, Nguyen C et al (2002) Demethylation of a hypermethylated P15/INK4B gene in patients with myelodysplastic syndrome by 5-aza-2′-deoxycytidine (decitabine) treatment. Blood 100:2957–2964

Davalos V, Esteller M (2010) MicroRNAs and cancer epigenetics: a macrorevolution. Curr Opin Oncol 22:35–45

Eisai, Inc (2009) Escalation study to determine bioavailability of a single oral dose of decitabine in patients with myelodysplastic syndrome (NCT00941109). http://clinicaltrials.gov

El-Osta A (2003) On the use of DNA methylation inhibitors and the reversal of transcriptional silencing. Blood 101:1656–1658

Estève PO, Chin HG, Smallwood A et al (2006) Direct interaction between DNMT1 and G9a coordinates DNA and histone methylation during replication. Genes Dev 15:3089–3103

Fandy TE, Herman JG, Kerns P (2009) Early epigenetic changes and DNA damage do not predict clinical response in an overlapping schedule of 5-azacytidine and entinostat in patients with myeloid malignancies. Blood 114:2764–2773

Fenaux P, Mufti GJ, Hellström-Lindberg E et al (2009) Efficacy of azacitidine compared with that of conventional care regimens in the treatment of higher-risk myelodysplastic syndromes: a randomised, open-label, phase III study. International Vidaza High-Risk MDS Survival Study Group. Lancet Oncol 10:223–232

Flotho C, Claus R, Batz C et al (2009) The DNA methyltransferase inhibitors azacitidine, decitabine and zebularine exert differential effects on cancer gene expression in acute myeloid leukemic cells. Leukemia 23:1019–1028

Fuks F, Burgers WA, Brehm A et al (2000) DNA methyltransferase dnmt1 associates with histone deacetylase activity. Nat Genet 24:88–91

Garcia-Manero G, Gore SD, Cogle C et al (2011) Phase I study of oral azacitidine in myelodysplastic syndromes, chronic myelomonocytic leukemia and acute myeloid leukemia. J Clin Oncol 29:2521–2527

Garcia-Manero G, Gore SD, Kambhampati S et al (2012) Safety and efficacy of oral azacitidine (CC-486) administered in extended treatment schedules to patients with lower-risk myelodysplastic syndromes. Blood 120:424

Glazer CA, Smith IM, Ochs MF et al (2009) Integrative discovery of epigenetically derepressed cancer testis antigens in NSCLC. PLoS One 4:e8189

Gore SD, Baylin S, Sugar E et al (2006) Combined DNA methyltransferase and histone deacetylase inhibition in the treatment of myeloid neoplasms. Cancer Res 66:6361–6369

Helm M (2006) Post-transcriptional nucleotide modification and alternative folding of RNA. Nucleic Acids Res 34:721–733

Herman JG, Gore SD, Mufti GJ et al (2009) Relationship among gene methylation, azacitidine treatment, and survival in patients with higher-risk myelodysplastic syndromes: results from the AZA-001 trial. 100th annual AACR meeting, Denver, CO. Abst 3394

Hernandez-Munoz I, Taghavi P, Kuijl C et al (2005) Association of BMI1 with polycomb bodies is dynamic and requires PRC2/EZH2 and the maintenance DNA methyltransferase DNMT1. Mol Cell Biol 25:11047–11058

Holliday R, Pukkila PJ, Dickson JM et al (1979) Cold Spring Harb Symp Quant Biol. 43 Pt 2: 1317–1323.

Hollenbach PW, Nguyen AN, Brady H et al (2010) A comparison of azacitidine and decitabine activities in acute myeloid leukemia cell lines. PLoS One 2;5(2):e9001

Israili ZH, Vogler WR, Mingioli ES et al (1976) The disposition and pharmacokinetics in humans of 5-azacytidine administered intravenously as a bolus or by continuous infusion. Cancer Res 36:1453–1461

Issa JP (2010) Epigenetic changes in the myelodysplastic syndrome. Hematol Oncol Clin North Am 24:317–330

Issa JP, Vertino PM, Wu J et al (1993) Increased cytosine DNA-methyltransferase activity during colon cancer progression. J Natl Cancer Inst 85:1235–1240

Jones PA, Taylor SM (1980) Cellular differentiation, cytidine analogs and DNA methylation. Cell 20:85–93

Jiemjit A, Fandy TE, Carraway H et al (2008) p21(WAF1/CIP1) induction by 5-azacytosine nucleosides requires DNA damage. Oncogene 5;27(25):3615–3623

Kantarjian H, Issa JP, Rosenfeld CS et al (2006) Decitabine improves patient outcomes in myelodysplastic syndromes: results of a phase III randomized study. Cancer 106:1794–1803

Kantarjian H, Oki Y, Garcia-Manero G, Huang X et al (2007) Results of a randomized study of 3 schedules of low-dose decitabine in higher-risk myelodysplastic syndrome and chronic myelomonocytic leukemia. Blood 109:52–57

Karon M, Sieger L, Leimbrock S et al (1973) 5-azacytidine: a new active agent for the treatment of acute leukemia. Blood 42:359–365

Karpf AR (2006) A potential role for epigenetic modulatory drugs in the enhancement of cancer/germ-line antigen vaccine efficacy. Epigenetics 1:116–120

Karpf AR, Moore BC, Ririe TO et al (2001) Activation of the p53 DNA damage response pathway following inhibition of DNA methyltransferase by 5-aza-2′-deoxycytidine. Mol Pharmacol 59: 751–757

Komashko VM, Farnham PJ (2010) 5-azacytidine treatment reorganizes genomic histone modification patterns. Epigenetics 5:229–240

Kong XB, Tong WP, Chou TC (1991) Induction of deoxycytidine kinase by 5-azacytidine in an HL-60 cell line resistant to arabinosylcytosine. Mol Pharmacol 39:250–257

Leone G, Voso MT, Teofili L et al (2003) Inhibitors of DNA methylation in the treatment of hematological malignancies and MDS. Clin Immunol 109:89–102

Li LH, Olin EJ, Buskirk HH et al (1970) Cytotoxicity and mode of action of 5-azacytidine on L1210 leukemia. Cancer Res 30:2760–2769

Li H, Rauch T, Chen Z-X, Szabo PE et al (2006) The histone methyltransferase SETDB1 and the DNA methyltransferase DNMT3A interact directly and localize to promoters silenced in cancer cells. J Biol Chem 281:19489–19500

Lin KT, Momparler RL, Rivard GE (1981) High-performance liquid chromatographic analysis of chemical stability of 5-aza-2′-deoxycytidine. J Pharm Sci 70:1228–1232

Link PA, Baer MR, James SR et al (2008) p53-inducible ribonucleotide reductase (p53R2/RRM2B) is a DNA hypomethylation-independent decitabine gene target that correlates with clinical response in myelodysplastic syndrome/acute myelogenous leukemia. Cancer Res 68:9358–9366

Loriot A, Reister S, Parvizi GK et al (2009) DNA methylation-associated repression of cancer-germline genes in human embryonic and adult stem cells. Stem Cells 27:822–824

Makos M, Nelkin BD, Lerman MI et al (1992) Distinct hypermethylation patterns occur at altered chromosome loci in human lung and colon cancer. Proc Natl Acad Sci USA 89:1929–1933

Marcucci G, Silverman L, Eller M et al (2005) Bioavailability of azacitidine subcutaneous versus intravenous in patients with myelodysplastic syndromes. J Clin Pharmacol 45: 597–602

Mayer RJ, Davis RB, Schiffer CA et al (1994) Intensive postremission chemotherapy in adults with acute myeloid leukemia. N Engl J Med 331:896–903

McCredie KB, Bodey GP, Burgess MA et al (1973) Treatment of acute leukemia with 5-azacytidine (NSC-102816). Cancer Chemother Rep 57:319–323

Momparler RL (2005) Pharmacology of 5-aza-2′-deoxycytidine (decitabine). Semin Hematol 42:S9–S16

Momparler RL, Derse D (1979) Kinetics of phosphorylation of 5-aza-2′-deoxyycytidine by deoxycytidine kinase. Biochem Pharmacol 28:1443–1444

Momparler RL, Gonzales FA (1978) Effect of intravenous infusions of 5-aza-2′-deoxycytidine on survival time of mice with L1210 leukemia. Cancer Res 38:2673–2678

Momparler RL, Siegel S, Avila F et al (1976) Effect of tRNA from 5-azacytidine-treated hamster fibrosarcoma cells on protein synthesis in vitro in a cell-free system. Biochem Pharmacol 25:389–392

Momparler RL, Momparler LF, Samson J (1984a) Comparison of the antileukemic activity of 5-aza-2′-deoxycytidine, 1-ß-D-arabinofuranosylcytosine and 5-azacytidine against L1210 leukemia. Leuk Res 8:1043–1049

Momparler RL, Samson J, Momparler LF et al (1984b) Cell cycle effects and cellular pharmacology of 5-aza-2′-deoxycytidine. Cancer Chemother Pharmacol 13:191–194

Momparler RL, Rivard GE, Gyger M (1985) Clinical trial on 5-aza-2′-deoxycytidine in patients with acute leukemia. Pharmacol Ther 30:277–286

Mund C, Hackanson B, Stresemann C (2005) Characterization of DNA demethylation effects induced by 5-aza-2′-deoxycytidine in patients with myelodysplastic syndrome. Cancer Res 65:7086–7090

Notari RE, DeYoung JL (1975) Kinetics and mechanisms of degradation of the antileukemic agent 5-azacytidine in aqueous solutions. J Pharm Sci 64:1148–1157

Palii SS, Van Emburgh BO, Sankpal UT et al (2008) DNA methylation inhibitor 5-Aza-2′-deoxycytidine induces reversible genome-wide DNA damage that is distinctly influenced by DNA methyltransferases 1 and 3B. Mol Cell Biol 28(2):752–771

Palm PE, Kensler CJ. (1971) Comparison of bulk 5-azacytidine (NSC 102816) and clinical formulation toxicity in hamster and dogs. Report to Laboratory of Toxicology National Cancer Institute, 29 Jan 1971 (PB 197 319 National Technical Information Service)

Piekarz RL, Bates SE (2009) Epigenetic modifiers: basic understanding and clinical development. Clin Cancer Res 15:3918–3926

Pliml I, Sorm F (1964) Synthesis of 2′-deoxy-D-ribofuranosyl-5-aza-cytosine. Collect Czech Chem Commun 29:2576–2578

Raj K, John A, Ho A et al (2007) CDKN2B methylation status and isolated chromosome 7 abnormalities predict responses to treatment with 5-azacytidine. Leukemia 21:1937–1944

Reichman M, Penman S (1973) The mechanism of inhibition of protein synthesis by 5-azacytidine in HeLa cells. Biochim Biophys Acta 324:282–289

Rivard GE, Momparler RL, Demers J et al (1981) Phase I study on 5-aza-2′-deoxycytidine in children with acute leukemia. Leuk Res 5:453–462

Robertson KD, Keyomarsi K, Gonzales FA et al (2000) Differential mRNA expression of the human DNA methyltransferases (DNMTs) 1,3a and 3b during the G(0)/G(1) to S phase transition in normal and tumor cells. Nucleic Acids Res 28:2108–2113

Roswell Park Cancer Institute (2009) Decitabine, vaccine therapy, and doxorubicin hydrochloride liposome in treating patients with recurrent ovarian epithelial cancer, fallopian Tube Cancer, or Primary Peritoneal Cancer (NCT00887796). http://clinicaltrials.gov

Rountree MR, Bachman KE, Baylin SB (2000) DNMT1 binds HDAC2 and a new co-repressor, DMAP1, to form a complex at replication foci. Nat Genet 25:269–277

Schaefer M, Hagemann S, Hanna K et al (2009) Azacytidine inhibits RNA methylation at DNMT2 target sites in human cancer cell lines. Cancer Res 2009:8127–8132

Shen L, Kantarjian H, Guo Y et al (2010) DNA methylation predicts survival and response to therapy in patients with myelodysplastic syndromes. J Clin Oncol 28:605–613

Sigalotti L, Altomonte M, Colizzi F et al (2003) 5-aza-2′-deoxycytidine (decitabine) treatment of hematopoietic malignancies: a multimechanism therapeutic approach? Blood 101:4644–4646

Silverman LR, Holland JF, Weeinberg RS et al (1993) Effects of treatment with 5-azacytidine on the in vivo and in vitro hematopoiesis in patients with myelodysplastic syndromes. Leukemia 7(Suppl 1):21–29

Silverman LR, Holland JF, Demakos EP et al (1994) Azacitidine in myelodysplastic syndromes: CALGB studies 8421 and 8921. Ann Hematol 68:A112

Silverman LR, Demakos EP, Peterson BL et al (2002) Randomized controlled trial of azacitidine in patients with the myelodysplastic syndrome: a study of the cancer and leukemia group B. J Clin Oncol 20:2429–2440

Skipper HE, Schabel FM, Wilcox WS (1967) Experimental evaluation of potential anticancer agents. XXI. Scheduling of arabinosylcytosine to take advantage of its S-phase specificity against leukemic cells. Cancer Chemother Rep 51:125–165

Smallwood A, Esteve PO, Pradhan S et al (2007) Functional cooperation between HP1 and DNMT1 mediates gene silencing. Genes Dev 21:1169–1178

Sorm F, Vesely J (1964) The activity of a new antimetabolite, 5-azacytidine, against lymphoid leukaemia in AK mice. Neoplasma 11:123–130

Steensma DP, Baer MR, Slack JL et al (2009) Multicenter study of decitabine administered daily for 5 days every 4 weeks to adults with myelodysplastic syndromes: the alternative dosing for outpatient treatment (ADOPT) trial. J Clin Oncol 27:3842–3848

Stegmann AP, Honders MW, Hagemeijer A et al (1995) In vitro-induced resistance to the deoxycytidine analogues cytarabine (AraC) and 5-aza-2′-deoxycytidine (DAC) in a rat model for acute myeloid leukemia is mediated by mutations in the deoxycytidine kinase (dck) gene. Ann Hematol 71:41–47

Stresemann C, Lyko F (2008) Modes of action of the DNA methyltransferase inhibitors azacytidine and decitabine. Int J Cancer 123:8–13

Tobey RA (1972) Effects of cytosine arabinoside, daunomycin, mithramycin, azacytidine, adriamycin, and camptothecin on mammalian cell cycle traverse. Cancer Res 32:2720–2725

Tomankova H, Zyka J (1980) Study of the time dependence of the stability of 5-aza-2′-deoxycytidine in acid medium. Microchem J 25:281–288

Toyota M, Issa JP (2005) Epigenetic changes in solid and hematopoietic tumors. Semin Oncol 32:521–530

Troetel WM, Weiss AJ, Stambaugh JE et al (1972) Absorption, distribution, and excretion of 5-azacytidine (NSC-102816) in man. Cancer Chemother Rep 56:405–411

Tsai KW, Kao HW, Chen HC et al (2009) Epigenetic control of the expression of a primate-specific microRNA cluster in human cancer cells. Epigenetics 4:587–592

Tsai HC, Li H, Van Neste L, Cai Y et al (2012) Transient low doses of DNA-demethylating agents exert durable antitumor effects on hematological and epithelial tumor cells. Cancer Cell 21:430–446

van Groeningen CJ, Leyva A, O'Brien AMP et al (1986) Phase I and pharmacokinetic study of 5-aza-2′-deoxycytidine (NSC127716) in cancer patients. Cancer Res 46:4831–4836

van Rompay AR, Norda A, Linden K et al (2001) Phosphorylation of uridine and cytidine nucleoside analogs by two human uridine-cytidine kinases. Mol Pharmacol 59:1181–1186

Vermeulen K, Van Bockstaele DR, Berneman ZN (2003) The cell cycle: a review of regulation, deregulation and therapeutic targets in cancer. Cell Prolif 36:131–149

Viré E, Brenner C, Deplus R et al (2006) The polycomb group protein EZH2 directly controls DNA methylation. Nature 439:871–874

von Hoff DD, Slavik M, Muggia FM (1976) 5-azacytidine. A new anticancer drug with effectiveness in acute myelogenous leukemia. Ann Intern Med 85:237–245

Weiss JW, Pitot HC (1974) Inhibition of ribosomal maturation by 5-azacytidine and 8-azaguanine in Novikoff hepatoma cells. Arch Biochem Biophys 160:119–129

Wiley JS, Jones SP, Sawyer WH et al (1982) Cytosine arabinoside influx and nucleoside transport sites in acute leukemia. J Clin Invest 69:479–489

Yang AS, Doshi KD, Choi SW et al (2006) DNA methylation changes after 5-aza-2′-deoxycytidine therapy in patients with leukemia. Cancer Res 66:5495–5503

Zhao M, Rudek MA, He P et al (2004) Quantification of 5-azacytidine in plasma by electrospray tandem mass spectrometry coupled with high-performance liquid chromatography. J Chromatogr B Analyt Technol Biomed Life Sci 813:81–88

Histone Methyltransferases: Opportunities in Cancer Drug Discovery

9

Richard Chesworth, Tim J. Wigle, Kevin W. Kuntz,
Jesse J. Smith, and Victoria M. Richon

9.1 Introduction

Posttranslational modifications on the core nucleosomal histones play an important role in the regulation of chromatin structure and function. These modifications include methylation of lysine and arginine residues, acetylation and ubiquitinylation of lysine residues, and phosphorylation of serine residues. The histone modifications are referred to as "marks," and the enzymes that catalyze the deposition of the marks are "writers," while the enzymes that remove the marks are "erasers." Proteins that recognize specific histone posttranslational marks or series of marks are referred to as "readers." Thus, the methyltransferases "write" the methyl marks on lysine and arginine residues. The methyl marks on lysine residues can exist in a mono-, di-, or trimethylation state, while arginine residues are either mono- or dimethylated, with the dimethylation existing in an asymmetrical or symmetrical state (Fig. 9.1a). Mass spectrometry studies have identified specific sites of lysine and arginine methylation found on histone H3 and histone H4 (Fig. 9.1b). The pattern of modifications present on the histones is associated with specific functional states of the chromatin. For example, trimethylation of histone H3 lysine 4 (H3K4me3) is found in areas of chromatin that are either poised for transcription or actively transcribed (Bernstein et al. 2005, 2006). H3K4me3 is found in combination with trimethylation of histone H3 lysine 27 (H3K27me3) in areas that are poised for transcription. Histone H3K27me3 is generally associated with transcriptional silencing. Our understanding of the role of

Richard Chesworth and Tim J. Wigle contributed equally to the chapter.

R. Chesworth • T.J. Wigle • K.W. Kuntz
Department of Molecular Discovery, 400 Technology Square 4th floor,
Cambridge, MA 02139, USA

J.J. Smith • V.M. Richon (✉)
Department of Biology, 400 Technology Square 4th floor,
Cambridge, MA 02139, USA
e-mail: vrichon@gmail.com

M. Lübbert, P.A. Jones (eds.), *Epigenetic Therapy of Cancer*,
DOI 10.1007/978-3-642-38404-2_9, © Springer-Verlag Berlin Heidelberg 2014

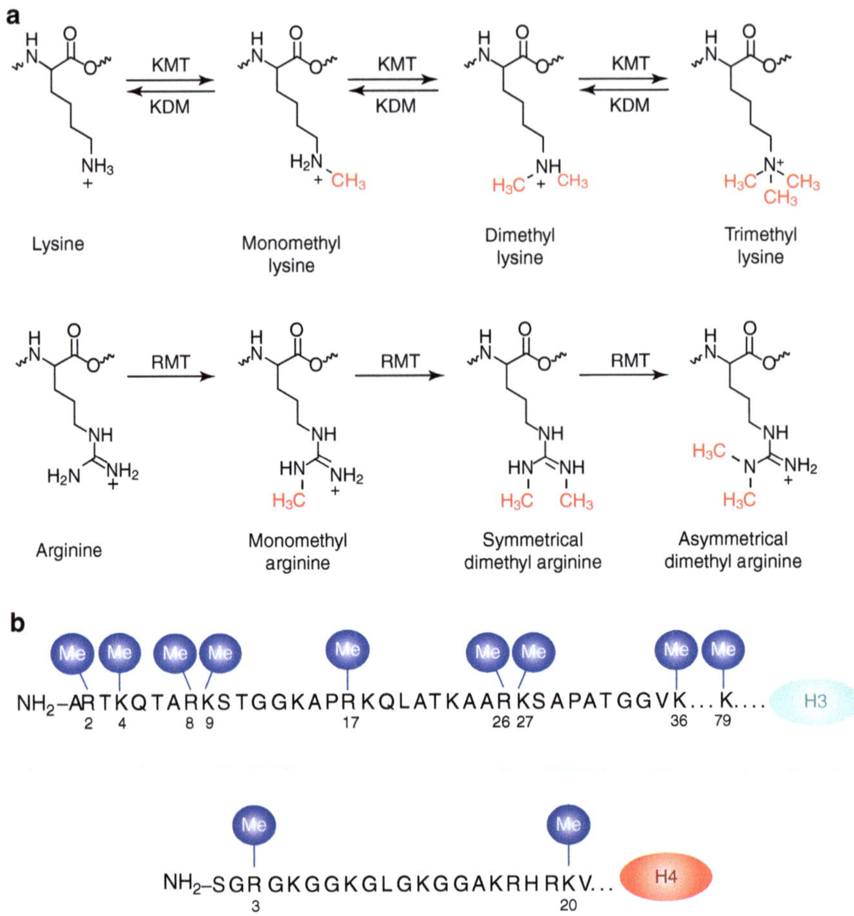

Fig. 9.1 Methylation of lysine and arginine residues in proteins. (**a**) Lysine methyltransferases mono-, di- or trimethylate lysine residues while lysine demethylases remove these modifications. Arginine methyltransferases monomethylate and asymmetrically or symmetrically dimethylate arginine residues and there are no known enzymes that directly remove these modifications. (**b**) Sequences of human histone H3 and H4 N-terminal tails and known sites of methylation

these posttranslational modifications of histones has increased tremendously in the past few years. The function and regulation of methyl marks on histone lysine and arginine residues are discussed in the sections in this review.

Histone methyltransferases are divided into two major families based upon their amino acid substrate: the lysine methyltransferases and arginine methyltransferases (Copeland et al. 2009; Bedford and Richard 2005; Richon et al. 2011). The lysine methyltransferases (KMTs) consist of over 50 enzymes, and all of the enzymes in this class share a common catalytic domain referred to as the Su(var)3–9, Enhancer of Zeste, Trithorax, or SET domain except for one enzyme, DOT1L. The catalytic domain of DOT1L shares structural homology with the arginine methyltransferases (RMTs), based on the observation that the cofactor S-adenosyl methionine (SAM) displays a common extended conformation in DOT1L and the RMTs (Richon et al. 2011). This is in contrast to the U shape conformation that SAM adopts in the catalytic domain of the SET domain KMTs (Schubert et al. 2003). Nine enzymes that catalyze arginine methylation have been described and include PRMT1, PRMT2, PRMT3, CARM1, PRMT5, PRMT6, PRMT7, PRMT8, and PRMT10 (Bedford and Richard 2005; Di Lorenzo and Bedford 2011). The RMTs are divided into two major groups. The type 1 enzymes (PRMT1, PRMT2, PRMT3, CARM1, PRMT6) catalyze either monomethylation or asymmetric dimethylation, and the type II enzymes catalyze symmetric dimethylation (PRMT5 and PRMT7). PRMT7 has also been shown to catalyze monomethylation of specific substrates and is the sole member of the type III enzyme group (Miranda et al. 2004). Two additional, related putative RMTs have been described (PRMT9 and PRMT11), but have not been biochemically characterized (Di Lorenzo and Bedford 2011). A systematic survey of the human genome for RMT-related enzymes was performed, and an additional 33 putative enzymes were identified that contained related methyltransferase domains (Richon et al. 2011).

Alterations in histone lysine and arginine methylation and associated protein methyltransferases have been observed in a wide variety of cancers (Table 9.1). These alterations include translocations, mutations, amplification, and aberrant recruitment of methyltransferases and demethylases. One example is EZH2, a histone H3K27 methyltransferase that is altered in several cancer types through a variety of different mechanisms that leads to increased H3K27me3 levels. The increase in H3K27me3 is associated with repression of gene expression that is believed to result in the development of cancer.

The identification of genetic alterations in methyltransferases in cancer leads to a strategy for targeting patient populations with these alterations using small molecules designed to selectively inhibit the oncogenic methyltransferase. Drug discovery efforts have been initiated, and several small molecule inhibitors of this class of enzymes have been identified. The current state of the development of the methyltransferase inhibitors is summarized in Sect. 4.

9.2 Histone Methylation, Methyltransferases, and Cancer Association

9.2.1 Lysine Methylation

9.2.1.1 H3K4 Methylation

The regulation of methylation on lysine 4 on histone H3 (H3K4) is complex, with at least 20 enzymes reported to catalyze the addition or removal of methylation at this site. Methylation of H3K4 is almost exclusively associated with transcriptionally active chromatin (Sims and Reinberg 2006; Strahl et al. 1999), and high levels of H3K4 mono-, di-, and trimethylation can be found at or near transcription start sites (Barski et al. 2007). There is a strong relationship between the state of methylation and transcription; trimethylation is found at the 5′ end of active genes and correlates positively with active transcription, RNA polymerase II occupancy, and histone acetylation (Bernstein et al. 2005; Santos-Rosa et al. 2002; Schneider et al. 2004).

Table 9.1 Examples of alterations of histone methyltransferases in cancer

Histone mark	Methyltransferase	Cancer association	References
Lysine			
H3K4	MLL	Translocated in *MLL-rearranged* leukemias; results in loss of SET domain	Hess (2004), Krivtsov and Armstrong (2007), Krivtsov et al. (2008)
	MLL4	Amplified in solid tumors	Hess (2004)
	SMYD3	Overexpressed in breast, liver, colon, and cervical cancer	Hamamoto et al. (2004, 2006), Luo et al. (2009), Wang et al. (2008a)
H3K9	G9a	Increased expression in transformed lung cell lines	Watanabe et al. (2008)
	SETDB1	Amplified and overexpressed in melanoma	Ceol et al. (2011)
H3K27	EZH2	Amplified and overexpressed in multiple solid tumors; mutated in lymphomas and MDS	Simon and Lange (2008), Sarma et al. (2008), Bracken et al. (2003), Cao et al. (2008b), Kirmizis et al. (2003), Kleer et al. (2003), van Haaften et al. (2009), Varambally et al. (2002), Morin et al. (2010), Sneeringer et al. (2010), Yap et al. (2011)
H3K36	WHSC1/NSD2, MMSET	Translocated and overexpressed in myeloma	Chesi et al. (1998), Lauring et al. (2008), Stec et al. (1998)
	WHSC1L1/NSD3	Amplified in lung cancer and breast cancer; translocation with NUP98	Angrand et al. (2001), Rosati et al. (2002)
H3K79	DOT1L	Mislocalized by *MLL* translocation in leukemia	Hess (2004), Krivtsov and Armstrong (2007), Krivtsov et al. (2008), Okada et al. (2005)
Arginine			
H4R3	PRMT1	Recruited to AML1-ETO oncogenic translocation in leukemia	Shia et al. (2012)
H3R8	PRMT5	PRMT5 and H3R8 methylation levels are elevated in lymphoid cancer cells	Pal et al. (2004, 2007)
H3R17	CARM1	Increased expression correlates with androgen independence in human prostate carcinoma, elevated expression in breast tumors	Frietze et al. (2008), El Messaoudi et al. (2006), Majumder et al. (2006)

Dimethylation of H3K4 often co-localizes with H3K4me3 in discrete zones 5–20 nucleosomes long proximal to actively transcribed genes. On its own, the dimethyl H3K4 mark has been found on genes that are maintained in a transcriptionally poised state (Bernstein et al. 2005; Schneider et al. 2004; Ruthenburg et al. 2007).

Unlike in yeast, where Set1 is the only H3K4 methyltransferase, humans have at least 13 confirmed or putative methyltransferases which regulate the addition of methyl groups at H3K4 (MLL1, MLL2, MLL3, MLL4, MLL5, Ash1, Set7/9, Set1A, Set1B, SMYD1, SMYD2, SMYD3, and PRDM9) (Ruthenburg et al. 2007; Abu-Farha et al. 2008; Hamamoto et al. 2004; Kouzarides 2007; Tan et al. 2006). Additionally, at least 7 H3K4 demethylases (LSD1, LSD2, JHMD1B, JARID1A, JARID1B, JARID1C, and JARID1D) have been reported to date (Kouzarides 2007; Lim et al. 2010a). The diverse array of human enzymes that have evolved to regulate the methylation status of the H3K4 indicates that exquisite control must be maintained over this mark in all cell types. In general, H3K4 methyltransferases are activators of gene expression, and H3K4 demethylases are repressors. The dynamic balance between these opposing classes of enzymes indicates the precision with which H3K4 methylation is regulated in diverse cell types.

While there is some overlap of function between H3K4 methyltransferases, the context-specific expression and activity of each enzyme is crucial to cell fate during differentiation and development (Eissenberg and Shilatifard 2010), cell functions, e.g., DNA repair, that maintain the status quo and in specialized processes, such as V(D)J recombination, which support physiological integrity (Shilatifard 2008). For example, the MLL family of H3K4 methyltransferases is known to exert control over the expression of *HOX* genes, and recent work from Shilatifard (2008) has described the phenomenon of redundancy versus specialization among this family in the activation of these gene clusters. Experiments performed using wild-type or *Mll1* knockout MEF cells indicate that of 10,041 genes associating with H3K4me3, only 5 % show a reduction in H3K4me3 in the *Mll1* knockout MEFs (Wang et al. 2009). Subsequent expression profiling indicated that the knockout of *Mll1* resulted in the enhanced expression of 2,265 genes and reduced expression of 2,459 or a positive or negative regulation of 3 % of all genes (Wang et al. 2009). Overall this analysis supported the concept that a substantial overlap in H3K4 methyltransferase activity does exist, but precise control over the expression of a small subset of genes is dependent on MLL. Cell-type-specific expression of MLL family methyltransferases has also been observed. For example, MLL3 and MLL4 are observed to have minimal roles in *HOX* gene regulation in fibroblasts (Wang et al. 2009). The methylation product of the methyltransferases also adds to the level of regulation of H3K4me3 observed; during oogenesis, MLL2 controls levels of trimethylation but has no effect on monomethylation, indicating that a different methyltransferase produces H3K4me1, and MLL2 activity is coordinated to catalyze the trimethyl state (Andreu-Vieyra et al. 2010). Similar target and product specificity exists among the H3K4 demethylases. LSD1 and LSD2 are observed to primarily act upon mono- and dimethylated H3K4, and JARID family demethylases are specific for di- and trimethyl H3K4 (Lim et al. 2010a). Beyond cell- and temporal-specific expression of H3K4 methyltransferases, another level of regulation may involve accessory proteins. For example, enzymatic activity may be nonexistent or greatly reduced when the SET domain-containing subunit is present on its own; however, activity is stimulated greatly when present as part of a complex. The identity of the other partners in the complex differs for each member of the MLL family and presumably dictates the specificity and the context in which methylation occurs at the target H3K4 residue (Eissenberg and Shilatifard 2010).

H3K4 methylation is associated with an open chromatin configuration which enables access of the chromatin to transcription factors and machinery. It is becoming apparent that protein modules capable of "reading" these methyl marks are responsible for attracting effector proteins containing these modules to chromatin sites bearing H3K4, leading to a variety of outcomes (Ruthenburg et al. 2007). Methyl-lysine binding modules are generally part of the Royal Family of proteins and include MBT, Agenet, Tudor, Chromo, and PWWP domains. Additionally, methyl-lysine recognition motifs can be found in the PHD family and WD40 repeat protein WRD5 (Maurer-Stroh et al. 2003). The key lysine methylation recognition features of these domains are an aromatic electron-rich cage, interacting with the lysine cation, with additional charge neutralization and H-bonding by 0–2 acidic functionalities depending on the methylation state of lysine (Guo et al. 2009; Kaustov et al. 2011). The number of proteins that contain H3K4 methyl-lysine recognition modules far outnumbers the enzymes that modulate methylation of this residue. The ING-family of proteins contain SHD fingers that preferentially recognize H3K4me2/3, and members of this family usually bind to and affect the activity of histone acetyltransferases and deacetylases (Adams-Cioaba and Min 2009; Feng et al. 2002). The recruitment of effector proteins to H3K4me3 often stimulates gene expression, as is the case for the PHD finger of human bromodomain and PHD domain transcription factor (BPTF), the largest subunit of the NURF complex, which is responsible for remodeling chromatin at active loci (Li et al. 2006; Wysocka et al. 2006). However, there are examples of H3K4me3 effector modules that repress gene expression upon recruitment. In response to DNA damage, the PHD finger of ING2, a critical component of the mSin3a-HDAC1 deacetylase complex, binds H3K4me3 in proximity to the promoters of proliferation genes and shuts off transcription (Shi et al. 2006). The binding of effector proteins to H3K4me3 can also impact other neighboring marks. The demethylases PHF8 and JHDM1D harbor a PHD finger, allowing them to dock onto the target nucleosome. However, the length and rigidity of a linker region separating the Jumonji domain from the PHD finger dictates whether the enzyme is a H3K9 (PHF8) or H3K27 (JHDM1D) demethylase (Horton et al. 2010). Unlike ING-family and BPTF PHD fingers, there are even recognition modules that selectively bind to unmodified lysine. A component of the LSD1 complex, BHC80, binds unmethylated H3K4, prevents remethylation and aids in the propagation of the H3K4 demethylation (Lan et al. 2007). Similarly, DNMT3L is recruited to unmethylated H3K4 by a PHD-like domain to maintain a repressive effect on gene expression at nucleosomes not demarcated by H3K4 methylation (Ooi et al. 2007).

Histone H3K4 methylation is associated with oncogenesis at multiple levels. However, given the complexity of enzymes that add or remove methyl groups from H3K4, and the diverse array of effector proteins that bind to H3K4, selecting the appropriate targets for initiating drug discovery is challenging (Copeland et al. 2009). SMYD3 is an example of a H3K4 methyltransferase where there appears to be a link between overexpression and tumor progression (Hamamoto et al. 2004). SMYD3 contains a SET domain and a MYND-type zinc-finger domain that is common among developmental proteins (Hamamoto et al. 2004). SMYD3 forms a complex with RNA Pol II (Hamamoto et al. 2004), and its overexpression is associated with increased expression of oncogenes (e.g., N-Myc, CrkL, Wnt10b, RIZ, and hTERT), cell cycle control genes (e.g., cyclin G1 and CDK2), and regulators of signal transduction (e.g., STAT1, MAP3K11, and PIK3CB) (Luo et al. 2009; Liu et al. 2007). SMYD3 has been shown to be overexpressed in hepatic, colorectal, cervical, and breast cancers (Hamamoto et al. 2004, 2006; Luo et al. 2009; Wang et al. 2008a). In the case of breast cancers, recent evidence suggests that SMYD3 directly interacts with the ligand-binding domain of the estrogen receptor α (ERα), enhancing the levels of di- and trimethylation of H3K4 at ERα target genes (Kim et al. 2009), ultimately increasing their expression. RNAi-mediated knockdown of the SMYD3 has been shown to decrease invasiveness and proliferation and in some cases induce apoptosis.

MLL is another example of an H3K4 methyltransferase implicated in cancer. Rearrangements of the *MLL* gene have been identified in both pediatric and adult leukemias and are correlated with poor prognosis (Hess 2004; Krivtsov and Armstrong 2007; Krivtsov et al. 2008). The *MLL* rearrangements result in loss of the SET or catalytic domain while retaining the DNA-targeting domain. The translocation results in aberrant expression of a subset of the *HOX* genes, causing a block of hematopoietic differentiation. Targeting of the fusion proteins or mediators of the fusion partners could represent a novel and effective way to treat these leukemias. Several MLL translocation partners (AF4, AF9, AF10, and ENL) recruit another lysine methyltransferase, DOT1L (Okada et al. 2005). DOT1L catalyzes methylation of histone H3K79 and is described in a subsequent section. In addition to alterations in *MLL*, amplification of *MLL4* is also observed in solid tumors (Hess 2004).

The histone H3K4 demethylases may also be important targets for therapeutic intervention using small molecules. LSD1 is overexpressed in prostate cancer, breast cancer, neuroblastoma and bladder cancer, and loss of H3K4me3 is postulated to result in the silencing of tumor suppressor gene expression (Lim et al. 2010a, b; Schulte et al. 2009; Shi and Whetstine 2007). Increasing local nonmethylated H3K4 not only impedes the recruitment of transcription factors but also enhances the activity of DNA methyltransferases proximal to the demethylated mark. Indeed, the use of LSD1 inhibitors in combination with a DNA methyltransferase inhibitor led to inhibition of the growth of human colon cancer xenografts (Huang et al. 2009). Similar to LSD1, JARID1B is found overexpressed in breast, testis, esophageal, and prostate cancers (Lim et al. 2010a; Barrett et al. 2007; Xiang et al. 2007). In addition to alterations in specific enzymes, alterations in H3K4 trimethylation have been described to be associated with cancer. For example, H3K4 trimethylation has been found to be associated with chromosome breakpoints in leukemia (Barski et al. 2007). While pursuing inhibitors of the reader domains that recognize H3K4 methylation is also a possibility (Kireev et al. 2010; Wigle et al. 2010), this chapter will focus on the opportunities presented by the histone methyltransferases.

9.2.1.2 H3K9 Methylation

Lysine methylation at H3K9 is generally associated with transcriptional silent chromatin and is an example of another mark where multiple enzymes regulate the methylation status. There are at least 7 methyltransferases (G9a, GLP, Suv39H1, Suv39H2, SETDB1, SETDB2, and PRDM2) and 7 demethylases (LSD1, JHDM2a, JHDM2b, JHDM3A, JMJD2B, JMJD2C, and JMJD2D) known to act upon this mark (Kouzarides 2007). Unlike H3K4, where there is no reported acetylation, the H3K9 mark is also prominently acetylated. Also, the serine (10) of histone H3 can become phosphorylated by the kinase Aurora B (Jeong et al. 2010).

Studies in organisms ranging from yeast to human show that H3K9 methylation is a hallmark of facultative and constitutive heterochromatin (Krishnan et al. 2011). High-resolution genomic mapping used to generate transcription start site (TSS) alignment has shown that both H3K9me2 and H3K9me3 were higher in chromatin of silent genes compared to transcriptionally active genes in a region of 10 kb surrounding the TSS. H3K9me1 localized to more active promoters surrounding the TSS (Barski et al. 2007). In addition, the di- and trimethylation states of H3K9 are implicated in the recruitment of DNA methyltransferases, which are also associated with areas of heterochromatin (Cheng and Blumenthal 2010).

Two of the most well-studied enzymes that catalyze methylation of H3K9 are G9a (also known as EHMT2) and G9a-like protein (GLP or EHMT1). G9a and GLP catalyze the mono- and dimethylation of H3K9 (Wu et al. 2010), but not trimethylation of H3K9. Unlike other methyltransferases, G9a and GLP do not rely on cross talk between neighboring marks to methylate H3K9, only the presence of a un- or monomethylated lysine (Rathert et al. 2008). DNA methyltransferases 3A and 3B are physically recruited to chromatin by G9a bound through its ankyrin repeats, facilitating the spread of heterochromatin (Xin et al. 2003). Functionally, G9a and GLP appear to be essential to early development, and knockouts of either in mouse embryos are lethal (Tachibana et al. 2002, 2005). In addition, G9a plays an essential role in embryonic stem cell differentiation through H3K9me2-mediated silencing of *Oct3/4* (Feldman et al. 2006). There is substantial redundancy between G9a and GLP target genes, but specialization does exist. G9a knockdown leads to a global reduction of H3K9me2 at 67 % of promoters (Wagschal et al. 2008).

The Suv39 family of methyltransferases catalyze di- and trimethylation of H3K9, and like G9a and GLP, they interact with DNA methyltransferases to facilitate the formation of heterochromatin (Loyola et al. 2009). Suv39 members are essential in recruiting Heterochromatin Protein 1 (HP1), a chromodomain-containing protein selectively recognizing trimethyl lysine that is essential in the stability of telomeres and centromeres. In addition to the Suv39 enzymes, SETDB1 has also been shown to catalyze di- and trimethylation of H3K9 (Schultz et al. 2002; Wang et al. 2003). The accessory protein mAM stimulates the conversion of di- to trimethylation of H3K9 by SETDB1 (Wang et al. 2003). SETDB1 is localized at the 3′ ends of zinc-finger genes and appears to play an important role in gene silencing induced at these promoters (Frietze et al. 2010). Demethylation of the H3K9 mark is carried out mainly by two families: JMJD1 family proteins are specific for H3K9 mono- and dimethylation and members of JMJD2 family demethylate di- and trimethylated H3K9 (Shi and Whetstine 2007; Cloos et al. 2006; Klose et al. 2006).

Overexpression of G9a, Suv39H1 and SETDB1 has been linked to oncogenic transformation in a variety of cancers, including lung and prostate cancer (Watanabe et al. 2008). However, despite reports of the overexpression of G9a in cancer, there is a lack of definitive proof to this end. Indeed, small molecules that are nanomolar or sub-nanomolar inhibitors of G9a and GLP (Kubicek et al. 2007; Liu et al. 2009a, 2010) can reverse H3K9me2 in cells and regulate G9a target gene expression; however, these changes do not correlate with inhibition of proliferation. G9a may also contribute to the development of cancer by methylating and inactivating the p53 tumor suppressor protein (Huang et al. 2010). Recently, it has been shown that Suv39H1 overexpression may be oncogenic through its association and recruitment of DNMT1 (Kang et al. 2007).

Recurrent amplification and overexpression of SETDB1 has been described in melanoma (Ceol et al. 2011). Ceol et al. show that enforced expression of SETDB1 can accelerate melanoma onset in a zebrafish model, thus supporting the role of SETDB1 as an oncogene in melanoma.

There are also genetic alterations in the H3K9 demethylases that have been described in cancer. For example, recurrent amplifications and overexpression of JMJD2C/GASC1 have been found in squamous cell cancer cell lines and the basal-like subtype of breast cancer (Cloos et al. 2006; Yang et al. 2000; Liu et al. 2009b). Liu et al. show that GASC1 induces transformed phenotypes and regulates the expression of genes critical for stem cell self-renewal when ectopically expressed in immortalized breast cells.

9.2.1.3 H3K27 Methylation

Methylation of lysine 27 on histone H3, in particular trimethylation, is associated with gene silencing. The deposition of methyl groups onto H3K27 is catalyzed by the Polycomb-Repressive Complexes 2 (PRC2) containing either EZH1 or EZH2 as the catalytic subunit of the complex. EZH2-PRC2 is noted for being the prominent complex in actively dividing cells, while EZH1-PRC2 is ubiquitously expressed (Margueron et al. 2008). The core PRC2 complex is composed of EED, RbAp48, Suz12, and EZH2 (Cao and Zhang 2004a). Demethylation of H3K27 is principally carried out by UTX and JMJD3 and results in the activation of gene expression (Agger et al. 2007).

PRC2 catalyzes the mono- through trimethylation of H3K27 (Margueron et al. 2008; Cao et al. 2002). In vivo, H3K27me2 is the most abundant form, accounting for roughly 50 % of H3K27 methylation, with H3K27me1 and H3K27me3 representing 10 and 35 % of H3K27 methylation, respectively (Peters et al. 2003). Of these methylation states, the trimethylation of H3K27 (H3K27me3) is associated with increased DNA methylation in proximity to nucleosomes bearing this mark. This leads to chromatin condensation and ultimately the repression of genes that are located in these heterochromatic regions (Schlesinger et al. 2007). The establishment of the H3K27me3 is important during processes such as X-inactivation, germline development, and stem cell pluripotency, which require sustained gene suppression (Cao and Zhang 2004b). PRC2 has important roles in stem cell biology; there is strong overlap between binding of PRC2 to regions that are populated by genes controlled by the transcription factors Oct4, Sox2, and Nanog, which are critical to pluripotent stem cell generation and maintenance (Boyer et al. 2005,

2006). Loss of PRC2 derepresses embryonic stem cell differentiation genes (Boyer et al. 2006), and knockdown of Oct4 disrupts PRC2 association with target genes (Squazzo et al. 2006), indicating that PRC2 activity is important in inhibiting differentiation. Interestingly, H3K27me3 can sometimes co-localize with H3K4me3, an activating mark. In this chromatin state, termed "bivalent chromatin," H3K27me3 is the dominant mark, and gene expression is repressed; however, the presence of the H3K4me3 is believed to maintain the genes in a poised state for activation of transcription upon demethylation by UTX or JMJD3 (Simon and Lange 2008).

The EED subunit of the PRC2 complex contains a WD40 domain that preferentially recognizes and binds to the higher methylation states of lysines in H3K9, H3K27, and H1K26, all of which contain a conserved ARKS sequence (Xu et al. 2010). Since H3K9me3 and H3K27me3 are repressive marks, their recognition by EED may facilitate the propagation of H3K27me3 across regions where gene expression is silenced. Additional proteins, such as PHF1, are not essential to EZH2 catalytic activity but may associate with PRC2 to enhance its activity. Loss of PHF1 correlates with a concomitant decrease in H3K27me3 at the HOXA6, HOXA9, and HOXA11 promoters. PHF1 contains a Tudor domain and two PHD fingers that most likely target PRC2 to discrete loci via recognition of adjacent methylated lysines (Cao et al. 2008a; Sarma et al. 2008). Also, it has been shown that large intervening noncoding RNAs (lincRNAs) interact with PRC2 and control the localization of H3K27 methylation via recognition of complementary DNA sequences (Gupta et al. 2010). The deposition of H3K27me3 is recognized by Polycomb-Repressive Complex 1 (PRC1), a complex with a core composition of Polycomb (PC), Polyhomeotic (PH), BMI-1, and RING1, which is thought to contribute to Polycomb silencing (Levine et al. 2002).

H3K27 trimethylation is strongly implicated in cancer, and several mechanisms leading to increased H3K27me3 (PRC2 overexpression, *UTX* loss of function mutations and PRC2 subunit overexpression) are associated with many human cancers (Simon and Lange 2008; Sarma et al. 2008; Bracken et al. 2003; Cao et al. 2008b; Kirmizis et al. 2003; Kleer et al. 2003; van Haaften et al. 2009; Varambally et al. 2002). As a result, PRC2, specifically its catalytic subunit EZH2, is one of the most pursued epigenetic targets. Overexpression and amplification of EZH2 (or other PRC2 subunits) is believed to silence genes that promote differentiation. One of the first reports of the involvement of PRC2 in cancer was a gene profiling study of metastatic and localized prostate cancer in which EZH2 scored as the most significant gene upregulated in metastatic cancer (Varambally et al. 2002). PRC2 correlates with poor outcome in prostate cancers and can be used as a prognostic indicator. Similarly, EZH2 overexpression in breast cancers is well documented and correlates with the aggressiveness of the tumor (Bracken et al. 2003; Kleer et al. 2003).

In addition to overexpression, somatic mutations in the catalytic domain of EZH2 have been described in diffuse large B-cell lymphoma (Morin et al. 2010). The mutations result in a single amino acid change in the catalytic SET domain of EZH2 at Y641 (Y641F, Y641N, Y641S, Y641H) in follicular lymphoma (FL) and germinal center B-cell-like (GCB) subtypes of diffuse large B-cell lymphoma (DLBCL). Initial biochemical experiments using recombinant PRC2 having these mutations demonstrated that mutant EZH2 complexes were unable to methylate a peptidic substrate corresponding to the H3K27 mark, while the wild-type enzyme methylated the same substrate. Morin et al. concluded, therefore, that the mutants appeared to be loss-of-function variants (Morin et al. 2010). However, subsequent studies using nucleosome, histone, and peptide substrates revealed that point mutations of Y641 to F, N, S, or H resulted in a change in the substrate specificity of EZH2 from unmethylated lysine to the dimethylated lysine. The Y641 mutants are much more proficient at catalyzing trimethylation than the wild-type enzyme (Sneeringer et al. 2010; Yap et al. 2011). Considering that these mutations were discovered as heterozygous, and both mutant and wild-type enzyme are expressed, it is believed that the coordinated activities of wild-type and mutant EZH2 drive H3K27 trimethylation and thus promote the development human lymphomas (Sneeringer et al. 2010; Yap et al. 2011). These findings suggest that lymphoma patients bearing the EZH2 mutation may be sensitive to small molecule inhibitors of EZH2. Ultimately, this may provide a framework for further genetic analysis of histone methyltransferase mutations, as catalytic site mutations that change the substrate specificity of the SET domain are not unprecedented (Wu et al. 2010; Del Rizzo et al. 2010).

9.2.1.4 H3K36 Methylation

H3K36 methylation is primarily an activating mark that is catalyzed by at least 6 methyltransferases (NSD1, NSD2, NSD3, SMYD2, SETD2, and SETMAR) and erased by at least 5 demethylases (JHDM1a, JHDM1b, JHDM3A, JMJD2B, and JMJD2C) (Kouzarides 2007; Lee et al. 2005; Li et al. 2009). Methylation at H3K36 competes with acetylation, as it is also recognized as a target for acetyltransferases. H3K36 trimethylation is generally observed downstream of transcriptional start sites, within the coding region of genes, and it peaks around the 3′ end (Barski et al. 2007). In yeast, H3K36 dimethylation is scarce or absent in upstream gene regulatory regions, telomeres, mating loci, and regions transcribed by RNA polymerase III and is predicted to be restricted to areas in contact with RNAP II. Localization of H3K36me2 is highly conserved from yeast to humans and is speculated to demarcate regulatory from coding regions in a similar fashion (Rao et al. 2005). It has been shown that SMYD2 associates with the Sin3A HDAC complex to generate H3K36me2 and restrain cell proliferation (Brown et al. 2006). WHSC1 (also known as NSD2) preferentially mono- and dimethylates H3K36 in the context of nucleosomes, but interestingly, in the absence of DNA, it can have its substrate preference changed to H4K44, a mark that has not been proven to exist in vivo (Li et al. 2009). While the NSD methyltransferases can only catalyze mono- or dimethylation, SETD2 can catalyze mono-, di-, and trimethylation (Yuan et al. 2009), and it is the key enzyme regulating trimethylation of H3K36.

Dysregulation of H3K36 methylation is a molecular determinant of several cancers. Overexpression of NSD3 (also known as WHSC1L1) resulting from amplification within chromosome 8p12 is observed in several tumor cell lines and breast carcinomas (Angrand et al. 2001). Chromosomal translocations that result in a fusion product of NSD methyltransferases to nucleoporin 98, NUP98-NSD1

(Jaju et al. 2001; Wang et al. 2007) or NUP98-NSD3 (Rosati et al. 2002), are defined genetic mutations associated with leukemogenesis. The NUP98-NSD1 fusion is believed to induce acute myeloid leukemia (AML) through the binding of genomic elements in proximity to Hox genes, maintaining H3K36 methylation and leading to overexpression of proto-oncogenes such as *HoxA7*, *HoxA9*, *HoxA10*, and *Meis1* (Wang et al. 2007). Inactivating mutations in the NSD SET domain of the NUP98 fusions abolished the oncogenic potential of the chimera (Wang et al. 2007). In myeloma, t(4:14) translocations have been found to drive overexpression of NSD2 leading cancer cell proliferation and adhesion (Chesi et al. 1998; Lauring et al. 2008; Stec et al. 1998). The alterations in the NSD proteins cause methylation of H3K36 in genomic regions which do not normally contain this modification, resulting in aberrant gene expression and transformation. Therefore, one can envision small molecules that inhibit the catalytic activity of NSD family methyltransferases being useful in the treatment of several hematological malignancies.

9.2.1.5 H3K79 Methylation

H3K79 methylation is catalyzed by DOT1L. Unlike other histone modifications that are situated in the accessible N-terminal histone tails, H3K79 methylation occurs on the core of histone H3. DOT1L is the only known lysine methyltransferase that lacks a canonical SET domain (Dillon et al. 2005; Gao and Liu 2007), and structurally, the catalytic domain of DOT1L is more closely related to arginine methyltransferases than to lysine methyltransferases (Richon et al. 2011; Wu et al. 2010; Min et al. 2003). The mechanism of depletion of the H3K79 methylation mark appears to require replacement of histone H3 since no H3K79 demethylases have been described. DOT1L was originally identified for its role in telomere silencing (Singer et al. 1998), and it was later discovered that it possessed H3K79 methylating activity (Ng et al. 2002a, b; van Leeuwen et al. 2002). DOT1L-mediated methylation of H3K79 is considered to enhance gene expression (Steger et al. 2008). The catalytic activity of DOT1L is highly dependent on the presented of ubiquitinylated histone H2B, and it is only active in the context of nucleosomal substrates (Ng et al. 2002b; Shahbazian et al. 2005).

DOT1L is linked to oncogenic transformation in MLL-rearranged leukemias. DOT1L is recruited by MLL fusion partners, resulting in the mis-targeting of DOT1L and aberrant H3K79 methylation. This leads to increased transcription of MLL fusion target genes which then block differentiation and promote proliferation (Krivtsov et al. 2008; Okada et al. 2005; Bitoun et al. 2007). *MLL* translocations are found in approximately 5–10 % of acute leukemias (Slany 2009) and involve fusion of the N-terminal domain of MLL to partners such as AF10, AF4, AF9, ENL, ELL, and AF6 (Krivtsov and Armstrong 2007). DOT1L associates with the MLL fusions through the partner-binding domains. In these fusions, the DNA binding of MLL is retained; however, it lacks the SET domain. This concept of MLL fusion-mediated DOT1L recruitment was reinforced by an artificial DOT1L-MLL fusion which also was capable of inducing leukemic transformation (Okada et al. 2005). Therefore, patients with *MLL*-rearranged leukemias capable of recruiting DOT1L are an example of a genetically defined cancer population that may be candidates for treatment with small molecule inhibitors of DOT1L (Barry et al. 2010).

9.2.1.6 H4K20 Methylation

Methylation of H4K20 is catalyzed by at least 4 enzymes (SETD8, Suv420H1, Suv420H2, and NSD1), and there are currently no known demethylases for this mark (Kouzarides 2007). Top-down mass spectrometry analysis has revealed that H4K20me2 is the dominant modification, with H4K20me1 and H4K20me3 being less abundant (Pesavento et al. 2008; Yang et al. 2008). H4K20me2 is widely distributed and is observed to be bound by the Tudor domain of 53BP1 (Botuyan et al. 2006), which is involved in initiating the DNA damage response (Yang et al. 2008; Sanders et al. 2004). H4K20me1, catalyzed by SETD8, is localized to the chromatin of active genes (Oda et al. 2009). H4K20me1, however, is a known target of malignant brain tumor domain proteins such as L3MBTL1, which result in chromatin compaction (Kalakonda et al. 2008). Additionally, monomethylation is seen in X-inactivation (Kohlmaier et al. 2004). H4K20me1 appears to be either activating or repressive depending on the context. H4K20me3, catalyzed primarily by Suv420H1 and Suv420H2, is found in pericentromeric chromatin and is thought to be a silencing mark (Schotta et al. 2004).

Several cancers have decreased H4K20 trimethylation. In non-small cell lung cancer, loss of H4K20me3 increases as the disease progresses, and this correlates negatively with survival (Van Den Broeck et al. 2008). Additionally, a study comparing a panel of normal cell lines to cancer cell lines found cancer cell lines displayed a loss of H4K20me3 (Tryndyak et al. 2006). Additionally, a mouse model of skin cancer indicates that this loss of H4K20me3 occurs early in tumorigenesis (Fraga et al. 2005). Therefore loss of H4K20me3 may serve as a biomarker in early cancer detection.

9.2.2 Histone Arginine Methylation

Methylated histone arginine residues have also been linked to oncogenic signaling events and cancer phenotypes. The next section outlines the roles of specific arginine methylation sites and their association with cancer.

9.2.2.1 H3R8me2s and H4R3me2s

The two most studied histone arginine methyl modifications linked to human cancer are H3R8me2s and H4R3me2s and both are catalyzed by PRMT5 (Pal et al. 2004). Arginine methylation at these sites is associated with transcriptional repression. In fact, PRMT5 can be recruited to specific promoters by a variety of transcriptional repressors, including Snail and AJUBA proteins (Hou et al. 2008). Hypermethylation of H3R8 and H4R3 has been observed in several lymphoid cancer cell lines, such as mantle cell lymphoma (MCL) and chronic lymphocytic leukemia (B-CLL), and in tumor samples from MCL patients. Furthermore, these methyl marks have been associated with the repression of multiple tumor suppressor genes, including ST7, NME1 (Pal et al. 2004, 2007), and RB family members (Wang et al. 2008b). Importantly, RNAi-mediated knockdown of PRMT5 in these lymphoid cancer cell lines reduced proliferation, diminished hypermethylation of H3R8 and H4R3, and restored expression of tumor suppressor genes.

The mechanism governing increased methylation of H3R8 and H4R3 in lymphomas and leukemias appears to be increased PRMT5 protein translation. Surprisingly, PRMT5 mRNA is generally lower in transformed lymphoid cancer cell lines when compared to "normal" cells of the same lineage. However, PRMT5 protein translation efficiency is greatly enhanced in transformed B cells and MCL cell lines due to aberrant expression of certain subsets of PRMT5-targeting microRNAs (miRNAs) (Pal et al. 2007). In addition to enhanced translational efficiency, PRMT5 enzymatic activity is regulated by phosphorylation of its co-stimulatory protein, MEP50. Increased phosphorylation of MEP50 by cyclin D1/cdk4 complexes is associated with increased PRMT5 activity. These data suggest that PRMT5 may play an important role in cyclin D1-driven cancers (Aggarwal et al. 2010).

9.2.2.2 H4R3me2a

Asymmetric dimethylation of histone H4 on Arg-3 (H4R3me2a) is generally associated with gene promoters undergoing active transcription. H4R3me3a formation is catalyzed by at least three different type I arginine methyltransferases, PRMT1, PRMT6, and PRMT8 (Di Lorenzo and Bedford 2011). Of these RMTs, PRMT1 is viewed to be the predominant cellular asymmetric arginine methyltransferase, accounting for as much 85 % of physiological protein arginine methylation (Tang et al. 2000).

H4R3me2a has been linked to oncogenic signaling in several contexts. Notably, PRMT1 has been reported to be a key component of a novel MLL oncogenic transcriptional complex, which includes MLL-EEN, CBP, and the bridging protein Sam68 (Cheung et al. 2007). Using chromatin immunoprecipitation, Cheung et al. demonstrated that H4R3me2a promoter levels correlate with the expression of key MLL-EEN target genes, such as HOXA9. Additionally, these authors directly fused PRMT1 to the MLL protein and demonstrated that this fusion product increased self-renewal potential in primary hematopoietic cells. However, an enzymatically inactive point mutant version of PRMT1 was not able to bolster self-renewal capacity in this assay. Finally, this group demonstrated that shRNA-mediated knockdown of PRMT1 abrogated MLL-EEN-mediated transformation of primary hematopoietic cells. In summary, these data support the link between the H4R3me2a mark and MLL-EEN-mediated oncogenic signaling.

Recently, PRMT1 was reported to interact with a splice isoform of the oncogenic fusion protein AML-ETO (AE9a), the characteristic translocation product of t(8;21)-positive acute myeloid leukemia (Shia et al. 2012). PRMT1 directly methylates AE9a on Arg-142 and is recruited to AE9a target gene promoters, where it increases methylation on H4R3 (H4R3me2a). Genetic knockdown of PRMT1 decreased the levels of H4R3me2a at AE9a target gene promoters in AML-ETO translocation-positive cell lines. Most notably, knockdown of PRMT1 also decreased the self-renewal capacity of AE9a in colony growth assays, consistent with an important role for PRMT1 and H4R3me2a in t(8;21) leukemogenesis.

Interestingly, dimethylation of H4R3 can repress or promote gene expression at the same promoter depending on whether the modification is symmetric or asymmetric.

Symmetric dimethylation of H4R3 by the type II protein arginine methyltransferase PRMT5 leads to recruitment of DNMT3A to the β-globin locus via direct binding of DNMT3A to H4R3me2s (Zhao et al. 2009). Subsequently, DNMT3A methylates CpG sites leading to transcriptional repression of the β-globin locus.

On the other hand, asymmetric methylation of H4R3 (H4R3me2a) by the type I protein arginine methyltransferase PRMT1 leads to repression of gene expression at the β-globin locus. The H4R3me2a mark, catalyzed by PRMT1, recruits the histone acetyltransferase KAT2B (PCAF) to the β-globin locus control region, and in turn, KAT2B acetylates H3K9 and K14 (Li et al. 2010). Acetylation of these sites is associated with increased transcription at the β-globin locus. Thus, the activities of PRMT5 and PRMT1 at the same histone H3 arginine residue have opposing functions on gene expression. Within the context of lymphomas, such as mantle cell and B-CLL, where the H4R3me2s mark is increased at key tumor suppressor promoters, it remains an open question as to whether H4R3me2a is concurrently downregulated.

9.2.2.3 H3R17me2a

Increased asymmetric dimethylation of H3R17, known to be catalyzed by CARM1, has been observed in breast (Frietze et al. 2008; El Messaoudi et al. 2006) and prostate (Majumder et al. 2006) cancers. CARM1 is recruited to nuclear hormone receptor complexes via interactions with members of the p160 steroid co-activator family (Chen et al. 1999). Upon hormone stimulation, CARM1 is recruited to p160-nuclear hormone receptor complexes and increases H3R17 dimethylation at androgen- and estrogen-responsive promoters. These signaling events lead to increased transcription of several proliferation genes, such as *E2F1*, *CCNA1*, *CCNE1*, *CCNE2*, and *CDC25A*. Disruption of CARM1 in both prostate and breast cancer cell lines decreases H3R17 methylation at hormone-responsive promoters and leads to decreased cancer cell proliferation. It should be noted that increased expression of nuclear CARM1 has been reported to correlate with the progression of prostate cancer malignancy (Majumder et al. 2006; Hong et al. 2004). However, these studies did not investigate whether H3R17me2a levels also correlate with disease progression.

9.2.2.4 H3R26me2a

Although not as well characterized as H3R17me2a, H3R26me2a is also generated by CARM1. This mark has been linked to oncogenic signaling by virtue of the observation that the CARM1/NCOA3 complex is recruited the promoters of a number of E2F-driven target genes, including CCNE1, DHFR, and CDC6 (El Messaoudi et al. 2006). Recruitment of the CARM1/NCOA3 complex to said promoters increases the levels of both H3R17me2a and H3R26me2a.

9.2.2.5 Nonhistone Substrates of Protein Arginine Methyltransferases in Cancer

The importance of nonhistone substrates in PRMT-mediated oncogenic signaling pathways is becoming increasingly clear. These substrates include a variety of signaling molecules such as transcription factors, transcriptional co-activators, chromatin modulating proteins, and other DNA-binding proteins. One of the most compelling examples of these nonhistone substrates is the tumor suppressor p53.

Jansson and colleagues identified in the oligomerization domain of p53 three arginine residues which appear to be methylated by PRMT5 (Jansson et al. 2008). Disruption of PRMT5 reduces methylation of these residues and promotes a p53-mediated apoptotic response following DNA damage. Thus, PRMT5 may have a role in regulating p53-mediated cell fate (cell cycle arrest versus apoptosis) following a DNA damage stimulus.

As mentioned previously, the CARM1 has been shown to be recruited to nuclear hormone receptors via its interaction with the p160 steroid co-activator family of proteins. As a part of these transcriptional complexes, CARM1 can methylate not only nucleosomes (H3R17) but also its p160-binding partner NCOA3 (Feng et al. 2006; Naeem et al. 2007). Interestingly, this methylation event, which is increased by hormone stimulation, leads to disassembly of the NCOA3 transcriptional complex and downregulation of hormone-dependent transcription. Thus, the role of CARM1 in nuclear hormone receptor signaling is complex, as CARM1 can activate proliferative transcriptional pathways via methylation of nucleosomes (H3R17), while simultaneously attenuating hormone-dependent transcription by methylating NCOA3. The question as to how the balance of these stimulatory and inhibitory pathways becomes shifted in favor of proliferation in certain types of breast and prostate cancer is an area for future investigation.

9.2.2.6 DNA Damage Response Machinery and PRMT1

PRMT1 has been linked to asymmetric arginine methylation of number of DNA damage checkpoint machinery proteins. Recently, it was reported that PRMT1 methylates BRCA1 in a region that contains multiple lysine and arginine methylation sites and that arginine methylation of BRCA1 can be detected in multiple breast cancer lines and breast tumor samples (Guendel et al. 2010). Knockdown of PRMT1 in breast cancer cell lines caused a change in the binding pattern of BRCA1 to target promoters. It remains unclear exactly how BRCA1 arginine methylation correlates with cancer phenotypes. PRMT1 has also been reported to methylate MRE11, a member of the DNA double-strand break repair complex (Boisvert et al. 2005a). While methylation of MRE11 did not appear to affect formation of the MRE11-RAD40-NBS1 complex, mutation of arginine residues in the GAR (glycine-arginine rich) domain diminished its exonuclease activity. Like MRE11, 53BP1 has also been reported to contain a GAR motif and to be methylated by PRMT1 (Boisvert et al. 2005b). Mutation of arginine residues within the 53BP1 GAR motif abrogated its ability to localize to sites of DNA damage. Taken together, these observations suggest a role for PRMT1 in regulating DNA damage pathways which have critical importance to oncogenic signaling.

9.3 Mechanism of Methyltransfer

The KMT and RMT share a common mechanism to transfer the methyl group from a universal methyl donor, S-adenosyl-L-methionine (SAM) to the nitrogen atom of lysine and arginine side chains, respectively (Fig. 9.1). The transfer of the methyl group results in the production of S-adenosyl-L-homocysteine (SAH).

9.3.1 SET Domain Lysine Methyltransferases

As discussed above, the SET domain class of lysine methyltransferases includes enzymes known to methylate several sites on histone H3 (K4, K9, K27 & K36) and at least one site on histone H4 (K20). The KMTs can transfer 1, 2, or 3 methyl groups to lysine utilizing SAM as a methyl donor. The mechanism for methyl transfer has been extensively studied, and several crystal structures of KMTs bound to SAM/SAH, and a peptide substrate have been solved. The substrate specificity of the KMTs is not only specific to the lysine site on the histone but also depends on the methylation state of the lysine. Mutations and different binding proteins can change the substrate preference of some of the KMTs.

The SET domain family of methyltransferases is reported to contain 51 human proteins (Copeland et al. 2009; Richon et al. 2011). Generally the SET methyltransferases are thought to function as part of larger complexes such as the PRC2 complex. The accessory proteins act to target and regulate activity while the SET methyltransferase is the catalytic engine of the complex.

The SAM-binding motif contained in the SET domain of the KMTs has both highly conserved and divergent regions. In the highly conserved region, a NHS sequence is maintained for the majority of SET proteins. The histidine backbone carbonyl accepts a hydrogen bond from the N-6 of SAM, while the backbone amine of the same histidine donates a hydrogen bond to the N-7 of SAM (Dillon et al. 2005). The interaction with the conserved histidine has been seen in all of the co-crystal structures of SET methyltransferases with SAM or SAH. The remaining SAM-binding pocket can vary significantly between subfamilies, but all contain interactions with the amino acid portion of SAM. It is worth noting that while the interactions vary, the 3-dimensional configuration of SAM/SAH in the SET methyltransferase co-crystals are superimposable on each other and completely distinct from any of the other SAM-utilizing methyltransferases.

One of the most studied KMT is SET7/9 (SETD7). It has been the focus of several mechanistic papers regarding the process of transferring a methyl group from SAM to the lysine. There is consensus that the reacting lysine is initially protonated when binding to the KMT. While some disagreement exists on the nature of the base, the mechanism involves the deprotonation of lysine to give the neutral amine which then attacks the methyl of SAM in a S_N2-like fashion. Guo et al. (Guo and Guo 2007) have suggested that the conserved tyrosine could be the base that deprotonates the lysine, while others have suggested water acts as the base. Xiao et al. (2005) pointed to bulk solvent to be the base, while Dirk et al. (2007) suggested a water molecule in the active site as the base. Zhang and Bruice (2007) favor the water being the base but point out that the water molecule in the active site is not basic enough to deprotonate the lysine and there is not access to bulk solvent in the active site. They indicate that a water channel forms upon binding the substrate, allowing the proton to be shuttled to bulk solvent. The water channel is proposed to form only when the lysine lacks a methyl group. Once the lysine is methylated, the methyl blocks the channel and prevents subsequent methylation, thus giving SET7/9 its specificity of catalyzing the 0–1 H3K4 methylation.

The lysine-binding portion of the active site of the SET domain has been shown to consist of an aromatic cage containing 1–3 tyrosine residues which can accept hydrogen bonds from the lysine. The aromatic cage stabilizes the charged species and lowers the pKa of the lysine, while the tyrosines play a role in proper alignment of lysine (Zhang and Bruice 2008). Mutational studies with GLP and G9a (Wu et al. 2010; Rathert et al. 2008) and with SET7/9 (Collins et al. 2005) have shown that mutation of one of the aromatic cage tyrosines to phenylalanine, and in one case to alanine, allows the enzyme to further methylate the lysine. Additionally for G9a, it was shown that mutating an aromatic cage phenylalanine to tyrosine restricted the number of methyl groups it could transfer, allowing only the unmethylated lysine to be an effective substrate. The two positions which control the ability of the SET to use methylated lysines as substrates have been termed the Phe/Tyr switch.

While initially these switches were identified by performing in vitro mutational studies, recently similar mutations have been described in follicular and germinal center B-derived diffuse large B-cell lymphomas (Morin et al. 2010). In these lymphomas, EZH2 was found to be mutated at Y641 (which corresponds to one of the residues identified previously as a Phe/Tyr switch) resulting in a change to several other amino acids (Morin et al. 2010). Enzymatic analysis of these mutant enzymes showed a change in substrate preference from H3K27me 0>1>2 for the wild-type enzyme to 2>1>0 for the Y641 mutants (Sneeringer et al. 2010; Yap et al. 2011). These change-of-function mutants led to elevated cellular levels of H3K27me3, which contributes to lymphomagenesis. Interestingly, all of the Y641 mutants displayed the same pattern of changes in substrate utilization, and all of the changes could be ascribed to transition state interactions with the enzyme (Sneeringer et al. 2010).

9.3.2 Arginine Methyltransferases

The arginine methyltransferases (RMTs) can be divided into two major subgroups, type I and II (Di Lorenzo and Bedford 2011). The type I RMTs consist of PRMT 1, 3, 4, 6, and 8 and type II of PRMT 5 and 7. Additionally, PRMT7 has been described to be a type III RMT on certain substrates (Fig. 9.2). The type I RMTs catalyze both the formation of monomethylated arginine (MMA) intermediates and asymmetrical dimethylated arginines. The type II RMTs catalyzes the formation of MMA and symmetrical dimethylated arginines. The type III RMT catalyzes only the formation of MMAs. In each case, SAM is utilized as the methyl donor as depicted in scheme A. The majority of methylated arginines found in vivo appear to be DMAs (dimethylated arginines) (Zhang and Cheng 2003).

A number of RMTs including PRMT1 and 3 and CARM1 (PRMT4) have been found to exist in dimeric or oligomeric states (Zhang and Cheng 2003); this has led groups to speculate on whether the in vivo observation of preponderant DMA versus MMA is due to the dimeric/oligomeric structure leading to a processive mechanism. Kolbel et al. (2009), however, have demonstrated that PRMT1 and PRMT3 act *via* a distributive mechanism (Fig. 9.3). This was based on the analysis of

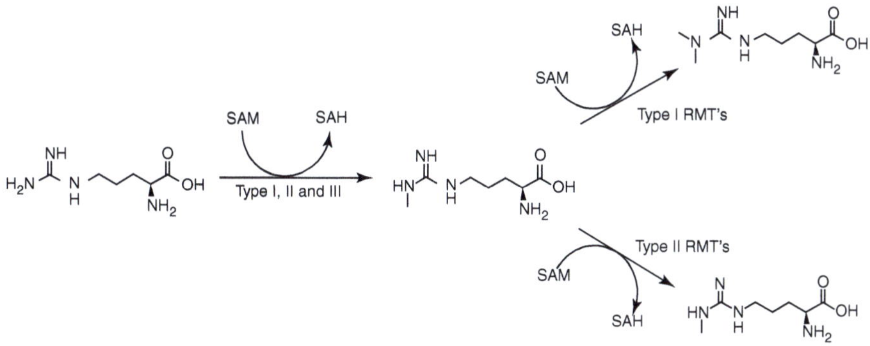

Fig. 9.2 Methylation of arginine residues by types I, II, and III RMTs

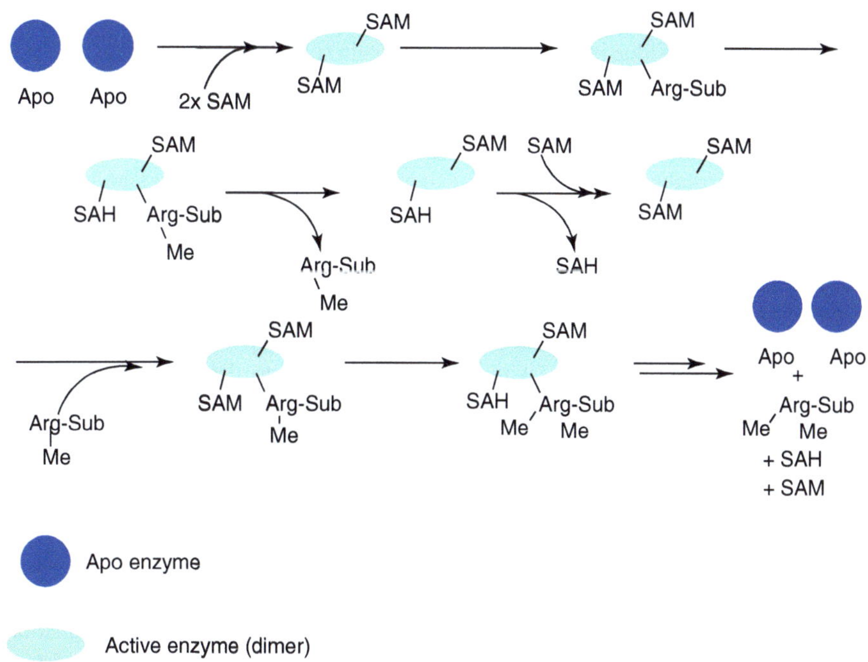

Fig. 9.3 Distributive mechanism of arginine methylation by type I RMTs

multiple kinetic experiments, including the observation of a Poisson product distribution highly indicative of a distributive mechanism whereas a processive mechanism should result in a product profile biased towards dimethylated species. The authors suggest that release of the methylated arginine substrate is obligatory and rate determining.

Additional work is necessary to understand why DMA products predominate in vivo as the distributive mechanism does not appear to account for this finding.

Experiments with peptide substrates suggest little change in Km and kcat values for MMA residues over the corresponding unmethylated counterparts, i.e., the MMA arginine residues are not preferred substrates; however, further work with physiological substrates is required. Alternative explanations include that the RMTs are components of multi-protein complexes, where the other proteins may influence the substrate specificity of the RMT. CARM1, for example, is found in a complex of at least ten proteins called the nucleosomal methylation activator complex (NUMAC) (Xu et al. 2004). Interestingly, recombinant CARM1 in the absence of some, if not all, of the other proteins of the NUMAC complex preferentially methylates free histone H3 rather than the nucleosome. CARM1 activity has also been reported to be modulated by phosphorylation resulting in a decrease in RMT activity (Higashimoto et al. 2007). Neighboring residues on histone H3, such as H3K18, have been demonstrated to affect the rate of methylation on H3R17 by CARM1. For example, CARM1 activity on H3R17 is increased when H3K18 is acetylated (~5×). This is due to an increase in kcat rather than Km (Daujat et al. 2002). It is interesting to note that for CARM1 substrates, the +1 residue is neutral in known protein substrates except for histone H3. For example, the following CARM1 substrates contain a neutral +1 residue; PABP1 R455, R460; HuR R206, R217; HuD R225, R236; p300 (KIX domain) R580, R604; and CBP (post-KIX domain) R714, R742, R768 (Yue et al. 2007). This suggests a potential electrostatic sensing mechanism to explain the preference of a DMA product on H3R17. However, this does not provide an explanation for other substrates of CARM1. This example also highlights the inherent complexity of histone modifications, as posttranslational modification of specific residues can affect the methylation status of other residues. This may be important for drug discovery as changes in methylation status may be gene-specific due to the effect of other posttranslation modifications of chromatin. Therefore, it may be very difficult to detect changes from a methyltransferase inhibitor when measuring global methylation levels.

9.3.2.1 Structure and Catalytic Mechanism of RMTs

The X-ray crystal structure of PRMT1, PRMT3, and CARM1 in various states has been obtained (Zhang and Cheng 2003; Yue et al. 2007; Zhang et al. 2000). The CARM1 X-ray structure was obtained in the presence and absence of SAH, and it was found that upon binding to SAH, significant structural reorganization of the protein occurs resulting in encapsulation of SAH (and presumably SAM) and the formation of the substrate-binding pocket. The authors conclude that the structure is consistent with an ordered mechanism in which SAM binding occurs first and the intermediate MMA must be released from the active site prior to the replenishing of SAM, an observation which is consistent with a distributive mechanism (Yue et al. 2007).

Insight from the structures of PRMT1, PRMT3, and CARM1 has led to the proposal of a catalytic mechanism (Fig. 9.4). When the substrate binds to the RMT-SAM complex, a conserved carboxylate (for CARM1, this is Glu 267, E153 in PRMT1, E355 in PRMT3) interacts with one of the nitrogen atoms in the guanidine group of the arginine residue, resulting in increased localization of positive charge on the Nη1 nitrogen allowing the Nη2 nitrogen to react with SAM (Zhang and Cheng 2003; Yue et al. 2007; Zhang et al. 2000). This carboxylate residue has been shown

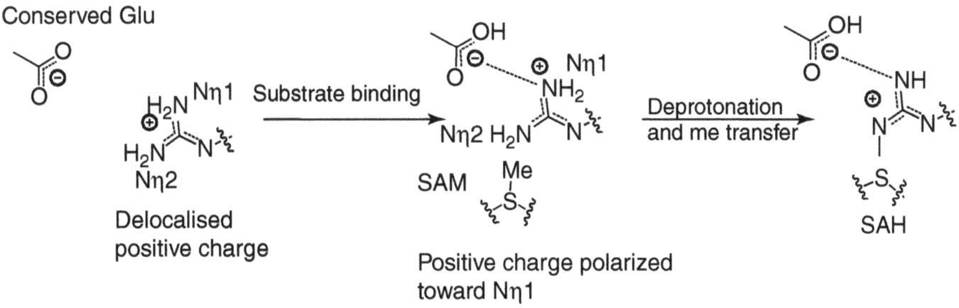

Fig. 9.4 Proposed catalytic mechanism of RMTs

to be critically important in catalysis, as the mutant Glu267Asn is catalytically inactive (Chen et al. 1999; Yue et al. 2007). It is likely, however, that the guanidine group is charged and needs to be deprotonated before reacting with SAM. The authors point out that the timing of the deprotonation step is unknown but is likely to occur *via* a His-Asp (CARM1-H415/D166, PRMT1-H476/D233) coupled proton relay similar to serine proteases (Zhang et al. 2000; Fersht and Sperling 1973). The His and Asp residues are also somewhat conserved throughout the RMTs (Zhang et al. 2000). It has been proposed that deprotonation is likely to be rate determining as in other S_N2 enzymatic reactions (Yue et al. 2007). If the His-Asp couple is involved in the rate-determining step, then it is likely to be highly sensitive to the electronic state of neighboring residues (e.g., difference in kcat for H3K18 and acetylated H3K18).

The protein crystal structures have also provided a hypothesis for the selectivity differences between type I and II RMTs. The type I RMTs produce asymmetric dimethylated arginine residues. One possible explanation for this is due to the sulfur atom of M337 (PRMT3), which is only 3.6 A away from Nη1, essentially sterically blocking this nitrogen. The Nη2 has space to accommodate a monomethyl group which allows for the asymmetrical DMA product formation (Zhang et al. 2000).

9.4 Inhibitors of Histone Methyltransferases

Despite the discovery of the first HMT over 10 years ago (Rea et al. 2000) and the description of close to 100 related proteins (Richon et al. 2011), there has been a paucity of literature describing potent and selective inhibitors not based on SAM, SAH, or Sinefungin (Table 9.2). The majority of reports have focused on inhibitors of CARM1, G9a, and GLP.

9.4.1 Lysine Methyltransferase Inhibitors

9.4.1.1 G9a (EHMT2) and GLP (EHMT1)

The majority of published work on chemical inhibitors of SET domain-containing HMTs has focused on GLP and G9a. The first drug-like small molecule inhibitor

Table 9.2 Lysine and arginine methyltransferase inhibitors: nucleoside analogs

Compound name	Compound structure	Primary target potency (IC_{50})	Comments
SAH	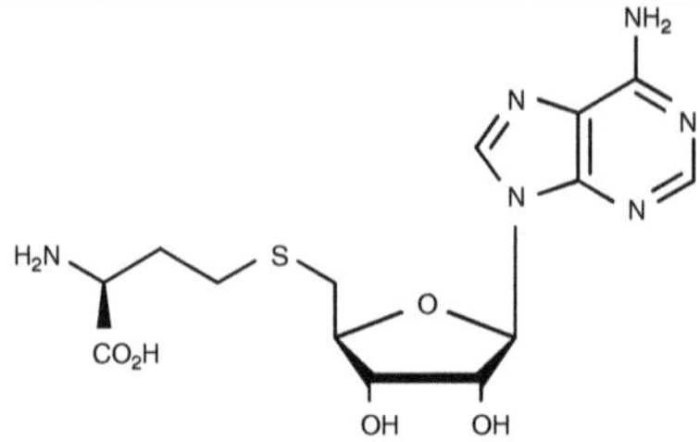	Product of reaction for all PMTs. IC_{50}s range from 0.1 to 20 μM	Nonselective
Sinefungin	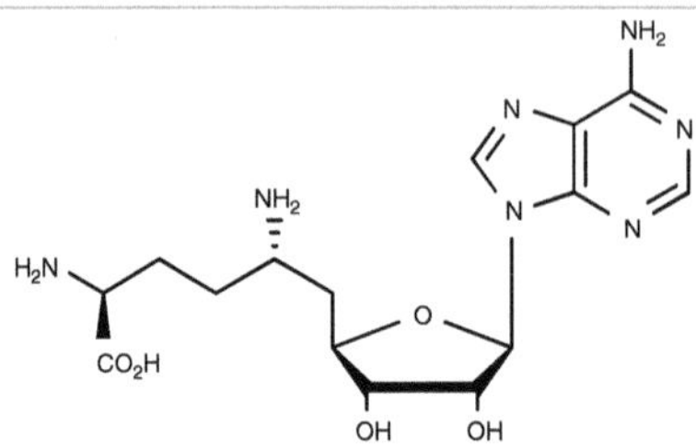	Natural product analog of SAM/SAH. IC_{50}s range from 0.1 to 20 μM	Nonselective
EPZ004777	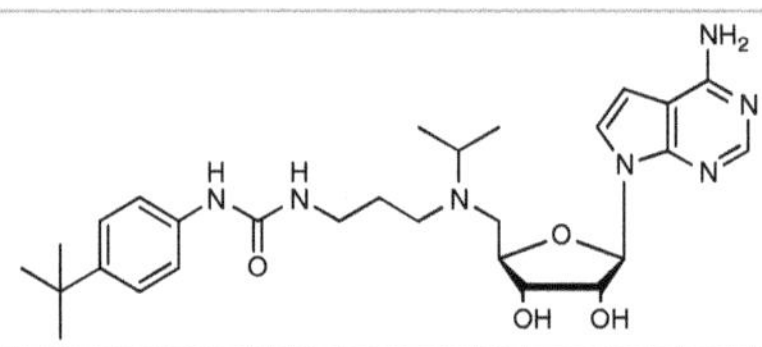	DOT1L inhibitor IC_{50} of 0.4 of nM; >1,000-fold selectivity against other PMTs	Selective DOT1L inhibitor

that acted on these two enzymes was Compound (I) and is known as BIX-01294 (Kubicek et al. 2007). Compound (I) was identified *via* high-throughput screening and is closely related to the α-adrenoceptor antagonist bunazosin (Weidinger 1995) (Table 9.3). Compound (I) demonstrated an IC_{50} of 1.7 μM for G9a and 38 μM for GLP. Two independent groups have replicated the IC_{50} for G9a but found the compound to be significantly more active at GLP with an IC_{50} ~ 0.7 μM (Liu et al. 2009a; Chang et al. 2010). The authors attribute the discrepancy to the fact that the original data was not performed under linear assay conditions. Compound (I) appears to be selective against other HMTs as only minimal activity was observed at PRMT1, ESET, SET7/9, Suv420H1, and SUV39H1.

Compound (I) is uncompetitive with SAM, suggesting that it only binds to the SAM-G9a complex and not the free enzyme. These data are consistent with the X-ray structure of Compound (I) bound to GLP (~80 % sequence similarity to G9a) where the small molecule is bound in the substrate-binding pocket and SAH is also bound (Chang et al. 2009).

In mouse embryonic stem cells treated with 4.1 μM of (I) the H3K9me2 mark was reduced by 20 % with a concomitant rise in unmethylated H3K9 and no change in H3K9me3 or H3K9me1 levels. No changes on the global methylation status of H3K27, H3K36, or H4K20 were observed indicating that the inhibitor selectively inhibits G9a/GLP in cells. The inhibitor (I) did reduce H3K9me2 in G9a null ES cells, and the authors ascribe this finding to the activity on GLP which also affects H3K9 methylation. This explanation is even more likely as the work of other groups has shown that Compound (I) is essentially equipotent against GLP. Therefore, the current evidence suggests that Compound (I) is a dual GLP/G9a inhibitor.

ChIP analysis demonstrated that Compound (I) affected H3K9me2 levels at target genes such as Mage-a2. Approximately 60 % loss of the H3K9me2 mark at the Mage-a2 promoter was observed in mouse ES cells that were treated with 4.1 μM Compound (I). This inhibition was reversible in that the mark returned to original levels within 48 h once the inhibitor was removed.

Two independent groups (Liu et al. 2009a; Chang et al. 2010) expanded upon the crystal structure findings of the GLP-Compound (I)-SAH complex, hypothesizing that an appropriately placed lysine mimic added to Compound (I) would result in improved activity at G9a and or GLP. The hypothesis was derived from the observation that when the X-ray structures of GLP-(I) and GLP-peptide substrate were compared, it was noted that Compound (I) resembled the bound conformation of histone H3 Lys4 to Arg8 but leaving the lysine-binding channel unoccupied. Using this observation, both Chang et al. and Liu et al. replaced the 7-OMe with an aminoalkoxy groups. The first result of the Lui et al. effort was UNC-0224 (III) which demonstrated improved potency compared to (I) (see Table 9.3). It was also found to be inactive in inhibiting other HMTs including SETD7, SET8/PreSET7, PRMT3, and the H3K9 demethylase JMJD2E.

A high-resolution (1.7Å) X-ray crystal structure of the G9a-UNC0224 (III) complex was obtained. On the basis of this structural information, the authors indicate the improved potency of UNC-0224/Compound (III) over Compound (I) is explained by interactions gained from the additional lysine mimetic moiety. In particular, the electrostatic interaction of the protonated dimethyl amine and Leu1086 and the π-cation interaction of the protonated dimethyl amine with Tyr 1154 add to the affinity.

Key structural insights were identified from this analysis, and these are illustrated in Fig. 9.5. Two features of particular note are that (1) the bulk of UNC-0224 (III) occupies the histone peptide-binding site as in the GLP-(I) structure and (2) the lysine-binding channel is not fully occupied by the amino-propoxy lysine mimic. This last observation suggested the potential for further improvement in potency with a longer lysine mimetic. This hypothesis was confirmed by the synthesis of Compound (IV) which shows improved potency against G9a (Table 9.3).

The inhibitor (IV) demonstrated a high Hill slope suggesting that the potency limit of the assays used had been reached (Liu et al. 2009a). Using microfluidic capillary electrophoresis, the Ki values of 2.6 nM and 63 pM were established for Compound (III)/UNC0224 and Compound (IV), respectively, compared to 16 nM for Compound (I). This analysis shows that Compound (IV) has greatly improved potency over both Compound (I)/BIX-01924 and Compound (III)/UNC0224.

Vedadi et al. describe the chemical probe UNC0638 (Vedadi et al. 2011) (Table 9.3). UNC0638 shares common features with (III)/UNC0224 and (IV) but interestingly the basic and polar 1-methyl-1,4-diazepane ring system has been replaced with the neutral and lipophilic cyclohexyl ring. This modification was presumably made in order

Table 9.3 Examples of G9a inhibitors

Compound name	Compound structure	Primary target potency (IC_{50})	Comments
Compound (I)/ BIX-01294	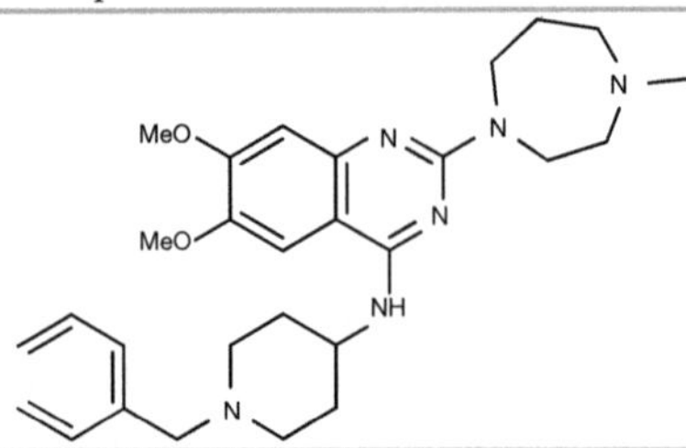	SAM noncompetitive inhibitor of G9a (0.2–1.7 μM) and GLP (0.03–38 μM)	
Compound (II) bunazosin	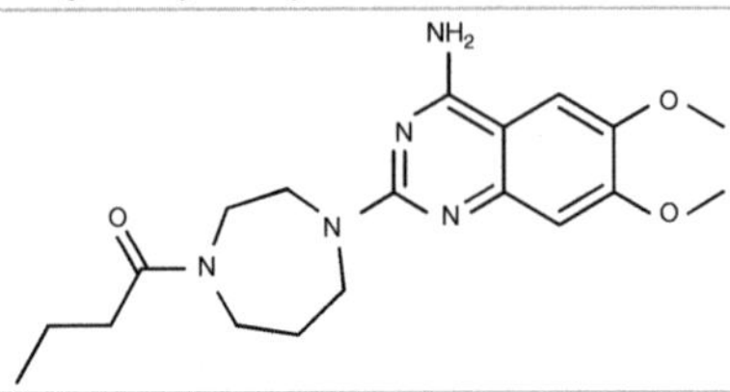		Alpha-adrenoceptor antagonist
Compound (III)/ UNC-0224	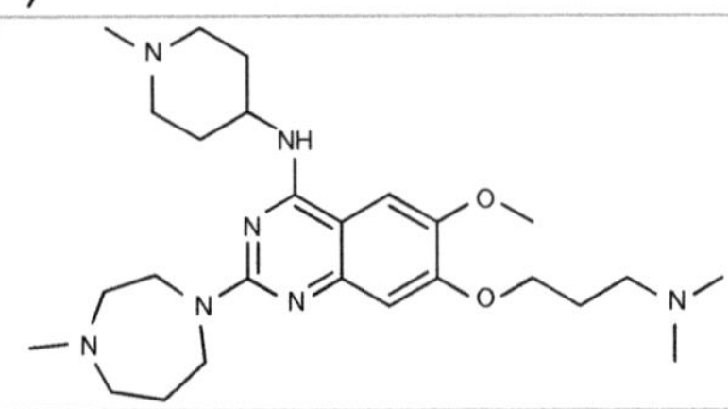	K_i 2.5 nM	Reported as essentially equipotent against GLP
Compound (IV)	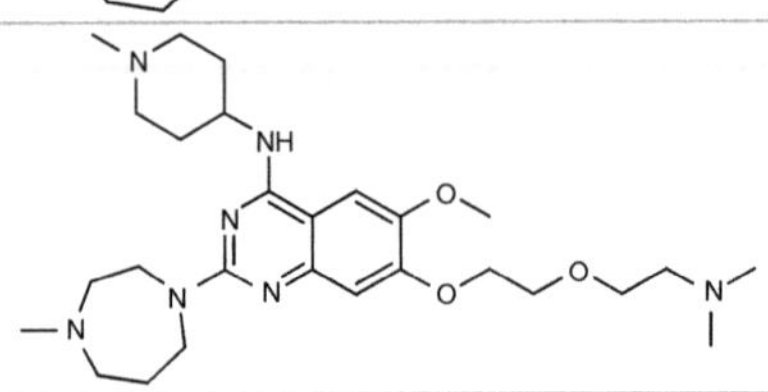	K_i 63 pM	Reported as essentially equipotent against GLP
Compound (V)/ UNC0638	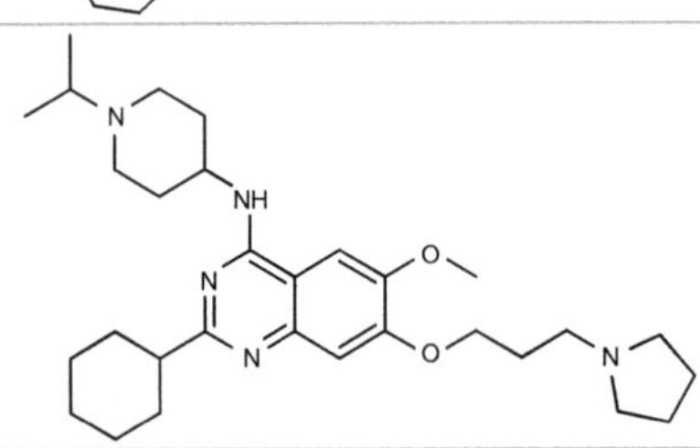	K_i 2.5 nM; G9a inhibitor (IC_{50} <15 nM)	Inhibitor reduces H3K9Me2 in MDA-MB231 cells with an IC_{50} of 81 nM
Compound (VI)	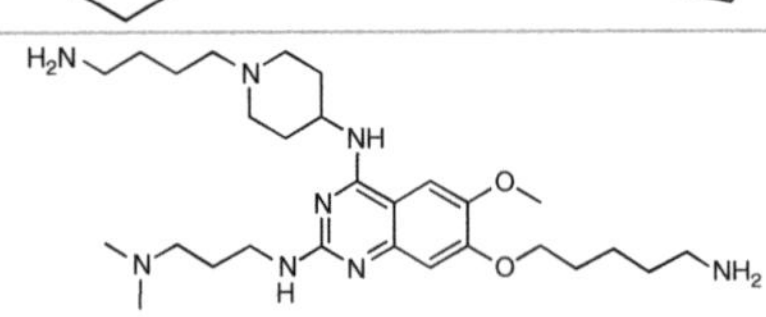	G9a inhibitor (IC_{50} 100 nM)	Essentially equipotent against GLP

to improve cell permeability. Indeed, Compound (V) showed reduction of H3K9me2 in MDA-MB-231 cells with an IC_{50} of 81 nM and with a better separation of methyl mark effects and cell toxicity compared to Compound (I).

Chang et al. (2010) also found that a longer chain at the seven position resulted in improved potency. This change combined with replacement of the diazepane ring and benzyl groups of Compound (I) with a 3-diemethylaminopropyl and a 5-aminopentyl chain, respectively, led to Compound (VI) (Table 9.3). The cumulative effect of these changes is 7-fold improvement in affinity for GLP relative to Compound (I) under identical assay conditions.

It was noted from the (VI)-GLP-SAH X-ray structure that the sulfur atom of SAH was only 4.7Å from the nitrogen of the lysine mimetic, very close to the distance seen in the GLP-SAH-H3K9me1peptide substrate structure of 4.2Å (Chang et al. 2010). Superposition of the (VI)/GLP complex with the GLP/H3K9me1 peptide side-chain complex suggested that the 5-aminopentoxy side chain was appropriately positioned to be a substrate for methylation. Mono-, di-, and trimethylated derivatives of (VI) were detected by mass spectrometry following overnight incubations of nearly equimolar ratio of (VI) and GLP. Despite the nonphysiological conditions of this experiment, it does provide evidence that the inhibitors may also be substrates.

9.4.1.2 DOT1L

EPZ004777 has been reported as a potent and selective inhibitor of DOT1L (Daigle et al. 2011). This molecule is an aminonucleoside analog that was shown to be SAM competitive with an IC_{50} of 0.4 nM for DOT1L biochemical activity and greater than 1,000-fold selectivity against other KMTs and RMTs (Table 9.2). EPZ004777 causes dose-dependent reduction of histone H3K79me2 in cultured cells and inhibits proliferation of leukemia cells bearing the *MLL* translocation. It is noteworthy that cells lacking the *MLL* translocation were insensitive with respect to antiproliferative effects despite undergoing a reduction in the H3K79me2 mark. EPZ004777 also demonstrated in vivo efficacy in a mouse model of disseminated *MLL-rearranged* leukemia, at doses that were well tolerated. These data demonstrate the high specificity of targeting DOT1L for *MLL*-rearranged leukemias.

9.4.2 Arginine Methyltransferase Inhibitors

9.4.2.1 CARM1

One of the first non-SAM like small molecule inhibitors of CARM1 was described by Purandare et al. (2008). High-throughput screening efforts identified Compound (VII) with a CARM1 IC_{50} of 1.8 μM (Table 9.4). Progression of this hit led to the identification of Compound (VIII) with a 10-fold improvement in CARM1 IC_{50}, 0.08 μM (Purandare et al. 2008). Compound (VIII) was also tested for activity against PRMT1 and PRMT3, and IC_{50} values of >25 μM were obtained for each enzyme. No cellular data was reported, presumably because the series was hampered by poor permeability. Compound (VIII) scored poorly in a PAMPA assay with a permeability of less than 0.015 mm/s. An improvement in the permeability was observed when the secondary amide was replaced with the bio-isosteric 1,3,4-oxadiazole ring. This change led to an increase of approximately 10-fold in permeability with no loss of CARM1 inhibitory activity.

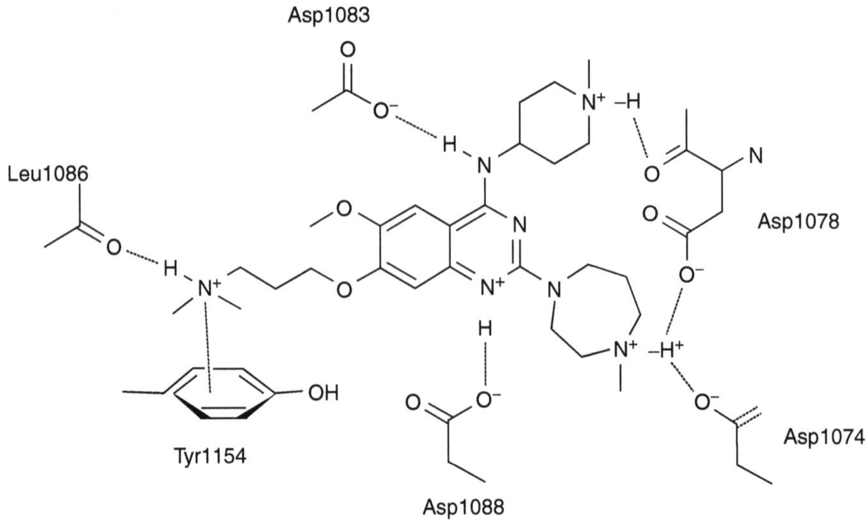

Fig. 9.5 Key interactions of compound (III)/UNC0224 with G9a

Further optimization of the oxadiazole (IX) led to the discovery of (X) which improved CARM1 potency (IC_{50} 0.04 μM) and permeability to 0.267 μm/s (Huynh et al. 2009) (Table 9.4). The compound was further characterized for ADMET properties and found to not inhibit P-450 enzymes (human hepatocyte assay-HHA) or to activate the human pregnane-X receptor (hPXR).

Allan et al. have also developed a related series of thienyl pyrazoles of which Compound (XI) is representative (Allan et al. 2009). They found that the series was of similar potency as earlier compounds described above. Compound (XI) was also selective over the RMT PRMT1 and the KMT SETD7 (IC_{50} >100 μM for each enzyme). Compound (XI), however, was reported to lack cellular activity in two different cell types after 48 h of exposure to the inhibitor at a concentration of 5 μM. A number of reasons for the lack of cell activity are possible, such as cell permeability (the authors report that the thienyl-amide series also possessed poor permeability similar to the phenyl-amide series (e.g., Compound (VIII)) (Huynh et al. 2009). It is also possible that the compounds lack sufficient biochemical potency to elicit cellular effects. Alternatively, the lack of changes in global levels of H3R26 methylation may be due to redundancy due to other RMTs. In light of this, Compounds (XI) and (XII) were evaluated in a series of functional assays. The assays targeted both estrogen dependent transcription, estrogen growth and androgen dependent transcription. Neither Compound (XI) nor (XIII) demonstrated any effect in these assays consistent with the lack of methylation changes observed previously.

Therrien et al. (2009) also noted the poor PK profile of the phenyl-amide and thienyl-amide series, low oral bioavailability in rats and low exposure in mice when dosed by intraperitoneal injection. Compound (XII) which is representative of the phenyl-amide series was characterized with extremely high clearance (1,433 ml/

min/kg) and a short $t_{1/2}$ (<0.25 h) when dosed by intravenous injection in rats. The high clearance precluded the accurate measurement of oral bioavailability, volume of distribution and half-life. Therrien et al. hypothesized that the high clearance was due to the presence of the (S)-alanine benzylamide present in both chemical series.

Table 9.4 Examples of CARM1 inhibitors

Compound name	Compound structure	Primary target potency (IC_{50})	Comments
Compound (VII)	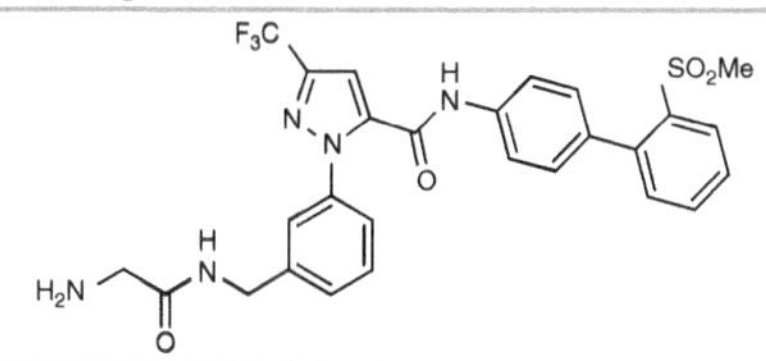	CARM1 IC_{50} 1.8 μM	
Compound (VIII)	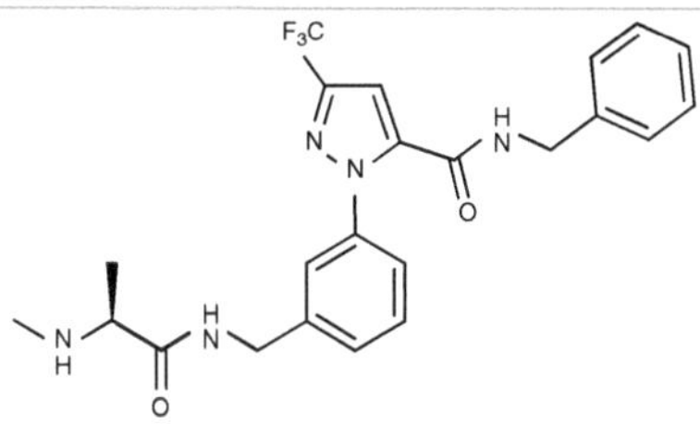	CARM1 IC_{50} 80 nM	PAMPA <15 nm/s
Compound (IX)	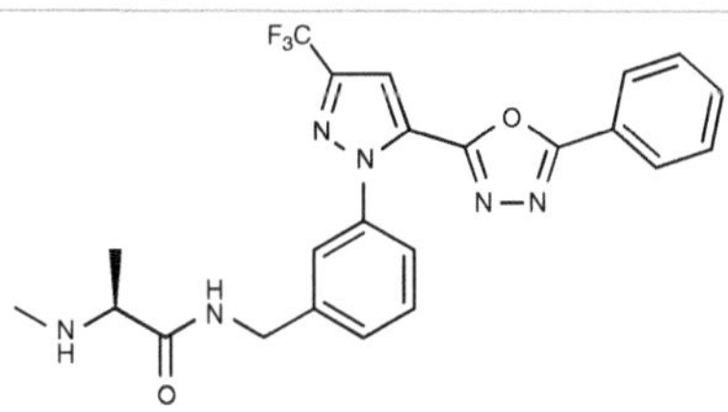	CARM1 IC_{50} 60 nM	PAMPA 106 nm/s
Compound (X)	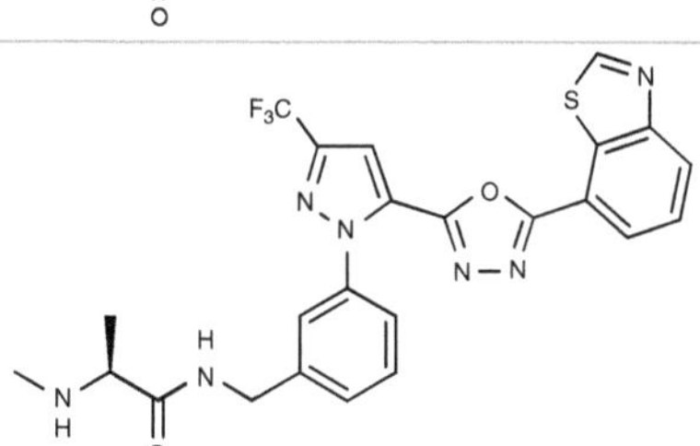	CARM1 IC_{50} 40 nM; >100-fold for PRMT1 and PRMT3	PAMPA 267 nm/s; hPXR (EC50) >25 μM; HHA IC_{50} >100 μM; improved permeability
Compound (XI)	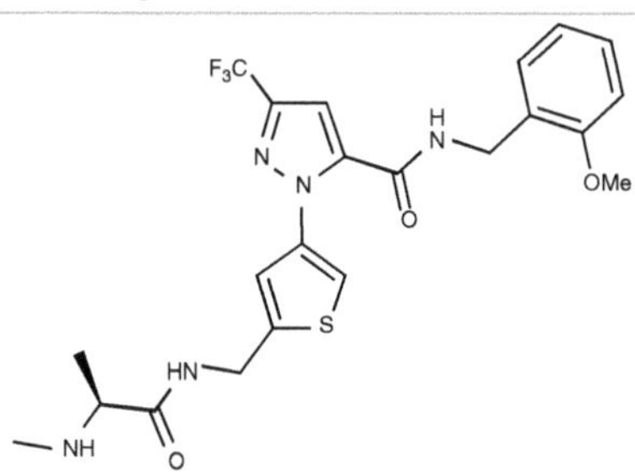	CARM1 IC_{50} 60 nM	

(continued)

Table 9.4 (continued)

Compound name	Compound structure	Primary target potency (IC_{50})	Comments
Compound (XII)	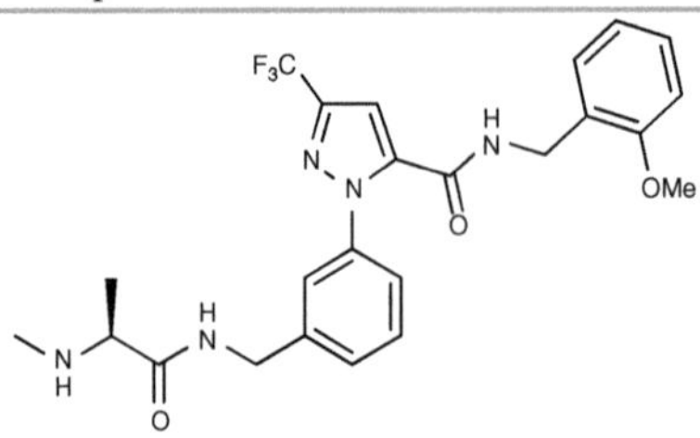	CARM1 IC_{50} 60 nM	Cl 1,433 ml/ min/kg
Compound (XIII)	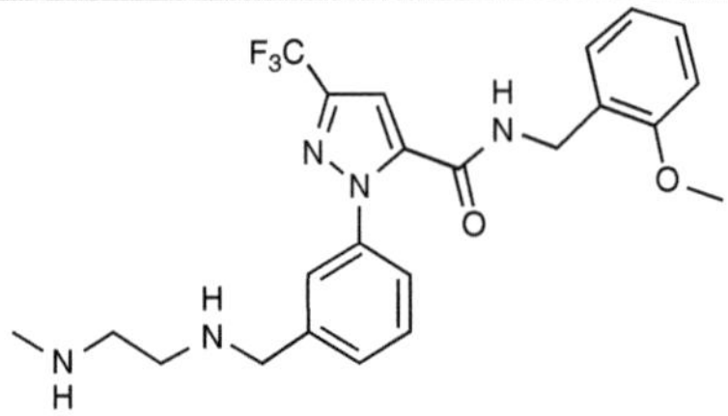	CARM1 IC_{50} 200 nM; >100 μM for PRMT1 and SET7/9	Cl 20 ml/min/ kg; Vdss 0.2 kg; $t_{1/2}$ 2.1 h; F4 %
Compound (XIV)	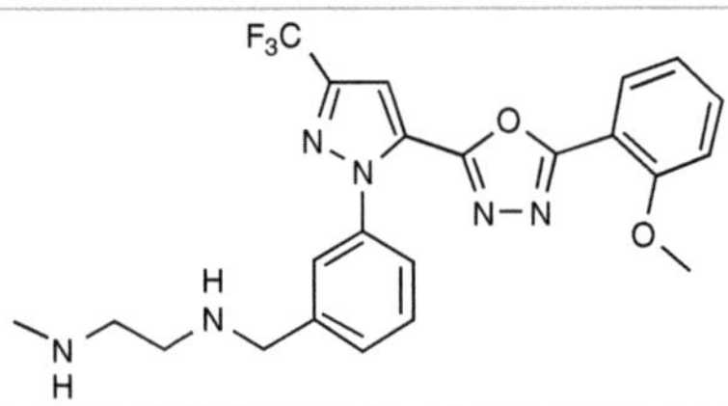	CARM1 IC_{50} 590 nM	Cl 37 ml/min/ kg; Vdss 0.6 kg/ $t_{1/2}$ 1.8 h; F3 %
Compound (XV)	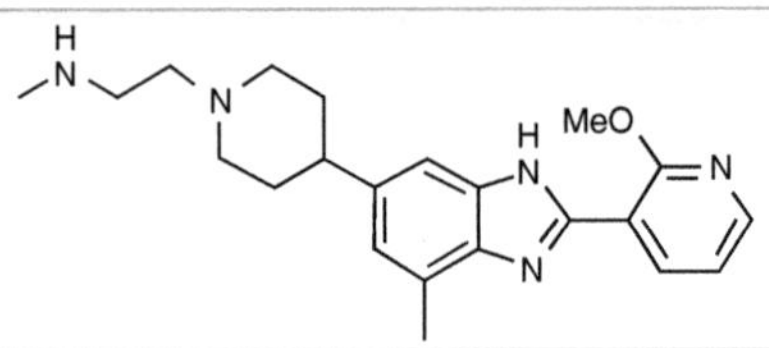	CARM1 IC_{50} 840 nM	X-ray complex of Sinefungin-CARM1-inhibitor
Compound (XVI)	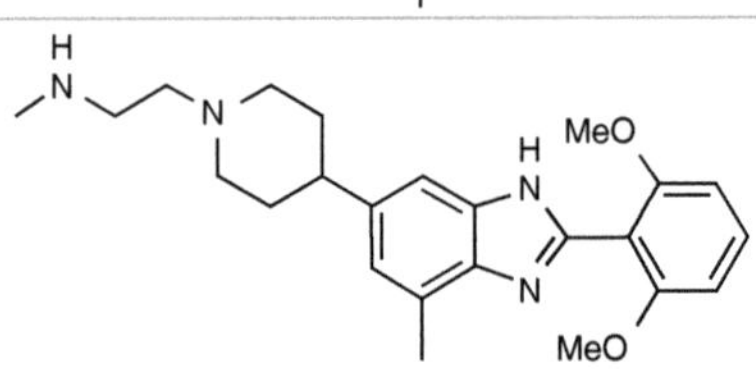	CARM1 IC_{50} 70 nM	>300-fold selective for CARM1 compared to PRMT1 and PRMT3
Compound (XVII)	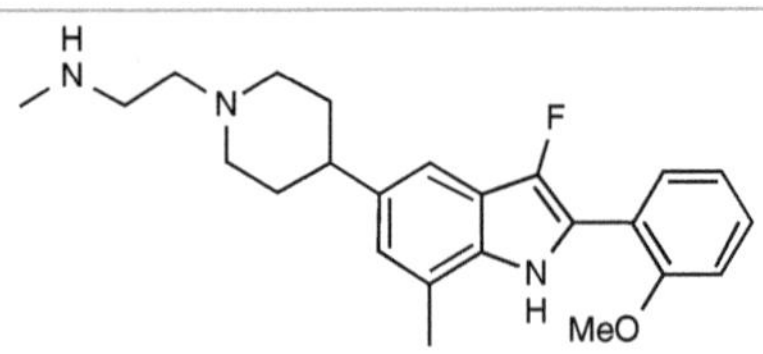	CARM1 IC_{50} 81 nM	>100-fold selective for CARM1 compared to PRMT1 and PRMT3

After SAR exploration into the replacement of this moiety, it was found that a N^1-benzyl-N^{2}methylethane-1,2 diamine unit could adequately replace the alanine amide group with minimal loss in CARM1 potency, as exemplified by Compound

(XIII). The PK profile of Compound (XIII) was evaluated in rats and was found to have a much reduced clearance (20 ml/min/kg) which resulted in an improved $t_{1/2}$ of 2.1 h. The volume of distribution and oral bioavailability, however, remained low: 1.4 l/kg and 4 %, respectively.

The low oral bioavailability may be due to the amide functionality, as both Therrien et al. (2009) and Huynh et al. (2009) indicate that this group confers low permeability in both the phenyl and thienyl series. To address these concerns, Therrien et al. (2009) synthesized Compound (XIV) with the 1,3,4-oxadiazole ring which had been shown to improve permeability (Huynh et al. 2009). As can be seen from Compound (XIV), bio-steric replacement did not improve oral bioavailability or increase the volume of distribution; however, no PAMPA data was reported for this analog, so it is unclear if this analog had improved permeability.

Troffer-Charlier et al. also proposed a binding mode based on docking (XIII) into a published X-ray structure of CARM1-SAH (Troffer-Charlier et al. 2007). A graphical representation of the critical interaction of the N^1-benzyl-N2methylethane-1,2 diamine group is shown schematically in Fig. 9.6. The diamine group is proposed to bind to a water molecule as well as the carboxylate group of Asp191 and the backbone carbonyl of Gly193. A significant SAR effort around the diamine side chain was undertaken, with small changes producing large changes in activity. It was proposed that the linker needs to be flexible in order to adopt the required conformation to interact with the water molecule, Asp 191 and Gly193, while avoiding a potentially energetically costly interaction with the positively charged Arg 169 (which interacts with the carboxylate of SAH). No kinetic or crystallographic data has been reported on this diamine series to date to support the idea that these compounds bind in the SAM-binding site.

Wan et al. also found a benzo[d]imidazole hit (XV) *via* high-throughput screening which inhibited CARM1 with an IC_{50} of 0.84 μM (Wan et al. 2009). This series also contains a diamine moiety similar to that in the Compounds (XIII) and (XIV), though in this series a tertiary amine is incorporated into the diamine, and no such corresponding analog was reported (Allan et al. 2009; Therrien et al. 2009). Therefore, it is unclear if the two series are related in regard to how they interact with CARM1.

Wan et al. performed a hit to lead effort on (XV) and found most changes to the molecule were detrimental (Wan et al. 2009). The C-2 substituent on the benzo[d]imidazole, however, proved to be a fruitful area to analog resulting in Compound (XVI) with over 10-fold improvement in CARM1 IC_{50}. Further studies from Wan et al. led to the discovery of the indole Compound (XVII) (presented at ACS Symposium, Boston, 2010). Compound (XVI) is a potent CARM1 inhibitor and inhibits histone H3 methylation (IC_{50} 0.081 μM). It was reported to inhibit the methylation of nonhistone CARM1 substrates (PABP and HuR) with similar potency. This group also performed additional pharmacology on the indole compound (XVII) and found that the compound is metabolically stable in mouse, rat, and human microsomes and displays no inhibition of P-450 enzymes but does, however, possess poor permeability as measured in Caco-2 and PAMPA experiments. The compound also is an hERG inhibitor which is likely due to the basic side chain

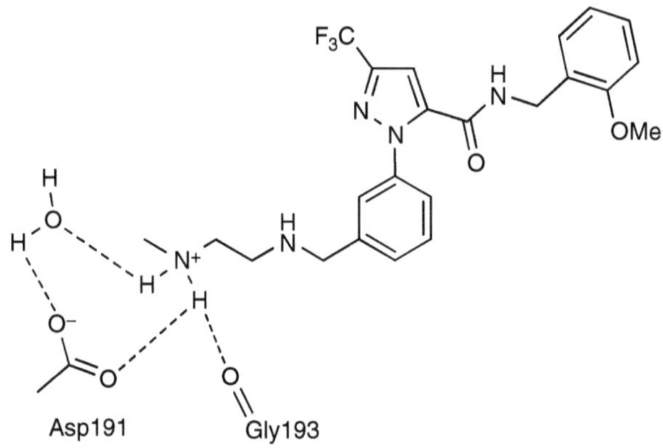

Fig. 9.6 Proposed binding of compound (XIII) in the SAM binding pocket of CARM1

coupled with high lipophilicity (clogP ~4.9). A co-crystal of Compound (XVII) with Sinefungin and CARM1 was also presented. Unlike the model proposed by Therrien et al. (2009), it was found that the inhibitor was bound in the substrate-binding pocket rather than the SAM-binding pocket which was occupied by Sinefungin.

No cellular data was reported for any of the new analogs. This remains an outstanding issue for the CARM1 inhibitors described to date, as poor permeability is observed in multiple series and until robust cellular effects are observed, it is unclear whether these compounds are appropriate tools for examining the role of CARM1 mediated biology.

9.5 Summary and Future Perspectives

The HMTs are a promising new class of targets for cancer. Members of the enzyme family have demonstrated strong cancer relevance, and recent genome studies have linked genetic alterations in members of this family with specific cancer indications. Until recently, very few small molecule inhibitors have been described, and currently the first inhibitors are entering evaluation in clinical trials. The field has begun identifying inhibitors of these novel enzymes, initially with nucleoside or natural product-derived inhibitors. The development of a rich set of selective inhibitors with diverse chemical properties will enable the field to evaluate the potential of these targets in both preclinical and ultimately clinical studies. Many question remain, but with the increasing biological understanding of these enzymes and their role in cancer and other diseases, it is likely that this field will rapidly evolve over the coming years to provide important new therapeutics for cancer treatment.

Acknowledgement We thank Dr. Robert A. Copeland for helpful discussions and careful reading of the Chapter.

References

Abu-Farha M et al (2008) The tale of two domains: proteomics and genomics analysis of SMYD2, a new histone methyltransferase. Mol Cell Proteomics 7(3):560–572

Adams-Cioaba MA, Min J (2009) Structure and function of histone methylation binding proteins. Biochem Cell Biol 87(1):93–105

Aggarwal P et al (2010) Nuclear cyclin D1/CDK4 kinase regulates CUL4 expression and triggers neoplastic growth via activation of the PRMT5 methyltransferase. Cancer Cell 18(4):329–340

Agger K et al (2007) UTX and JMJD3 are histone H3K27 demethylases involved in HOX gene regulation and development. Nature 449(7163):731–734

Allan M et al (2009) N-Benzyl-1-heteroaryl-3-(trifluoromethyl)-1H-pyrazole-5-carboxamides as inhibitors of co-activator associated arginine methyltransferase 1 (CARM1). Bioorg Med Chem Lett 19(4):1218–1223

Andreu-Vieyra CV et al (2010) MLL2 is required in oocytes for bulk histone 3 lysine 4 trimethylation and transcriptional silencing. PLoS Biol 8(8):e1000453

Angrand PO et al (2001) NSD3, a new SET domain-containing gene, maps to 8p12 and is amplified in human breast cancer cell lines. Genomics 74(1):79–88

Barrett A et al (2007) Breast cancer associated transcriptional repressor PLU-1/JARID1B interacts directly with histone deacetylases. Int J Cancer 121(2):265–275

Barry ER, Corry GN, Rasmussen TP (2010) Targeting DOT1L action and interactions in leukemia: the role of DOT1L in transformation and development. Expert Opin Ther Targets 14(4):405–418

Barski A et al (2007) High-resolution profiling of histone methylations in the human genome. Cell 129(4):823–837

Bedford MT, Richard S (2005) Arginine methylation: an emerging regulator of protein function. Mol Cell 18:263–272

Bernstein BE et al (2005) Genomic maps and comparative analysis of histone modifications in human and mouse. Cell 120(2):169–181

Bernstein BE et al (2006) A bivalent chromatin structure marks key developmental genes in embryonic stem cells. Cell 125(2):315–326

Bitoun E, Oliver PL, Davies KE (2007) The mixed-lineage leukemia fusion partner AF4 stimulates RNA polymerase II transcriptional elongation and mediates coordinated chromatin remodeling. Hum Mol Genet 16(1):92–106

Boisvert FM et al (2005a) Arginine methylation of MRE11 by PRMT1 is required for DNA damage checkpoint control. Genes Dev 19(6):671–676

Boisvert FM et al (2005b) The GAR motif of 53BP1 is arginine methylated by PRMT1 and is necessary for 53BP1 DNA binding activity. Cell Cycle 4(12):1834–1841

Botuyan MV et al (2006) Structural basis for the methylation state-specific recognition of histone H4-K20 by 53BP1 and Crb2 in DNA repair. Cell 127(7):1361–1373

Boyer LA et al (2005) Core transcriptional regulatory circuitry in human embryonic stem cells. Cell 122(6):947–956

Boyer LA et al (2006) Polycomb complexes repress developmental regulators in murine embryonic stem cells. Nature 441(7091):349–353

Bracken AP et al (2003) EZH2 is downstream of the pRB-E2F pathway, essential for proliferation and amplified in cancer. EMBO J 22(20):5323–5335

Brown MA et al (2006) Identification and characterization of Smyd2: a split SET/MYND domain-containing histone H3 lysine 36-specific methyltransferase that interacts with the Sin3 histone deacetylase complex. Mol Cancer 5:26

Cao R, Zhang Y (2004a) SUZ12 is required for both the histone methyltransferase activity and the silencing function of the EED-EZH2 complex. Mol Cell 15(1):57–67

Cao R, Zhang Y (2004b) The functions of E(Z)/EZH2-mediated methylation of lysine 27 in histone H3. Curr Opin Genet Dev 14(2):155–164

Cao R et al (2002) Role of histone H3 lysine 27 methylation in Polycomb-group silencing. Science 298(5595):1039–1043

Cao R et al (2008a) Role of hPHF1 in H3K27 methylation and Hox gene silencing. Mol Cell Biol 28(5):1862–1872

Cao Q et al (2008b) Repression of E-cadherin by the polycomb group protein EZH2 in cancer. Oncogene 27(58):7274–7284

Ceol CJ et al (2011) The histone methyltransferase SETDB1 is recurrently amplified in melanoma and accelerates its onset. Nature 471(7339):513–517

Chang Y et al (2009) Structural basis for G9a-like protein lysine methyltransferase inhibition by BIX-01294. Nat Struct Mol Biol 16(3):312–317

Chang Y et al (2010) Adding a lysine mimic in the design of potent inhibitors of histone lysine methyltransferases. J Mol Biol 400(1):1–7

Chen D et al (1999) Regulation of transcription by a protein methyltransferase. Science 284(5423):2174–2177

Cheng X, Blumenthal RM (2010) Coordinated chromatin control: structural and functional linkage of DNA and histone methylation. Biochemistry 49(14):2999–3008

Chesi M et al (1998) The t(4;14) translocation in myeloma dysregulates both FGFR3 and a novel gene, MMSET, resulting in IgH/MMSET hybrid transcripts. Blood 92(9):3025–3034

Cheung N et al (2007) Protein arginine-methyltransferase-dependent oncogenesis. Nat Cell Biol 9(10):1208–1215

Cloos PA et al (2006) The putative oncogene GASC1 demethylates tri- and dimethylated lysine 9 on histone H3. Nature 442(7100):307–311

Collins RE et al (2005) In vitro and in vivo analyses of a Phe/Tyr switch controlling product specificity of histone lysine methyltransferases. J Biol Chem 280(7):5563–5570

Copeland RA, Solomon ME, Richon VM (2009) Protein methyltransferases as a target class for drug discovery. Nat Rev Drug Discov 8(9):724–732

Daigle SR et al (2011) Selective killing of mixed lineage leukemia cells by a potent small-molecule DOT1L inhibitor. Cancer Cell 20(1):53–65

Daujat S et al (2002) Crosstalk between CARM1 methylation and CBP acetylation on histone H3. Curr Biol 12(24):2090–2097

Del Rizzo PA et al (2010) SET7/9 catalytic mutants reveal the role of active site water molecules in lysine multiple methylation. J Biol Chem 285(41):31849–31858

Di Lorenzo A, Bedford MT (2011) Histone arginine methylation. FEBS Lett 585(13):2024–2031

Dillon SC et al (2005) The SET-domain protein superfamily: protein lysine methyltransferases. Genome Biol 6(8):227

Dirk LM et al (2007) Kinetic manifestation of processivity during multiple methylations catalyzed by SET domain protein methyltransferases. Biochemistry 46(12):3905–3915

Eissenberg JC, Shilatifard A (2010) Histone H3 lysine 4 (H3K4) methylation in development and differentiation. Dev Biol 339(2):240–249

El Messaoudi S et al (2006) Coactivator-associated arginine methyltransferase 1 (CARM1) is a positive regulator of the Cyclin E1 gene. Proc Natl Acad Sci USA 103(36):13351–13356

Feldman N et al (2006) G9a-mediated irreversible epigenetic inactivation of Oct-3/4 during early embryogenesis. Nat Cell Biol 8(2):188–194

Feng X, Hara Y, Riabowol K (2002) Different HATS of the ING1 gene family. Trends Cell Biol 12(11):532–538

Feng Q et al (2006) Signaling within a coactivator complex: methylation of SRC-3/AIB1 is a molecular switch for complex disassembly. Mol Cell Biol 26(21):7846–7857

Fersht AR, Sperling J (1973) The charge relay system in chymotrypsin and chymotrypsinogen. J Mol Biol 74(2):137–149

Fraga MF et al (2005) Loss of acetylation at Lys16 and trimethylation at Lys20 of histone H4 is a common hallmark of human cancer. Nat Genet 37(4):391–400

Frietze S et al (2008) CARM1 regulates estrogen-stimulated breast cancer growth through up-regulation of E2F1. Cancer Res 68(1):301–306

Frietze S et al (2010) ZNF274 recruits the histone methyltransferase SETDB1 to the 3′ ends of ZNF genes. PLoS One 5(12):e15082

Gao WL, Liu HL (2007) DOT1: a distinct class of histone lysine methyltransferase. Yi Chuan 29(12):1449–1454

Guendel I et al (2010) Methylation of the tumor suppressor protein, BRCA1, influences its transcriptional cofactor function. PLoS One 5(6):e11379
Guo HB, Guo H (2007) Mechanism of histone methylation catalyzed by protein lysine methyltransferase SET7/9 and origin of product specificity. Proc Natl Acad Sci USA 104(21):8797–8802
Guo Y et al (2009) Methylation-state-specific recognition of histones by the MBT repeat protein L3MBTL2. Nucleic Acids Res 37(7):2204–2210
Gupta RA et al (2010) Long non-coding RNA HOTAIR reprograms chromatin state to promote cancer metastasis. Nature 464(7291):1071–1076
Hamamoto R et al (2004) SMYD3 encodes a histone methyltransferase involved in the proliferation of cancer cells. Nat Cell Biol 6(8):731–740
Hamamoto R et al (2006) Enhanced SMYD3 expression is essential for the growth of breast cancer cells. Cancer Sci 97(2):113–118
Hess JL (2004) Mechanisms of transformation by MLL. Crit Rev Eukaryot Gene Expr 14(4):235–254
Higashimoto K et al (2007) Phosphorylation-mediated inactivation of coactivator-associated arginine methyltransferase 1. Proc Natl Acad Sci USA 104(30):12318–12323
Hong H et al (2004) Aberrant expression of CARM1, a transcriptional coactivator of androgen receptor, in the development of prostate carcinoma and androgen-independent status. Cancer 101(1):83–89
Horton JR et al (2010) Enzymatic and structural insights for substrate specificity of a family of jumonji histone lysine demethylases. Nat Struct Mol Biol 17(1):38–43
Hou Z et al (2008) The LIM protein AJUBA recruits protein arginine methyltransferase 5 to mediate SNAIL-dependent transcriptional repression. Mol Cell Biol 28(10):3198–3207
Huang Y et al (2009) Novel oligoamine analogues inhibit lysine-specific demethylase 1 and induce reexpression of epigenetically silenced genes. Clin Cancer Res 15(23):7217–7228
Huang J et al (2010) G9a and Glp methylate lysine 373 in the tumor suppressor p53. J Biol Chem 285(13):9636–9641
Huynh T et al (2009) Optimization of pyrazole inhibitors of Coactivator Associated Arginine Methyltransferase 1 (CARM1). Bioorg Med Chem Lett 19(11):2924–2927
Jaju RJ et al (2001) A novel gene, NSD1, is fused to NUP98 in the t(5;11)(q35;p15.5) in de novo childhood acute myeloid leukemia. Blood 98(4):1264–1267
Jansson M et al (2008) Arginine methylation regulates the p53 response. Nat Cell Biol 10(12):1431–1439
Jeong YS et al (2010) Phosphorylation of serine-10 of histone H3 shields modified lysine-9 selectively during mitosis. Genes Cells 15(3):181–192
Kalakonda N et al (2008) Histone H4 lysine 20 monomethylation promotes transcriptional repression by L3MBTL1. Oncogene 27(31):4293–4304
Kang MY et al (2007) Association of the SUV39H1 histone methyltransferase with the DNA methyltransferase 1 at mRNA expression level in primary colorectal cancer. Int J Cancer 121(10):2192–2197
Kaustov L et al (2011) Recognition and specificity determinants of the human cbx chromodomains. J Biol Chem 286(1):521–529
Kim H et al (2009) Requirement of histone methyltransferase SMYD3 for estrogen receptor-mediated transcription. J Biol Chem 284(30):19867–19877
Kireev D et al (2010) Identification of non-peptide malignant brain tumor (MBT) repeat antagonists by virtual screening of commercially available compounds. J Med Chem 53(21):7625–7631
Kirmizis A, Bartley SM, Farnham PJ (2003) Identification of the polycomb group protein SU(Z)12 as a potential molecular target for human cancer therapy. Mol Cancer Ther 2(1):113–121
Kleer CG et al (2003) EZH2 is a marker of aggressive breast cancer and promotes neoplastic transformation of breast epithelial cells. Proc Natl Acad Sci USA 100(20):11606–11611
Klose RJ et al (2006) The transcriptional repressor JHDM3A demethylates trimethyl histone H3 lysine 9 and lysine 36. Nature 442(7100):312–316
Kohlmaier A et al (2004) A chromosomal memory triggered by Xist regulates histone methylation in X inactivation. PLoS Biol 2(7):E171

Kolbel K et al (2009) Type I arginine methyltransferases PRMT1 and PRMT-3 Act distributively. J Biol Chem 284(13):8274–8282

Kouzarides T (2007) Chromatin modifications and their function. Cell 128(4):693–705

Krishnan S, Horowitz S, Trievel RC (2011) Structure and function of histone H3 lysine 9 methyltransferases and demethylases. Chembiochem 12(2):254–263

Krivtsov AV, Armstrong SA (2007) MLL translocations, histone modifications and leukaemia stem-cell development. Nat Rev Cancer 7(11):823–833

Krivtsov AV et al (2008) H3K79 methylation profiles define murine and human MLL-AF4 leukemias. Cancer Cell 14(5):355–368

Kubicek S et al (2007) Reversal of H3K9me2 by a small-molecule inhibitor for the G9a histone methyltransferase. Mol Cell 25(3):473–481

Lan F et al (2007) Recognition of unmethylated histone H3 lysine 4 links BHC80 to LSD1-mediated gene repression. Nature 448(7154):718–722

Lauring J et al (2008) The multiple myeloma associated MMSET gene contributes to cellular adhesion, clonogenic growth, and tumorigenicity. Blood 111(2):856–864

Lee SH et al (2005) The SET domain protein Metnase mediates foreign DNA integration and links integration to nonhomologous end-joining repair. Proc Natl Acad Sci USA 102(50): 18075–18080

Levine SS et al (2002) The core of the polycomb repressive complex is compositionally and functionally conserved in flies and humans. Mol Cell Biol 22(17):6070–6078

Li H et al (2006) Molecular basis for site-specific read-out of histone H3K4me3 by the BPTF PHD finger of NURF. Nature 442(7098):91–95

Li Y et al (2009) The target of the NSD family of histone lysine methyltransferases depends on the nature of the substrate. J Biol Chem 284(49):34283–34295

Li X et al (2010) H4R3 methylation facilitates beta-globin transcription by regulating histone acetyltransferase binding and H3 acetylation. Blood 115(10):2028–2037

Lim S et al (2010a) Epigenetic regulation of cancer growth by histone demethylases. Int J Cancer 127(9):1991–1998

Lim S et al (2010b) Lysine-specific demethylase 1 (LSD1) is highly expressed in ER-negative breast cancers and a biomarker predicting aggressive biology. Carcinogenesis 31(3):512–520

Liu C et al (2007) The telomerase reverse transcriptase (hTERT) gene is a direct target of the histone methyltransferase SMYD3. Cancer Res 67(6):2626–2631

Liu F et al (2009a) Discovery of a 2,4-diamino-7-aminoalkoxyquinazoline as a potent and selective inhibitor of histone lysine methyltransferase G9a. J Med Chem 52(24):7950–7953

Liu G et al (2009b) Genomic amplification and oncogenic properties of the GASC1 histone demethylase gene in breast cancer. Oncogene 28(50):4491–4500

Liu F et al (2010) Protein lysine methyltransferase G9a inhibitors: design, synthesis, and structure activity relationships of 2,4-diamino-7-aminoalkoxy-quinazolines. J Med Chem 53(15):5844–5857

Loyola A et al (2009) The HP1alpha-CAF1-SetDB1-containing complex provides H3K9me1 for Suv39-mediated K9me3 in pericentric heterochromatin. EMBO Rep 10(7):769–775

Luo XG et al (2009) Effects of SMYD3 overexpression on transformation, serum dependence, and apoptosis sensitivity in NIH3T3 cells. IUBMB Life 61(6):679–684

Majumder S et al (2006) Involvement of arginine methyltransferase CARM1 in androgen receptor function and prostate cancer cell viability. Prostate 66(12):1292–1301

Margueron R et al (2008) Ezh1 and Ezh2 maintain repressive chromatin through different mechanisms. Mol Cell 32(4):503–518

Maurer-Stroh S et al (2003) The Tudor domain 'Royal Family': Tudor, plant Agenet, Chromo, PWWP and MBT domains. Trends Biochem Sci 28(2):69–74

Min J et al (2003) Structure of the catalytic domain of human DOT1L, a non-SET domain nucleosomal histone methyltransferase. Cell 112(5):711–723

Miranda TB et al (2004) PRMT7 is a member of the protein arginine methyltransferase family with a distinct substrate specificity. J Biol Chem 279(22):22902–22907

Morin RD et al (2010) Somatic mutations altering EZH2 (Tyr641) in follicular and diffuse large B-cell lymphomas of germinal-center origin. Nat Genet 42(2):181–185

Naeem H et al (2007) The activity and stability of the transcriptional coactivator p/CIP/SRC-3 are regulated by CARM1-dependent methylation. Mol Cell Biol 27(1):120–134

Ng HH et al (2002a) Lysine methylation within the globular domain of histone H3 by Dot1 is important for telomeric silencing and Sir protein association. Genes Dev 16(12):1518–1527

Ng HH et al (2002b) Ubiquitination of histone H2B by Rad6 is required for efficient Dot1-mediated methylation of histone H3 lysine 79. J Biol Chem 277(38):34655–34657

Oda H et al (2009) Monomethylation of histone H4-lysine 20 is involved in chromosome structure and stability and is essential for mouse development. Mol Cell Biol 29(8):2278–2295

Okada Y et al (2005) hDOT1L links histone methylation to leukemogenesis. Cell 121(2):167–178

Ooi SK et al (2007) DNMT3L connects unmethylated lysine 4 of histone H3 to de novo methylation of DNA. Nature 448(7154):714–717

Pal S et al (2004) Human SWI/SNF-associated PRMT5 methylates histone H3 arginine 8 and negatively regulates expression of ST7 and NM23 tumor suppressor genes. Mol Cell Biol 24(21):9630–9645

Pal S et al (2007) Low levels of miR-92b/96 induce PRMT5 translation and H3R8/H4R3 methylation in mantle cell lymphoma. EMBO J 26(15):3558–3569

Pesavento JJ et al (2008) Certain and progressive methylation of histone H4 at lysine 20 during the cell cycle. Mol Cell Biol 28(1):468–486

Peters AH et al (2003) Partitioning and plasticity of repressive histone methylation states in mammalian chromatin. Mol Cell 12(6):1577–1589

Purandare AV et al (2008) Pyrazole inhibitors of coactivator associated arginine methyltransferase 1 (CARM1). Bioorg Med Chem Lett 18(15):4438–4441

Rao B et al (2005) Dimethylation of histone H3 at lysine 36 demarcates regulatory and nonregulatory chromatin genome-wide. Mol Cell Biol 25(21):9447–9459

Rathert P et al (2008) Protein lysine methyltransferase G9a acts on non-histone targets. Nat Chem Biol 4(6):344–346

Rea S et al (2000) Regulation of chromatin structure by site-specific histone H3 methyltransferases. Nature 406(6796):593–599

Richon VM et al (2011) Chemogenetic analysis of human protein methyltransferases. Chem Biol Drug Des 78(2):199–210

Rosati R et al (2002) NUP98 is fused to the NSD3 gene in acute myeloid leukemia associated with t(8;11)(p11.2;p15). Blood 99(10):3857–3860

Ruthenburg AJ, Allis CD, Wysocka J (2007) Methylation of lysine 4 on histone H3: intricacy of writing and reading a single epigenetic mark. Mol Cell 25(1):15–30

Sanders SL et al (2004) Methylation of histone H4 lysine 20 controls recruitment of Crb2 to sites of DNA damage. Cell 119(5):603–614

Santos-Rosa H et al (2002) Active genes are tri-methylated at K4 of histone H3. Nature 419(6905):407–411

Sarma K et al (2008) Ezh2 requires PHF1 to efficiently catalyze H3 lysine 27 trimethylation in vivo. Mol Cell Biol 28(8):2718–2731

Schlesinger Y et al (2007) Polycomb-mediated methylation on Lys27 of histone H3 pre-marks genes for de novo methylation in cancer. Nat Genet 39(2):232–236

Schneider R et al (2004) Histone H3 lysine 4 methylation patterns in higher eukaryotic genes. Nat Cell Biol 6(1):73–77

Schotta G et al (2004) A silencing pathway to induce H3-K9 and H4-K20 trimethylation at constitutive heterochromatin. Genes Dev 18(11):1251–1262

Schubert HL, Blumenthal RM, Cheng X (2003) Many paths to methyltransfer: a chronicle of convergence. Trends Biochem Sci 28(6):329–335

Schulte JH et al (2009) Lysine-specific demethylase 1 is strongly expressed in poorly differentiated neuroblastoma: implications for therapy. Cancer Res 69(5):2065–2071

Schultz DC et al (2002) SETDB1: a novel KAP-1-associated histone H3, lysine 9-specific methyltransferase that contributes to HP1-mediated silencing of euchromatic genes by KRAB zinc-finger proteins. Genes Dev 16(8):919–932

Shahbazian MD, Zhang K, Grunstein M (2005) Histone H2B ubiquitylation controls processive methylation but not monomethylation by Dot1 and Set1. Mol Cell 19(2):271–277

Shi Y, Whetstine JR (2007) Dynamic regulation of histone lysine methylation by demethylases. Mol Cell 25(1):1–14

Shi X et al (2006) ING2 PHD domain links histone H3 lysine 4 methylation to active gene repression. Nature 442(7098):96–99

Shia WJ et al (2012) PRMT1 interacts with AML1-ETO to promote its transcriptional activation and progenitor cell proliferative potential. Blood 119(21):4953–4962

Shilatifard A (2008) Molecular implementation and physiological roles for histone H3 lysine 4 (H3K4) methylation. Curr Opin Cell Biol 20(3):341–348

Simon JA, Lange CA (2008) Roles of the EZH2 histone methyltransferase in cancer epigenetics. Mutat Res 647(1–2):21–29

Sims RJ 3rd, Reinberg D (2006) Histone H3 Lys 4 methylation: caught in a bind? Genes Dev 20(20):2779–2786

Singer MS et al (1998) Identification of high-copy disruptors of telomeric silencing in Saccharomyces cerevisiae. Genetics 150(2):613–632

Slany RK (2009) The molecular biology of mixed lineage leukemia. Haematologica 94(7): 984–993

Sneeringer CJ et al (2010) Coordinated activities of wild-type plus mutant EZH2 drive tumor-associated hypertrimethylation of lysine 27 on histone H3 (H3K27) in human B-cell lymphomas. Proc Natl Acad Sci USA 107(49):20980–20985

Squazzo SL et al (2006) Suz12 binds to silenced regions of the genome in a cell-type-specific manner. Genome Res 16(7):890–900

Stec I et al (1998) WHSC1, a 90 kb SET domain-containing gene, expressed in early development and homologous to a Drosophila dysmorphy gene maps in the Wolf-Hirschhorn syndrome critical region and is fused to IgH in t(4;14) multiple myeloma. Hum Mol Genet 7(7):1071–1082

Steger DJ et al (2008) DOT1L/KMT4 recruitment and H3K79 methylation are ubiquitously coupled with gene transcription in mammalian cells. Mol Cell Biol 28(8):2825–2839

Strahl BD et al (1999) Methylation of histone H3 at lysine 4 is highly conserved and correlates with transcriptionally active nuclei in Tetrahymena. Proc Natl Acad Sci USA 96(26): 14967–14972

Tachibana M et al (2002) G9a histone methyltransferase plays a dominant role in euchromatic histone H3 lysine 9 methylation and is essential for early embryogenesis. Genes Dev 16(14):1779–1791

Tachibana M et al (2005) Histone methyltransferases G9a and GLP form heteromeric complexes and are both crucial for methylation of euchromatin at H3-K9. Genes Dev 19(7):815–826

Tan X et al (2006) SmyD1, a histone methyltransferase, is required for myofibril organization and muscle contraction in zebrafish embryos. Proc Natl Acad Sci USA 103(8):2713–2718

Tang J, Kao PN, Herschman HR (2000) Protein-arginine methyltransferase I, the predominant protein-arginine methyltransferase in cells, interacts with and is regulated by interleukin enhancer-binding factor 3. J Biol Chem 275(26):19866–19876

Therrien E et al (2009) 1,2-Diamines as inhibitors of co-activator associated arginine methyltransferase 1 (CARM1). Bioorg Med Chem Lett 19(23):6725–6732

Troffer-Charlier N et al (2007) Functional insights from structures of coactivator-associated arginine methyltransferase 1 domains. EMBO J 26(20):4391–4401

Tryndyak VP, Kovalchuk O, Pogribny IP (2006) Loss of DNA methylation and histone H4 lysine 20 trimethylation in human breast cancer cells is associated with aberrant expression of DNA methyltransferase 1, Suv4-20h2 histone methyltransferase and methyl-binding proteins. Cancer Biol Ther 5(1):65–70

Van Den Broeck A et al (2008) Loss of histone H4K20 trimethylation occurs in preneoplasia and influences prognosis of non-small cell lung cancer. Clin Cancer Res 14(22):7237–7245

van Haaften G et al (2009) Somatic mutations of the histone H3K27 demethylase gene UTX in human cancer. Nat Genet 41(5):521–523

van Leeuwen F, Gafken PR, Gottschling DE (2002) Dot1p modulates silencing in yeast by methylation of the nucleosome core. Cell 109(6):745–756

Varambally S et al (2002) The polycomb group protein EZH2 is involved in progression of prostate cancer. Nature 419(6907):624–629

Vedadi M et al (2011) A chemical probe selectively inhibits G9a and GLP methyltransferase activity in cells. Nat Chem Biol 7(8):566–574

Wagschal A et al (2008) G9a histone methyltransferase contributes to imprinting in the mouse placenta. Mol Cell Biol 28(3):1104–1113

Wan H et al (2009) Benzo[d]imidazole inhibitors of Coactivator Associated Arginine Methyltransferase 1 (CARM1)–Hit to Lead studies. Bioorg Med Chem Lett 19(17): 5063–5066

Wang H et al (2003) mAM facilitates conversion by ESET of dimethyl to trimethyl lysine 9 of histone H3 to cause transcriptional repression. Mol Cell 12(2):475–487

Wang GG et al (2007) NUP98-NSD1 links H3K36 methylation to Hox-A gene activation and leukaemogenesis. Nat Cell Biol 9(7):804–812

Wang SZ et al (2008a) Knockdown of SMYD3 by RNA interference inhibits cervical carcinoma cell growth and invasion in vitro. BMB Rep 41(4):294–299

Wang L, Pal S, Sif S (2008b) Protein arginine methyltransferase 5 suppresses the transcription of the RB family of tumor suppressors in leukemia and lymphoma cells. Mol Cell Biol 28(20):6262–6277

Wang P et al (2009) Global analysis of H3K4 methylation defines MLL family member targets and points to a role for MLL1-mediated H3K4 methylation in the regulation of transcriptional initiation by RNA polymerase II. Mol Cell Biol 29(22):6074–6085

Watanabe H et al (2008) Deregulation of histone lysine methyltransferases contributes to oncogenic transformation of human bronchoepithelial cells. Cancer Cell Int 8:15

Weidinger G (1995) Pharmacokinetic and pharmacodynamic properties and therapeutic use of bunazosin in hypertension. A review. Arzneimittelforschung 45(11):1166–1171

Wigle TJ et al (2010) Screening for inhibitors of low-affinity epigenetic peptide-protein interactions: an AlphaScreen-based assay for antagonists of methyl-lysine binding proteins. J Biomol Screen 15(1):62–71

Wu H et al (2010) Structural biology of human H3K9 methyltransferases. PLoS One 5(1):e8570

Wysocka J et al (2006) A PHD finger of NURF couples histone H3 lysine 4 trimethylation with chromatin remodelling. Nature 442(7098):86–90

Xiang Y et al (2007) JARID1B is a histone H3 lysine 4 demethylase up-regulated in prostate cancer. Proc Natl Acad Sci USA 104(49):19226–19231

Xiao B et al (2005) Specificity and mechanism of the histone methyltransferase Pr-Set7. Genes Dev 19(12):1444–1454

Xin Z et al (2003) Role of histone methyltransferase G9a in CpG methylation of the Prader-Willi syndrome imprinting center. J Biol Chem 278(17):14996–15000

Xu W et al (2004) A methylation-mediator complex in hormone signaling. Genes Dev 18(2):144–156

Xu C et al (2010) Binding of different histone marks differentially regulates the activity and specificity of polycomb repressive complex 2 (PRC2). Proc Natl Acad Sci USA 107(45):19266–19271

Yang ZQ et al (2000) Identification of a novel gene, GASC1, within an amplicon at 9p23-24 frequently detected in esophageal cancer cell lines. Cancer Res 60(17):4735–4739

Yang H et al (2008) Preferential dimethylation of histone H4 lysine 20 by Suv4-20. J Biol Chem 283(18):12085–12092

Yap DB et al (2011) Somatic mutations at EZH2 Y641 act dominantly through a mechanism of selectively altered PRC2 catalytic activity, to increase H3K27 trimethylation. Blood 117(8):2451–2459

Yuan W et al (2009) Heterogeneous nuclear ribonucleoprotein L Is a subunit of human KMT3a/Set2 complex required for H3 Lys-36 trimethylation activity in vivo. J Biol Chem 284(23):15701–15707

Yue WW et al (2007) Insights into histone code syntax from structural and biochemical studies of CARM1 methyltransferase. EMBO J 26(20):4402–4412

Zhang X, Bruice TC (2007) Histone lysine methyltransferase SET7/9: formation of a water channel precedes each methyl transfer. Biochemistry 46(51):14838–14844

Zhang X, Bruice TC (2008) Enzymatic mechanism and product specificity of SET-domain protein lysine methyltransferases. Proc Natl Acad Sci USA 105(15):5728–5732

Zhang X, Cheng X (2003) Structure of the predominant protein arginine methyltransferase PRMT1 and analysis of its binding to substrate peptides. Structure 11(5):509–520

Zhang X, Zhou L, Cheng X (2000) Crystal structure of the conserved core of protein arginine methyltransferase PRMT3. EMBO J 19(14):3509–3519

Zhao Q et al (2009) PRMT5-mediated methylation of histone H4R3 recruits DNMT3A, coupling histone and DNA methylation in gene silencing. Nat Struct Mol Biol 16(3):304–311

Histone Deacetylase (HDAC) Inhibitors in Recent Clinical Trials for Cancer Therapy

10

Kristina Keller and Manfred Jung

Abbreviations

bid	Two times daily
CPT-11	Irinotecan
CR	Complete response
CTCL	Cutaneous T-cell lymphoma
DLT	Dose-limiting toxicity
EIAEDs	Enzyme-inducing antiepileptic drugs
FDA	Food and Drug Administration
HDAC	Histone deacetylase
HDACi	Histone deacetylase inhibitor
HI	Haematological improvement
MTD	Maximum tolerated dose
MWF	Monday, Wednesday, Friday
ORR	Overall response rate
OS	Overall survival
PBMC	Peripheral blood mononuclear cell
PFS	Progression free survival
PR	Partial response
qd	Once daily
RP2D	Recommended phase II dose
SD	Stable disease

K. Keller • M. Jung (✉)
Institute of Pharmaceutical Sciences,
Albert-Ludwigs-Universität Freiburg,
Albertstr. 25, Freiburg, 79104, Germany
e-mail: manfred.jung@pharmazie.uni-freiburg.de, http://jungm.de

M. Lübbert, P.A. Jones (eds.), *Epigenetic Therapy of Cancer*,
DOI 10.1007/978-3-642-38404-2_10,

10.1 Reversible Histone Acetylation and Histone Deacetylases

One of the pivotal modifications associated with epigenetic gene regulation is the acetylation of histone proteins within chromatin. Two enzymes are responsible for the maintenance of the acetylation equilibrium. Histone acetyltransferases (HATs) mediate the transfer of an acetyl group to the ε-amino group of lysine residues in histones and other proteins by using the cofactor acetyl-CoA. Histone deacetylases (HDACs) catalyse the removal of the acetyl group. Upon acetylation, the positive charge of lysines is neutralised, and in the case of histones, the interaction with the negatively charged DNA backbone is diminished. This leads to a more open chromatin (euchromatin) that is available for binding of proteins like transcription factors. Deacetylation restores the positive charge, and the intensified interaction with the DNA backbone is leading to a more condensed form of the chromatin (heterochromatin). Generally, acetylation is associated with transcriptional activation, whereas deacetylation is associated with gene repression (Latham and Dent 2007). However, it was shown that HDACs are also located at active genes to reset the acetylation state in active genes and maintain an adequate level of histone acetylation (Wang et al. 2009).

Histone deacetylases can be divided into four classes based on phylogenetic comparison with yeast enzymes. The classes I, II and IV comprises zinc-dependent deacetylases (HDACs), whereas the class III enzymes have a NAD^+-dependent mechanism and are generally referred to as sirtuins because of their homology to the yeast-silencing protein Sir2 (Sauve et al. 2006). Because of the different catalytic mechanism, clinically relevant inhibitors that are active on class I, II and IV HDACs do not target sirtuins and vice versa. Class I consists of HDAC 1, 2, 3 and 8 and is homologous to the yeast enzyme rpd3, and its members are predominantly located in the nucleus. Class II can be further subdivided into class IIa and class IIb. The isotypes 4, 5, 7 and 9 constitute the HDACs of class IIa, and the subtypes 6 and 10 belong to class IIb. HDAC 6 and 10 have two catalytic domains, and there is conflicting evidence on the relevance for in vivo enzyme activity. While some reports indicated that both are required for enzymatic activity (Verdin et al. 2003; Zhang et al. 2006), there is also evidence for the activity of only one site (Zou et al. 2006). The enzymes of class II are homologous to the yeast protein hda1 (Verdin et al. 2004) and shuttle between the cytoplasm and the nucleus (Yoo and Jones 2006). The only member of class IV is HDAC 11 which is located in the nucleus.

Besides histones many other proteins have been recognised as substrates for HDACs (Choudhary et al. 2009). Examples are transcription factors, hormone receptors, signal transducers, chaperones and proteins of the cytoskeleton. Protein acetylation and deacetylation influence a lot of processes besides transcription. An important example is protein stability via the non-histone substrates tubulin, which affects the aggresome pathway of protein degradation (Hideshima et al. 2005), and the chaperone hsp90 (Bali et al. 2005). Most of the non-histone proteins, e.g. the tumour suppressor p53 (Luo et al. 2000), are deacetylated by class I HDACs. α-Tubulin and hsp90 are targets of HDAC 6. Because of the many non-histone targets, HDACs are sometimes referred to as protein or lysine deacetylases (KDACs) rather than histone deacetylases. The application of subtype-specific HDACi might help to address the relevance of the different substrates in mechanistic studies, and the investigation of unselective inhibitors in comparison to selective inhibitors in the clinic will help to understand the underlying mechanisms (Glozak et al. 2005; Buchwald et al. 2009).

10.2 HDACs and Disease

In recent years HDACs have emerged as potential therapeutic targets because their inhibitors are able to reverse dysregulated epigenetic states associated with disease, esp. cancer. It could be shown that there is aberrant acetylation and altered expression of HDACs in cancer cells and tumour tissue (Bolden et al. 2006). Oncogenic fusion proteins, present in some forms of leukaemia, recruit HDAC-containing repressor complexes that constitutively repress expression of specific target genes. In acute promyelocytic leukaemia, fusion proteins of the retinoic acid receptor-α with other proteins that block transcription via recruitment of HDACs are responsible for pathogenesis of the disease on a molecular level (Lin et al. 2001; Pandolfi 2001). In diffuse large B-cell lymphomas, the transcription factor B-cell lymphoma 6 (BCL6) is highly overexpressed. BCL6 itself is hypoacetylated by HDACs and recruits HDAC 2 to repress growth-regulatory target genes. Treatment of this disease with HDACi results in hyperacetylation of BCL6, release of HDAC 2, reactivation of repressed target genes and tumour cell apoptosis (Pasqualucci et al. 2003). Overexpression of different HDACs has been reported in several cancers. In general, it was found that class I expression was high in advanced, strongly proliferating tumours and thus associated with negative prognosis in certain tumours. Class II HDACs were found to be downregulated in human tumours, and high expression predicted better outcome. These findings have to be further investigated because information about the acetylation status and HDAC expression in tumours compared to normal tissue might be an important marker of prognosis and response to treatment (Weichert 2009).

Several other diseases are associated with HDAC activity. HDACi might be able to overcome HIV latency by activation of HIV production from latently infected cells and thereby enhance elimination of these cells (Wightman et al. 2012). HDACs are also implicated to play a crucial role in cardiovascular diseases (Ohtani and Dimmeler 2011). HDAC inhibitors have been shown to be efficacious in preclinical models of heart failure (McKinsey 2012). Furthermore, altered histone acetylation is involved in neurodegeneration (Fischer et al. 2010). HDACi have shown neuroprotection in models for neurodegenerative diseases like Huntington's disease or spinocerebellar ataxias (Gottesfeld and Pandolfo 2009).

Overall, HDACs play an important role in processes like apoptosis, differentiation and autophagy. Inhibitors targeting these enzymes are valuable to treat diseases that underlie a dysregulation in acetylation. Thus, a lot of effort has been put in the development of HDACi in the last few years. The preclinical pharmacology has been reviewed broadly, elsewhere (Khan and La Thangue 2012), and we will only highlight selected findings and focus mainly on the clinical studies.

10.3 HDAC Inhibitors (HDACi)

Originally, some HDACi have been discovered initially as inducers of cell differentiation (Leder et al. 1975; Riggs et al. 1977). They are able to cause cell cycle arrest in G1 and/or G2 phase, leading to inhibition of cell growth (Bolden et al. 2006). HDACi are also able to induce apoptosis by activating extrinsic (death receptor) and intrinsic (mitochondrial) pathways (Ma et al. 2009). The advantage of HDACi is that they show a high sensitivity towards transformed cells compared to normal cells (Parsons et al. 1997).

Because of these findings, the development of HDACi has become a major goal especially since clinical efficacy could be demonstrated for vorinostat and romidepsin (see below). So far inhibitors of four structurally different classes are in clinical development. All of them have a functional group that is responsible for chelating the zinc ion in the active centre and hence enzyme inactivation (see Fig. 10.1). Structural differences among the inhibitors lead to different HDAC subtype selectivity profiles. So far it is not clear whether pan-inhibitors or subtype-selective compounds are better for cancer treatment. This may vary with the disease indication. Additionally, it remains to be determined whether the chemical classification is associated with certain benefits or risks for one chemical group or the other.

One group is the cyclic peptides like romidepsin (Istodax®). Romidepsin, a natural product isolated from *Chromobacterium violaceum*, is a prodrug that is activated in the cell by reduction of the disulfide and is a class I-selective inhibitor (Furumai et al. 2002). Romidepsin inhibits tumour growth in mouse models and humans (Ueda et al. 1994) and was approved by the FDA in 2009 for the treatment of refractory cutaneous T-cell lymphoma. Another important structural group is the hydroxamic acids. The first compound found to inhibit HDACs was the natural product trichostatin A (Yoshida et al. 1990). Further compounds like vorinostat, panobinostat, belinostat, givinostat and SB939 have shown great inhibitory activity and are currently under clinical investigation. Vorinostat (Zolinza®) was the first HDACi to be approved by the FDA for the treatment of cutaneous T-cell lymphoma in 2006. It has been shown that vorinostat is able to induce differentiation, cell growth arrest and apoptosis in numerous cancer cell lines at low micromolar concentrations and inhibits tumour growth with little toxicity in a wide range of animal models (Jones 2009). Panobinostat, an orally available HDACi, shows antiproliferative and cytotoxic activity in a variety of cancer cell lines and induces hyperacetylation of histone H3 and H4 (Atadja 2009). Belinostat is a potent (IC_{50} 27 nM) HDACi that induces apoptosis in human tumour cell lines and xenografts (Plumb et al. 2003). Pracinostat (SB939) is a novel HDACi with improved pharmacokinetic properties. It shows a fourfold improved bioavailability and a threefold increased plasma half-life over vorinostat and accumulates in tumour tissue (Novotny-Diermayr et al. 2010). Furthermore quisinostat (JNJ-26481585), a hydroxamic acid-containing inhibitor with potent antitumoural activity and favourable pharmacodynamic properties was developed and is currently investigated in clinical studies (Arts et al. 2009). New pyrimidine hydroxamates with potent protein inhibition have been synthesised with CHR-3996 being

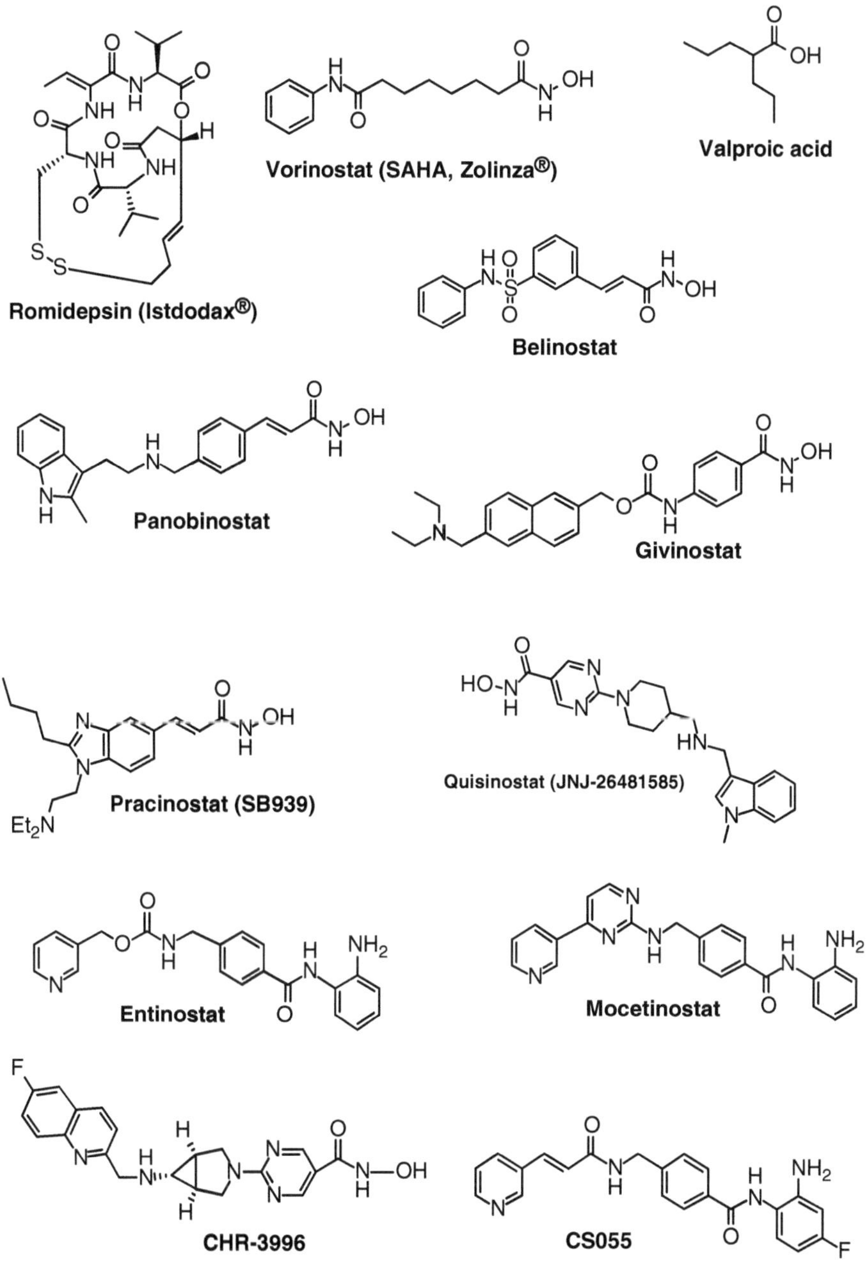

Fig. 10.1 HDAC inhibitors currently investigated in clinical trials

the most promising one. CHR-3996 shows class I subtype selectivity, and good oral bioavailability as well as complete inhibition of growth in human tumour xenografts is described (Moffat et al. 2010). Another structurally different class of

HDACi are the short-chain fatty acids like valproic acid and phenylbutyrate. These compounds show only low inhibitory (100–1000-fold weaker than romidepsin or vorinostat) effects but are applied already in the clinic for other indications. Valproic acid is already approved for the use as an antiepileptic drug and induces differentiation and hyperacetylation of histones (Göttlicher et al. 2001). Because of its well-characterised pharmacodynamic and pharmacokinetic profile and manageable side effects, it is investigated in different trials as antileukaemic agent, usually in combination with other drugs.

Benzamides like entinostat, mocetinostat and CS055 are another class of HDACi. Here the amino anilide group is responsible for enzyme inhibition and also confers a selectivity to class I HDACs (Bressi et al. 2010). Entinostat and mocetinostat are class I-selective inhibitors and cause cell cycle arrest and hyperacetylation of histone H4. Entinostat inhibits cell proliferation and growth in human tumour xenografts (Saito et al. 1999). Mocetinostat induces histone hyperacetylation and apoptosis and shows antiproliferative activities against several human cancer cell lines and xenografts (Fournel et al. 2008). CS055 has a similar chemical structure like entinostat. However, it displays lower toxicity, better tolerance and higher stability during administration to animals. It is a class I-selective inhibitor and induces growth arrest, apoptosis and differentiation of leukaemia cells (Gong et al. 2012).

HDACi are investigated in several clinical trials in haematological and solid malignancies as single agents, but in quite a number of cases, the efficacy was not satisfying. Therefore, in many studies HDACi are used in combination with other anticancer agents. The epigenetic combination HDACi and DNA-methyltransferase inhibitors like azacytidine in haematological malignancies is supported by the fact that in these malignancies, abnormal recruitment of HDACs to nuclear protein complexes takes place (Khan and La Thangue 2012). Furthermore, as outlined above there is a role of HDAC6 in protein degradation, and therefore, it was logic to combine HDACi with proteasome inhibitors that target the other major protein degradation pathway. This combination has shown efficacy, even in patients with relapsed/refractory disease who have previously received proteasome inhibitor treatment (Jagannath et al. 2010). In the light of the differentiation inducing abilities of HDACi, another obvious combination is one with other differentiating agents, such as retinoids. Additionally, many other mechanistically different agents are investigated. Also a combination with radiotherapy is based on preclinical evidence (Kim et al. 1999) and is applied clinically (see below).

Besides the question of mono- versus combination therapy, the question of class selectivity has to be addressed. It has to be proven whether class-specific HDACi will reveal greater clinical benefit or if pan-HDAC inhibition has greater efficacy. Due to the presence of HDACi in multi-protein complexes, there is also evidence for a complex rather than subtype selectivity of HDAC inhibitors (Bantscheff et al. 2011). A thorough overview of clinical trials of HDACi has been reported by us a few years ago (Wagner et al. 2010). Here we provide an update of the clinical trials reported between 2010 and the middle of 2012.

10.4 Clinical Trials of Vorinostat

Vorinostat was approved by the FDA for the treatment of refractory cutaneous T-cell lymphoma. It was the first HDACi to be approved and is currently under investigation in clinical trials as monotherapy as well as in combination with several other antitumour agents for various cancers (see Table 10.1).

Recently, five trials of vorinostat as single-agent therapy have been reported. In a phase I trial, the effect of vorinostat in patients suffering from advanced solid tumours and hepatic dysfunction was investigated. Fifty-seven patients were enrolled of which 42 had hepatic dysfunction. The recommended phase II dose for patients with mild, moderate and severe hepatic dysfunction was determined to be 300, 200 and 100 mg/day. Twelve patients experienced stabilisation of disease. Of five patients with adenoid cystic carcinoma, one patient had a partial response, and four patients had stable disease. As adenoid cystic carcinoma is usually refractory to chemotherapy, treatment with vorinostat is a concept to be further investigated in future trials (Ramalingam et al. 2010). In a phase I/II study, the impact of UDP-glucuronyltransferase 2B17 genotype on vorinostat metabolism and clinical outcome in Asian women with breast cancer was investigated. UGT2B17 is a key enzyme in the metabolism of vorinostat (Balliet et al. 2009). Vorinostat is glucuronidated by UGT2B17 and thereby inactivated. Patients received 400 mg/day vorinostat in a lead-in phase I followed by a phase II study. Patients were genotyped for UGT2B17 null genotype (UGT2B17*2), a deletion variant that reduced vorinostat glucuronidation. Wild-type homozygotes (UGT2B17*1/*1), heterozygotes (UGT2B17*1/*2) and homozygotes (UGT2B17*2/*2) for the deletion were compared. Patients who carried at least one copy of a functional UGT2B7 variant were expected to have clinically relevant enzymatic activity (UGT2B17*1/*1 or *1/*2), whereas patients who were homozygous for the null variant (UGT2B17*2/*2) were expected to possess minimal enzyme activity. UGT2B17*2 homozygotes were more likely to experience a serious adverse event, to derive clinical benefit and have longer progression-free survival compared to those who carried at least one copy of UGT2B17*1, although these differences were not statistically significant due to the small patient population. Twenty-six patients received treatment, one patient achieved a partial response and six patients had stable disease lasting for 12 weeks or more (Wong et al. 2011). Another phase I study of 16 patients with gastrointestinal cancer was reported. They were treated with vorinostat 300 mg bid for three consecutive days followed by four rest days per cycle or vorinostat 400 mg qd for 21 consecutive days per cycle. Five patients taking 300 mg bid and two patients taking 400 mg qd maintained stable disease for more than 8 weeks. The 300 mg bid dosing regimen was better tolerated in regard to hematologic toxicities. The most common drug-related adverse events were anorexia, nausea, fatigue and hyperglycaemia (Doi et al. 2013). In a phase II study, 35 patients with relapsed or refractory indolent non-Hodgkin's lymphoma and mantle cell lymphoma were treated with vorinostat at a dose of 200 mg twice daily on days 1 through 14 of a 21-day cycle. Five patients had complete responses and five partial responses (Kirschbaum et al. 2011). In another phase II study, 25 patients with relapsed/refractory Hodgkin

Table 10.1 Vorinostat trials reported in the years 2007–2012

Combination therapy	Type of cancer	Phase	Patients number	Outcome	Literature
None	Advanced solid tumours, hepatic dysfunction	I	57	12 SD	Ramalingam et al. (2010)
None	Breast cancer	I/II	26	1 PR 6 SD	Wong et al. (2011)
None	Gastrointestinal cancer	I	16	5 SD	Doi et al. (2013)
None	Relapsed or refractory indolent non-Hodgkin's lymphoma, mantle cell lymphoma	II	35	5 CR 5 PR	Kirschbaum et al. (2011)
None	Relapsed or refractory Hodgkin lymphoma	II	25	1 PR 12 SD	Kirschbaum et al. (2012)
None	Cutaneous T-cell lymphoma	II	33	8 PR	Duvic et al. (2007)
None	Cutaneous T-cell lymphoma	IIb	74	1 CR, 22 PR	Olsen et al. (2007)
Marizomib	Melanoma, pancreatic and lung cancer	I	22	11 SD	Millward et al. (2012)
Vinorelbine	Advanced cancers	I	7	MDT=200 mg once daily	Gandia et al. (2011)
Decitabine	Solid tumours, non-Hodgkin's lymphomas	I	43	MTD=200 mg twice a day 11 SD	Stathis et al. (2011)
Tamoxifen	Hormone therapy-resistant breast cancer	II	43	Response rate 19 %	Munster et al. (2011)
5-Fluorouracil Leucovorin	Refractory solid tumours	I	43	21 SD 1 PR	Fakih et al. (2010)
5-Fluorouracil Leucovorin	Refractory colorectal cancer	II	58	1,400 mg/day PFS=2.9 OS=6.7 800 mg/day PFS=2.4 month OS=6.5 month	Fakih et al. (2012)
Bevacizumab Irinotecan	Recurrent glioblastoma	I	19	MTD=400 mg	Chinnaiyan et al. (2012)
Bortezomib	Recurrent glioblastoma	II	37	No response	Friday et al. (2012)
Bortezomib	Myeloma	I	23	Response rate 42 %	Badros et al. (2009)
Bexarotene	Cutaneous T-cell lymphoma	I	23	4 PR 15 SD	Dummer et al. (2012)
Gemtuzumab ozogamicin	Acute myeloid leukaemia	II	31	6 CR	Walter et al. (2012)

In all tables only papers that have not already been mentioned in Wagner et al. (2010)

lymphoma received oral vorinostat, 200 mg twice daily, for 14 days on a 21-day cycle. The overall response rate was 4 %. One patient had a partial response and 12 had stable disease, seven of them remaining progression-free for more than a year (Kirschbaum et al. 2012). Taken together vorinostat as a single agent is well tolerated but shows in many cases only weak clinical activity, especially in solid tumours. Further studies of vorinostat in combination with other active agents will investigate the beneficial effect of a combination therapy. In the last few years, a lot of trials of vorinostat combination therapy for various cancers have been reported.

A phase I study of vorinostat combined with the proteasome inhibitor marizomib in patients with melanoma, pancreatic and lung cancer was conducted. Twenty-two patients received weekly marizomib in combination with 300 mg vorinostat daily for 16 days in 28-day cycles. No confirmed responses were reported, but of 18 evaluable patients, 11 had stable disease (61 %, all having melanoma). Combining marizomib with vorinostat in patients was seen to be feasible and tolerable (Millward et al. 2012). The MTD of vorinostat in combination with vinorelbine was investigated in a phase I study. Seven patients with advanced cancers were treated with a starting dose of 200 mg oral vorinostat once daily for 7 days every 21 days in combination with a weekly infusion of vinorelbine (25 mg/m^2). This dosing was determined to be the MTD (Gandia et al. 2011). The safety, tolerability, pharmacokinetics and preliminary efficacy of vorinostat in combination with the DNA-methyltransferase inhibitor decitabine were also investigated in a phase I study in patients with advanced solid tumours and non-Hodgkin lymphomas. Forty-three patients were treated in a sequential or a concurrent dose schedule. Intravenous decitabine was administered on days 1–5 combined with oral vorinostat in a sequential (vorinostat starting on day six) or a concurrent schedule (vorinostat starting on day three), in 28-day cycle. The recommended phase II dose is decitabine 10 mg/m^2/day on days 1–5 with 200 mg vorinostat twice daily on days 6–12 on a sequential schedule. The most frequent adverse events were neutropenia and thrombocytopenia. Of 38 patients evaluable for response, 11 had stable disease for 4 or more cycles of treatment (Stathis et al. 2011). The effect of vorinostat in combination with tamoxifen for the treatment of patients with hormone therapy-resistant breast cancer was studied in a phase II trial. Tamoxifen has antiproliferative effects on cancer cells. In combination with an HDACi, it could be shown that tamoxifen induces apoptosis rather than growth inhibition. Data from preclinical models suggest that the combination of tamoxifen with an HDACi resensitises hormone therapy-resistant breast cancer cells. Forty-three patients with ER-positive metastatic breast cancer progressing on endocrine therapy were enrolled and treated with 400 mg of vorinostat daily for 3 of 4 weeks and 20 mg tamoxifen daily, continuously. Eight patients had objective responses and nine patients had stable disease for more than 24 weeks. Histone H4 hyperacetylation in PBMCs was measured, and it was found that patients with a response or stable disease showed pronounced histone H4 hyperacetylation compared to nonresponders. This trial demonstrates that the combination of vorinostat and tamoxifen in patients with hormone receptor-positive breast cancer results in tumour regression or prolonged disease stabilisation in patients who had progressed on prior therapy and is worth to be further investigated (Munster et al. 2011). Two studies evaluated the effect of vorinostat in combination with 5-fluorouracil and leucovorin in patients with refractory solid tumours. A phase I study determined the MTD of daily or twice daily vorinostat on 3 days when combined with fixed doses of 5-fluorouracil and leucovorin every 2 weeks. Forty-three patients were treated and the MTD of vorinostat in this combination was found to be 1,700 mg orally once daily on three consecutive days or 600 mg orally twice daily on three consecutive days every 2 weeks. Of 38 patients with 5-fluorouracil-refractory colorectal cancer, 21 had stable disease and one had a partial response (Fakih et al. 2010). In a phase II study, it was investigated whether the combination of relatively high doses of intermittent vorinostat overcomes resistance to 5-fluorouracil in refractory metastatic colorectal cancer. Fifteen patients received high-dose (1,400 mg) vorinostat, and 43 received low-dose (800 mg) vorinostat. The median progression-free survival and overall survival on the high-dose arm were 2.9 and 6.7 months, compared to 2.4 and 6.5 months on the low-dose arm, respectively. Accrual on the high-dose arm had to be halted because the number of patients without progression at 2 months did not reach the threshold. On the low-dose arm, one patient had a partial response and eight patients had stable disease. However, the progression-free survival rate did not reach the prespecified threshold of 27 out of 43 patients, and the combination was not deemed interesting enough for further evaluation (Fakih et al. 2012). Two trials have been reported using vorinostat in combination therapy for the treatment of recurrent glioblastoma. In a phase I trial, vorinostat was combined with bevacizumab and CPT-11. Nineteen patients were treated. The MTD of vorinostat was established at 400 mg on days 1–7 and 15–21 every 28 days when combined with bevacizumab and CPT-11. The median progression-free survival (PFS) among patients receiving higher-dose vorinostat had an improved response, although not statistically significant (Chinnaiyan et al. 2012). Furthermore, a phase II trial of vorinostat in combination with bortezomib was conducted. Thirty-seven patients were treated with vorinostat at a dose of 400 mg daily for 14 days of a 21-day cycle, and bortezomib was administered at a dose of 1.3 mg/m^2 intravenously on days 1, 4, 8 and 11 of the cycle. The trial failed to meet the interim analysis threshold for continuation. None of the 34 patients were progression-free at 6 months (Friday et al. 2012). Another phase I trial was reported to investigate the MTD of vorinostat in combination with bexarotene in patients with advanced (stage IB or higher) CTCL who were refractory to at least one prior systemic treatment and were suitable for bexarotene therapy. The study was divided into two parts. For patients enrolled in part I, up to three dose levels of vorinostat (200, 300 and 400 mg daily) and up to three dose levels of bexarotene (150, 225 and 300 mg/m^2) were tested. For patients enrolled in part II, dosing began at dose level 6 with vorinostat at 400 mg once daily and bexarotene at 150 mg once daily. Four patients had partial responses and 15 patients had stable disease. The MTD of part I was established at vorinostat 200 mg/day plus bexarotene 300 mg/m^2/day. The MTD for part II was not reached; a result of early study termination due to low enrolment. The efficacy of vorinostat and the retinoid bexarotene at an optimum dose and schedule could not be fully explored in patients with advanced CTCL because of the aggressive nature of the underlying disease. Furthermore, the number of patients treated in this study was small, and thus no general conclusions are possible regarding efficacy (Dummer et al. 2012). A phase II trial of vorinostat in combination with gemtuzumab ozogamicin (GO), as induction and post-remission therapy in older adults with previously untreated acute myeloid leukaemia, has been conducted. Patients received vorinostat 400 mg orally once daily on days 1–9 and GO 3 mg/m^2 on day 8. Hydroxyurea was given to reduce the white blood cells to less than 10×10^9/L before treatment with vorinostat. Thirty-one patients have been enrolled of which six achieved complete remission and one achieved complete remission with incomplete platelet recovery. Four patients are in ongoing remission after 455, 496, 956 and 988 days (Walter et al. 2012). As already reviewed in (Wagner et al. 2010), vorinostat was also investigated in combination with radiotherapy (Ree et al. 2010).

10.5 Clinical Trials of Panobinostat

Panobinostat is a highly potent HDACi with antitumour activities at low nanomolar concentrations in several preclinical studies, and its clinical efficacy is currently under investigation in several clinical trials (see Table 10.2). There are several trials investigating the effect of panobinostat as single agent. In two phase I trials, the safety and tolerability of intravenous and oral panobinostat in solid tumours are studied. In a multicenter phase I dose-escalation study, 14 patients received intravenous panobinostat on days 1 and 8 of a 21-day cycle. Stable disease for more than 4 months was observed in six patients, and the MTD of 20 mg/m^2 was thought to be safe and potentially effective in patients with advanced solid tumours (Morita et al. 2012). In another phase I, open-label, dose-escalation study, panobinostat was administered orally once daily on MWF weekly on a 28-day cycle to 13 patients with advanced solid tumours or CTCL. Seven patients had stable disease but the MTD was not reached (Fukutomi et al. 2012). The most frequently reported adverse event in both trials was thrombocytopenia, which could be observed for several other HDACi. Panobinostat was also administered as single agent in a phase II trial of patients with refractory metastatic renal cell carcinoma. Patients received 45 mg panobinostat twice a week. After 8 weeks of treatment, 12 patients had progressed disease, and because of the lack of efficacy, the trial was closed (Hainsworth et al. 2011). A phase II study of panobinostat in patients with low- or intermediate-risk myelodysplastic syndrome was conducted. Thirteen patients were treated to determine the clinical efficacy, safety and tolerability of oral panobinostat at a dose of 20 mg three times a week followed by 1 week of rest. One patient achieved a haematological improvement, and six patients had stable disease for a median duration of 6 months. Treatment was well tolerated but overall the study showed only limited clinical activity and was closed to further patient entry (Dimicoli et al. 2012). In a phase II study in patients with relapsed and/or refractory Hodgkin's lymphoma after autologous stem-cell transplantation, the activity of panobinostat was examined. One hundred and twenty-nine patients were treated with 40 mg panobinostat orally three times per week in a 21-day cycle. Reductions in tumour size were observed in 74 % of the patients with

Table 10.2 Panobinostat trials reported in the years 2010–2013

Combination therapy	Type of cancer	Phase	Patients number	Outcome	Literature
None	Solid tumours	I	14	6 SD MDT = 20 mg/m^2	Morita et al. (2012)
None	Solid tumours	I	13	7 SD MTD not reached	Fukutomi et al. (2012)
None	Refractory metastatic renal cell carcinoma	II	20	No response	Hainsworth et al. (2011)
None	Myelodysplastic syndrome	II	13	1 HI 6 SD	Dimicoli et al. (2012)
None	Relapsed/refractory Hodgkin's lymphoma	II	129	5 CR 30 PR	Younes et al. (2012)
None	Cutaneous T-cell lymphoma	II	139	Response rate 17.3 %	Duvic et al. (2013)
None Docetaxel	Castration-resistant prostate cancer	I	16	None: no response Docetaxel: 2 PR 4 SD	Rathkopf et al. (2010)
Lenalidomide Dexamethasone	Relapsed/refractory multiple myeloma	Ib	46	1 CR,8 PR,7 SD	Mateos et al. (2010)
Gemcitabine	Solid tumours	I	17	5 SD	Jones et al. (2011)
Bevacizumab Everolimus	Advanced solid tumours	I	12	1 PR 3 SD	Strickler et al. (2012)
Bevacizumab	High-grade glioma	I	12	3 PR 7 SD	Drappatz et al. (2012)
Bortezomib	Pancreatic cancer	II	7	No response	Wang et al. (2012)
Melphalan Thalidomide Prednisone	Relapsed/refractory multiple myeloma	II	31	12 PR 2 CR 11 SD	Offidani et al. (2012)

5 patients having complete response and 30 patients having a partial response lasting for 6.9 months in the median. Panobinostat monotherapy in patients who were heavily pretreated demonstrated antitumour activity, resulting in durable responses. This promising data suggest that further investigation especially in combination with other agents might be valuable to improve therapy (Younes et al. 2012). In a phase I study, treatment of patients with castration-resistant prostate cancer with panobinostat as single agent in comparison to panobinostat in combination with docetaxel was investigated. Eight patients received 20 mg panobinostat on 3 days a week for two consecutive weeks followed by a 1-week break. Eight patients received 15 mg panobinostat on the same schedule in combination with 75 mg/m^2 docetaxel every 3 weeks and 5 mg prednisone orally twice a day. None of the patients in the panobinostat monotherapy arm responded. In the combination arm, 2 of 7 evaluable patients had a partial response and four patients had stable disease (Rathkopf et al. 2010). Thus,

also panobinostat as a single agent shows limited clinical response so far. Therefore, panobinostat is also investigated in several trials in combination with various other antitumour agents.

In a phase Ib study, the safety, tolerability and preliminary efficacy of panobinostat in combination with the immune modulator lenalidomide plus dexamethasone in patients with relapsed or refractory multiple myeloma were evaluated. Forty-six patients have been treated of which 30 were evaluable for response. One patient had a partial response, 7 had stable disease and 6 progressed on treatment. Some safety concerns were identified, but as preliminary efficacy was very encouraging, further studies with a lower dexamethasone dose and a noncontinuous panobinostat dosing schedule will be conducted (Mateos et al. 2010). A phase I study investigated the effect of panobinostat in combination with the nucleoside analogue gemcitabine in the treatment of solid tumours. Seventeen patients were enrolled, and after several dose de-escalations because of myelosuppression, the recommended doses for further studies were found to be intermittent oral panobinostat administered at a dose of 10 mg three times weekly for 2 weeks in combination with 800 mg/m^2 gemcitabine administered intravenously on days 1 and 8 every 21 days. One patient with ovarian cancer had an unconfirmed partial response, and five patients had stable disease lasting more than 4 cycles (Jones et al. 2011). The combination of bevacizumab, everolimus and panobinostat was investigated in a phase I trial of 12 patients with advanced solid tumours. Patients received 10 mg of panobinostat three times weekly, 5 or 10 mg everolimus daily and bevacizumab at 10 mg/kg every 2 weeks. One patient with breast cancer had a partial response lasting for 2 months, and three patients with metastatic colorectal cancer had stable disease. HDAC activity of PBMCs was evaluated on day 1 and 15, but no significant difference was detected. These findings support 20 mg three times per week as the minimum dose level to ensure consistent HDAC inhibition. The addition of panobinostat to the combination bevacizumab/everolimus revealed added toxicity which compromised the tolerability of the full combination (Strickler et al. 2012). Panobinostat in combination with bevacizumab for the treatment of recurrent high-grade glioma was investigated in a phase I trial. Twelve patients received 10 mg/kg bevacizumab every 2 weeks and panobinostat at different dose levels. Three patients had partial response and 7 had stable disease. Although the MTD could not be found, a 30 mg dose in combination with bevacizumab was deemed to represent the maximum feasible dose (Drappatz et al. 2012). A phase II study to examine the efficacy and safety of panobinostat and bortezomib in patients with pancreatic cancer progressing on gemcitabine-based therapy was conducted. Patients received 1.3 mg/m^2 bortezomib twice weekly and 20 mg panobinostat three times weekly during the first 2 weeks, followed by 9 days of rest. Seven patients were enrolled but the study had to be closed due to lack of treatment responses and early treatment-related toxicity (Wang et al. 2012). Panobinostat in combination with melphalan, thalidomide and prednisone was investigated in a phase II study in patients with relapsed and or refractory multiple myeloma. Thirty-one patients received a fixed dose of melphalan, thalidomide and prednisone with escalating doses of panobinostat three times weekly for 3 weeks, followed by a 9-day rest period. Two patients achieved a complete response, 12 patients achieved a partial response and 11 had stable disease, but 8 progressed on treatment. This study suggests that the combination of panobinostat plus melphalan, thalidomide and prednisone at this dose and schedule has no therapeutic benefit compared to the combination without HDACi but is more toxic. However, further studies with an improved dose schedule might improve efficacy (Offidani et al. 2012).

10.6 Clinical Trials of Romidepsin

Romidepsin was the second HDACi approved in 2009 by the FDA for the treatment of CTCL of patients who had received at least one systemic therapy. Besides this application, the effect of romidepsin is investigated in the last years in several trials against other haematologic cancers and solid tumours primarily as single agent (see Table 10.3).

A phase II study was conducted to confirm the efficacy of romidepsin in patients with treatment refractory cutaneous T-cell lymphoma. Ninety-six patients were treated with romidepsin as an intravenous infusion at a dose of 14 mg/m^2 on days 1, 8 and 15 every 28 days. The overall response was 34 % with six patients having complete response. This study showed that romidepsin has significant activity as a single agent with durable responses in patients with refractory CTCL with an acceptable safety profile and is a valuable therapeutic agent for these patients (Whittaker et al. 2010). Two phase II studies investigated romidepsin in the treatment of patients with peripheral T-cell lymphoma. Piekarz et al. reported the treatment of 45 patients with 14 mg/m^2 romidepsin on days 1, 8 and 15 of a 28-day cycle. Eight patients experienced complete responses and nine patients experienced partial responses (Piekarz et al. 2011). A further trial confirmed the efficacy of romidepsin in patients with relapsed or refractory peripheral T-cell lymphoma. One hundred and thirty patients received 14 mg/m^2 romidepsin on days 1, 8 and 15 every 28 days. The overall response rate (ORR) was 25 % with 19 patients having complete response and 3 having stable disease (Coiffier et al. 2012). Furthermore, a phase II study was conducted investigating the efficacy of romidepsin in patients with multiple myeloma. Thirteen patients were treated with 13 mg/m^2 romidepsin on days 1, 8 and 15 every 28 days. Five patients showed clinical benefit and two patients showed reduction of pain, but no patient achieved an objective response (Niesvizky et al. 2011). A phase II study investigated the effect of romidepsin in patients suffering from relapsed small-cell lung cancer. Sixteen patients were enrolled and received weekly infusions of romidepsin at 13 mg/m^2 on days 1, 8 and 15 on a 4-week schedule. The best response seen was stable disease in three patients. The study was closed because it did not reach the target response rate (Otterson et al. 2010). Haigentz et al. reported a phase II trial of romidepsin in patients with recurrent/metastatic head and neck cancer. Fourteen patients were treated with 13 mg/m^2 romidepsin on days 1, 8 and 15 of 28-day cycles. The best response seen was stable disease in two patients. Because the study lacked efficacy, it was terminated early (Haigentz et al. 2012). In a phase I/II trial, the effect of romidepsin in 50 patients with recurrent malignant glioma was studied. In phase I of the study, the maximum tolerated dose in patients receiving strong CYP3A4-inducing antiepileptic drugs (EIAEDs) was determined. Romidepsin is metabolised by cytochromes

Table 10.3 Romidepsin trials reported in the years 2009–2012

Combination therapy	Type of cancer	Phase	Patients number	Outcome	Literature
None	Cutaneous T-cell lymphoma	II	96	34 % ORR 6 CR	Whittaker et al. (2010)
None	Peripheral T-cell lymphoma	II	45	8 CR 9 PR	Piekarz et al. (2009)
None	Peripheral T-cell lymphoma	II	130	25 % ORR	Coiffier et al. (2012)
None	Multiple myeloma	II	13	No response	Niesvizky et al. (2011)
None	Small-cell lung cancer	II	16	3 SD	Otterson et al. (2010)
None	Head and neck cancer	II	14	2 SD	Haigentz et al. (2012)
None	Glioma	I/II	50	1 PFS >6 months	Iwamoto et al. (2011)
None	Cutaneous T-cell lymphoma	II	71	4 CR, 20 PR	Piekarz et al. (2009)
Gemcitabine	Solid tumours	I	36	MTD = 12 mg/m^2	Jones et al. (2012)

CYP3A4 and CYP3A514, and EIAEDs potently induce CYP3A4. It could be shown that EIAEDs did not affect romidepsin exposure. Because of the potential cardiotoxicity with doses of more than 17.7 mg/m^2, the MTD for patients receiving EIAEDs was not defined. In phase II the PFS at 6 months was investigated. Phase II patients were treated with romidepsin at dosage of 13.3 mg/m^2/day on days 1, 8 and 15 of each 28-day cycle. Among the 35 patients receiving romidepsin in phase II, one had progression-free survival for more than 6 months but developed tumour progression at 32 weeks. The trial showed that romidepsin had no significant clinical activity as a single agent in patients with recurrent glioma (Iwamoto et al. 2011).

A phase I trial of romidepsin in combination with gemcitabine in patients with advanced solid tumours was reported in 2012. Thirty-six patients with solid tumours were treated, and the MTD of 12 mg/m^2 romidepsin and 800 mg/m^2 gemcitabine was determined. Twenty-seven patients were evaluable of which 2 had a partial response and 14 had stable disease (Jones et al. 2012). The outcome of the described studies showed that the treatment with romidepsin is also effective in patients with peripheral T-cell lymphoma. However, in solid tumours a combination therapy with other agents might be valuable to improve efficacy.

10.7 Clinical Trials of Valproic Acid

Valproic acid is a well-tolerated drug already used in the treatment of epilepsy with a good characterised safety profile. Although it shows a 1,000-fold lesser HDAC activity compared to other HDACi like vorinostat, it is successfully applied in several trials against different cancers (see Table 10.4).

Table 10.4 Valproic acid trials reported in the years 2010–2012

Combination therapy	Type of cancer	Phase	Patients number	Outcome	Literature
None	Neuroendocrine carcinoma	II	8	5 SD	Mohammed et al. (2011)
Cytarabine	Acute myeloid leukaemia Refractory anaemia with excess of blasts	II	31	8 CR	Corsetti et al. (2011)
AraC	Acute myeloid leukaemia		15	No response	Lane et al. (2012)
Hydralazine	Myelodysplastic syndrome	II	12	6 OR 1 CR 1PR	Candelaria et al. (2011)
Hydralazine	Chronic myeloid leukaemia		8	2 CR 3 SD	Cervera et al. (2012)
ATRA-IV	Solid tumour	I	9	1 SD MTD could not be established	David et al. (2010)
Doxorubicin	Mesothelioma	II	45	7 PR	Scherpereel et al. (2011)

Preclinical data showed that Notch1 is a tumour suppressor in neuroendocrine tumours. Notch1 signalling is very minimal or nonexistent in neuroendocrine tumours, and the activation of Notch1 signalling leads to a decrease in tumour growth. Valproic acid has been shown to activate the Notch1 signalling pathway leading to a decrease in tumour markers. Because of these data, a phase I study to evaluate the effects of valproic acid on tumour marker production, tumour response, survival and Notch1 signalling has been conducted. Eight patients received a valproic acid dose of 500 mg orally, two times a day with a goal target serum level between 50 and 100 g/mL. Five patients had stable disease over the course of the treatment. It could be shown that the majority of patients experienced an improvement in their tumour markers and after treatment there was a tenfold induction of Notch1 mRNA compared to pretreatment levels (Mohammed et al. 2011).

In several trials valproic acid is applied in combination with other therapeutic agents. Two studies in combination with cytarabine in acute myeloid leukaemia were conducted. A phase II study investigated the effect of valproate in acute myeloid leukaemia (AML) and refractory anaemia with excess of blasts (RAEB). Thirty-one patients were treated with subsequent courses of low-dose cytarabine (20 mg) twice daily for 8 days and valproic acid with a starting dose of 5 mg/kg. Dose escalation of valproic acid was performed according to patient tolerance until the therapeutic range of 50–100 μg/mL was reached. Eight patients had complete response, with nearly complete clearing of marrow blasts and normalisation of blood counts at a median of 5 months. Three patients showed haematologic improvement. It could be shown that low-dose cytarabine in combination with valproic acid is well tolerated and shows good therapeutic activity in elderly patients with AML/RAEB (Corsetti et al. 2011). In another trial 15 patients were treated with a starting dose of 200 mg valproic acid three times a day. The dose was increased according to patient tolerance to achieve serum valproate levels of 50–100 μg/mL. Additionally, patients received 10 mg/m^2 cytarabine daily for the first 14 days of therapy. In contrast to the study mentioned before, no responses were observed (Lane et al. 2012). A possible explanation might be that the dose of valproic acid could not be escalated due to poor tolerance of this patient population. In the trial reported by Corsetti et al., the patients received a higher dose of cytarabine with a longer duration, and the patients had a better prognosis at the time of inclusion of the study. In a phase II study, valproate in combination with the DNA-methyltransferase inhibitor hydralazine was investigated in 12 patients with myelodysplastic syndrome. Patients received 83/182 mg hydralazine and 30 mg/kg valproic acid on a daily schedule. Overall response was seen in six patients, including 1 complete response and 1 partial response and 4 haematological improvements. A follow-up after about 14 months showed that only two patients progressed to AML. Overall this study shows that the combination of valproate and hydralazine may be an effective and safe combination in the treatment of MDS; however, so far only a small number of patients were treated (Candelaria et al. 2011). In another trial valproate in combination with hydralazine was administered to eight patients with chronic myeloid leukaemia who were refractory to imatinib. Patients received 83/182 mg hydralazine and 30 mg/kg valproic acid on a daily schedule and continued receiving imatinib at the same dose they were receiving at the time of progression. Two patients had a complete response and 3 had stable disease and only 1 did not respond. This trial gives evidence that therapy using an epigenetic agent can overcome imatinib resistance. However, the number of patients in this study is too small to make a clear statement (Cervera et al. 2012).

Besides haematological malignancies, the efficacy of valproic acid was studied in two trials in solid tumours. In a phase I study, valproic acid in combination with ATRA-IV is investigated in solid tumours refractory to prior therapy. One patient had stable disease lasting for 16 weeks. The MTD of both drugs in combination could not be established due to early closure of the trial (David et al. 2010). In another trial the combination of valproic acid with doxorubicin in patients with mesothelioma was examined. In the phase II trial, 45 patients were treated with oral valproic acid until a serum valproate level of 50–100 μg/mL was reached. Then patients were treated additionally with doxorubicin at 60 mg/m^2 every 3 weeks. Valproic acid administration continued during the whole treatment. Seven patients had a partial response. In recurrent mesothelioma after first-line cisplatin-based chemotherapy, this treatment regimen seems to be effective and warrants further trials (Scherpereel et al. 2011).

10.8 Clinical Trials of Belinostat

Belinostat is a hydroxamic acid-based HDACi that is currently investigated in clinical trials (see Table 10.5).

Two trials investigated the efficacy of belinostat as single agent. Cashen et al. reported the application of belinostat in the treatment of myelodysplastic syndrome.

Table 10.5 Belinostat trials reported in the years 2010–2012

Combination therapy	Type of cancer	Phase	Patients number	Outcome	Literature
None	Myelodysplastic syndrome	II	21	1 CR	Cashen et al. (2012)
None	Thymic epithelial tumours	II	41	2 PR 25 SD	Giaccone et al. (2011)
Carboplatin and/or paclitaxel	Solid tumours	I	23	2 PR 6 SD	Lassen et al. (2010)
Carboplatin	Platinum-resistant ovarian, fallopian tube or primary peritoneal carcinoma	II	27	1 CR 1 PR 12 SD	Dizon et al. (2012a)
Carboplatin Paclitaxel	Ovarian cancer	II	35	3 CR 12 PR	Dizon et al. (2012b)

Twenty-one patients were enrolled and treated with 1,000 mg/m^2 belinostat on days 1–5 of a 21-day cycle. One patient received a partial response lasting for 2.1 months. The study was closed after the first stage of enrolment (Cashen et al. 2012).

Another trial using belinostat as single agent was reported in 2011 by Giaccone et al. In this phase II study, patients with recurrent or refractory advanced thymic epithelial tumours were treated with 1 g/m^2 on days 1–5 of a 21-day cycle. Forty-one patients were enrolled of which 25 had thymoma and 16 had thymic carcinoma. Two patients achieved a partial response and 25 had stabilisation of disease lasting for 5.8 months (median), and treatment was well tolerated. In general, patients with thymic carcinoma had significantly shorter survival than those with thymoma. Protein hyperacetylation was analysed, but no correlation between hyperacetylation and response could be found (Giaccone et al. 2011). Several studies describe the combination of belinostat with other agents in solid tumours. In a phase I study, the combination of belinostat with carboplatin and/or paclitaxel was investigated in patients having solid tumours. Belinostat was administered in escalating doses of 600, 800 and 1,000 mg/m^2/day on days 1–5 of a 21-day cycle. Carboplatin and paclitaxel were administered on day 3. Treatment was well tolerated and the recommended dose of belinostat was 1,000 mg/m^2/day. The pharmacokinetics of belinostat, paclitaxel and carboplatin were unaltered by the concurrent administration. There was one complete CA-125 response, two patients had a partial response and six patients had stable disease for more than 6 months (Lassen et al. 2010). Another phase II study investigated the effect of the combination belinostat and carboplatin in the treatment of recurrent or persistent platinum-resistant ovarian, fallopian tube or primary peritoneal carcinoma. Twenty-seven patients received belinostat in a dose of 1,000 mg/m^2 for 5 days every 3 weeks and carboplatin on day 3. There was one complete response, one partial response and 12 patients had stable disease. Because the overall response rate did not meet the criteria for further development, the study was closed at the first stage (Dizon et al. 2012a).

The activity of belinostat, carboplatin, and paclitaxel in women with previously treated ovarian cancer was also investigated by Dizon et al. Thirty-five patients were treated with belinostat (1,000 mg/m^2) daily for 5 days; carboplatin and paclitaxel were given on day 3 of a 21-day cycle. Three patients had a complete response, and 12 had a partial response. The overall response rate among resistant patients was 44 and 63 % among sensitive patients. This study could show that the addition of belinostat to standard therapy could enhance the outcome and is worth to be further investigated (Dizon et al. 2012b).

10.9 Clinical Trials of Mocetinostat

Preclinical data have shown that mocetinostat, an oral class I-selective HDAC inhibitor, has potent antiproliferative activity against a wide range of cancers (Fournel et al. 2008). To investigate its clinical efficacy, several clinical trials for haematologic malignancies and solid tumours were conducted (Wagner et al. 2010). In the last year a phase II trial of mocetinostat in patients with relapsed Hodgkin's lymphoma was reported (see Table 10.6). Fifty-one patients were treated with Mocetinostat three times a week and a dose of 85 mg was found to be the best tolerated. Two patients had a complete response, 12 had a partial response and one had stable disease. These results show that mocetinostat has significant clinical efficacy and its use either as single agent or in combination should be further investigated (Younes et al. 2011).

Table 10.6 Other HDACi trials reported in the years 2010–2012

Study medication	Type of cancer	Phase	Patients number	Outcome	Literature
Mocetinostat	Hodgkin's lymphoma	II	51	2 CR 12 PR 1 SD	Younes et al. (2011)
Entinostat 13-*cis* retinoic acid	Solid tumours	I	19	MTD=4 mg/m^2 No response	Pili et al. (2012)
Givinostat	Chronic myeloproliferative neoplasms	II	29	3 CR 6 PR	Rambaldi et al. (2010)
CS055	Solid tumours and lymphomas	I	31	5 PR 11 SD	Dong et al. (2012)
SB939	Refractory solid malignancies	I	30	MTD=80 mg/day 5 SD	Yong et al. (2011)
SB939	Advanced solid tumours	I	38	RP2D=60 mg on five consecutive days every 2 weeks	Razak et al. (2011)
CHR-3996	Solid tumours	I	39	RP2D=40 mg/day 1 PR 9 SD	Banerji et al. (2012)

10.10 Clinical Trials of Entinostat

The ability of HDACi to resensitise tumour cells to retinoids was investigated in a phase I trial of entinostat in combination with 13-*cis* retinoic acid in patients with solid tumours (see Table 10.6). Nineteen patients were treated with entinostat orally once a week and 13-*cis* retinoic acid orally twice a day (1 mg/kg) for 21 days every 4 weeks. The MTD was determined at 4 mg/m^2 entinostat. There were no complete or partial responses. However, seven patients had stable disease (Pili et al. 2012).

10.11 Clinical Trials of Givinostat

The safety and efficacy of givinostat in the treatment of JAK2V617F-positive chronic myeloproliferative neoplasms, including polycythaemia vera, essential thrombocythaemia and myelofibrosis, was studied in a phase II trial (see Table 10.6). Twenty-nine patients received oral givinostat for 24 weeks at a dose of 50 mg twice daily. Among the patients having polycythaemia vera or essential thrombocythaemia, one patient had a complete haematological response, and six patients had a partial response. Furthermore, complete control of pruritus was observed in all but one patient. Among the patients having myelofibrosis, three patients had achieved a complete response. JAK2V617F tumour allele burden was monitored during treatment and a progressive decrease of the JAK2V617F mutated allele during treatment could be found. The treatment was well tolerated with the most common side effects being mild gastrointestinal disorders like diarrhoea, nausea and gastric or abdominal pain. This study confirmed that givinostat shows clinical activity. In vitro experiments implied that the efficacy of givinostat could be improved by combining it with hydroxycarbamide or other JAK2V617F inhibitors (Rambaldi et al. 2010).

10.12 Clinical Trials of Chidamide

Chidamide is a new orally available benzamide-containing HDACi. Preclinical data have shown that chidamide has in vitro and in vivo antitumour activity against several cancer cell lines. In a phase I trial, tolerability and dose-limiting toxicities of chidamide in patients with advanced solid tumours or lymphomas were determined (see Table 10.6). Thirty-one patients received oral doses of 5, 10, 17.5, 25, 32.5 or 50 mg chidamide either twice (BIW) or three times (TIW) per week for four consecutive weeks every 6 weeks. Five patients had a partial response and 11 patients had stable disease. Chidamide is well tolerated, exhibited a relatively long half-life of 17–18 h and showed a long-lasting histone H3 acetylation (Dong et al. 2012). This data suggest that chidamide is a promising new HDACi and its clinical efficacy should be further evaluated.

10.13 Clinical Trials of Pracinostat (SB939)

Because of the favourable preclinical pharmacological properties of pracinostat, the maximum tolerated dose, the pharmacokinetics, the pharmacodynamics and preliminary efficacy of pracinostat in patients with advanced solid malignancies were investigated in a phase I trial (see Table 10.6). Thirty patients received oral pracinostat (10–80 mg/day) three times a week for 3 weeks in a 4-week cycle. Five patients had stable disease. The maximum tolerated dose using this regimen was determined at 80 mg/day, and the recommended dose for phase II studies is 60 mg/day. Although no partial responses were seen, prolonged nonprogression of breast cancer, follicular thyroid carcinoma, neuroblastoma and hepatocellular carcinoma were promising observations and should be further evaluated (Yong et al. 2011).

Another phase I trial was reported by Razak et al. 38 patients received oral pracinostat. The maximal administered dose was 90 mg, and the recommended phase II dose was 60 mg given five consecutive days every 2 weeks. No objective tumour responses were observed, but ten patients showed stable disease for 5.7 months (median) (Razak et al. 2011).

The most common adverse events were toxicities that included fatigue, nausea, vomiting, anorexia and diarrhoea and are common among HDACi application.

10.14 Clinical Trials of CHR-3996

CHR-3996 is a new, orally available, class I-selective HDACi that has shown promising activity against a wide range of cancer cell lines. In a phase I study, the pharmacokinetics and pharmacodynamics of CHR-3996 were investigated in patients with refractory solid tumours (see Table 10.6). Thirty-eight patients received CHR-3996 (5–160 mg) once a day. One patient had a partial response and nine patients had stable disease. The recommended phase II dose was 40 mg/day. The most common seen DLTs were thrombocytopenia, fatigue and elevated plasma creatinine. Because of the manageable toxicity profile and favourable pharmacokinetic and pharmacodynamic properties, CHR-3996 should be investigated in further studies (Banerji et al. 2012).

Conclusions

HDACi are antiproliferative agents with manageable side effects, successfully applied in the clinic for the treatment of mainly haematological diseases. Besides vorinostat and romidepsin which are already approved by the FDA, several other potent HDACi are currently investigated for their clinical efficacy in the treatment of cancer.

Even though some promising results could be observed, especially in combination with other anticancer agents, the treatment of solid malignancies with HDACi remains to be unsatisfactory and has to be further investigated in clinical trials. Several trials could demonstrate that HDACi can be administered in combination with standard therapy without decrease of the doses and without additional side effects. Improvement of the dosing and the schedule as well as the optimisation of combination therapies might help to achieve an increased response especially in solid tumours.

Especially interesting in that regard is the question of surrogate biomarkers for HDAC inhibitor dosing. Diagnostic as well as prognostic biomarkers are valuable tools to optimise therapy and improve safety. Although biomarkers like the acetylation of tumour tissue and PBMCs to correlate treatment and response are used in many trials, a clear correlation could not be verified yet. Standard procedures are the analysis of histone hyperacetylation by western blotting, ELISA or mass spectrometry (Chung et al. 2006) Alternatively, total cellular histone deacetylase activity measured with a cell-permeable small molecule substrate has been suggested (Hoffmann et al. 1999; Bonfils et al. 2008).

Another question that has to be addressed is if class-selective inhibitors can increase efficacy or reduce side effects. To answer that, more information about the role of specific isoforms and their function in cancer is needed. Some experiments using knockout mice have been done to elucidate this (Haberland et al. 2009), but a lot still needs to be learned to fully understand the distinct roles of the HDAC subtypes. In this context the role of protein versus histone acetylation and the clinical application has to be investigated. This will be especially true for the planned clinical development of HDAC6-selective inhibitors.

Altogether, despite many years of HDAC research, there are still many fundamental issues that we have to understand better. Still, HDAC inhibitors are already used in the clinic with some success, and we expect to exploit their potential even better in the upcoming years.

Acknowledgments The authors thank the Deutsche Forschungsgemeinschaft for funding (Ju 295/9-1 within the priority programme SPP1463 Epigenetic regulation of normal hematopoiesis and its dysregulation in myeloid neoplasia; coordinators M. Lübbert, Freiburg, C. Plass, Heidelberg).

References

Arts J, King P, Marien A, Floren W, Belien A, Janssen L, Pilatte I, Roux B, Decrane L, Gilissen R, Hickson I, Vreys V, Cox E, Bol K, Talloen W, Goris I, Andries L, Du Jardin M, Janicot M, Page M, van Emelen K, Angibaud P (2009) JNJ-26481585, a novel "second-generation" oral histone deacetylase inhibitor, shows broad-spectrum preclinical antitumoral activity. Clin Cancer Res 15:6841–6851

Atadja P (2009) Development of the pan-DAC inhibitor panobinostat (LBH589): successes and challenges. Cancer Lett 280:233–241

Badros A, Burger AM, Philip S, Niesvizky R, Kolla SS, Goloubeva O et al (2009) Phase I study of vorinostat in combination with bortezomib for relapsed and refractory multiple myeloma. Clin Cancer Res 15:5250–5257

Bali P, Pranpat M, Bradner J, Balasis M, Fiskus W, Guo F, Rocha K, Kumaraswamy S, Boyapalle S, Atadja P, Seto E, Bhalla K (2005) Inhibition of histone deacetylase 6 acetylates and disrupts the chaperone function of heat shock protein 90: a novel basis for antileukemia activity of histone deacetylase inhibitors. J Biol Chem 280:26729–26734

Balliet RM, Chen G, Gallagher CJ, Dellinger RW, Sun D, Lazarus P (2009) Characterization of UGTs active against SAHA and association between SAHA glucuronidation activity phenotype with UGT phenotype. Cancer Res 69:2981–2989

Banerji U, van Doorn L, Papadatos-Pastos D, Kristeleit R, Debnam P, Tall M, Stewart A, Raynaud F, Garrett MD, Toal M, Hooftman L, De Bono JS, Verweij J, Eskens FA (2012) A phase I pharmacokinetic and pharmacodynamic study of CHR-3996, an oral class I selective histone deacetylase inhibitor in refractory solid tumors. Clin Cancer Res 18:2687–2694

Bantscheff M, Hopf C, Savitski MM, Dittmann A, Grandi P, Michon AM, Schlegl J, Abraham Y, Becher I, Bergamini G, Boesche M, Delling M, Dumpelfeld B, Eberhard D, Huthmacher C, Mathieson T, Poeckel D, Reader V, Strunk K, Sweetman G, Kruse U, Neubauer G, Ramsden NG, Drewes G (2011) Chemoproteomics profiling of HDAC inhibitors reveals selective targeting of HDAC complexes. Nat Biotechnol 29:255–265

Bolden JE, Peart MJ, Johnstone RW (2006) Anticancer activities of histone deacetylase inhibitors. Nat Rev Drug Discov 5:769–784

Bonfils C, Kalita A, Dubay M, Siu LL, Carducci MA, Reid G, Martell RE, Besterman JM, Li Z (2008) Evaluation of the pharmacodynamic effects of MGCD0103 from preclinical models to human using a novel HDAC enzyme assay. Clin Cancer Res 14:3441–3449

Bressi JC, Jennings AJ, Skene R, Wu Y, Melkus R, De Jong R, O'Connell S, Grimshaw CE, Navre M, Gangloff AR (2010) Exploration of the HDAC2 foot pocket: synthesis and SAR of substituted N-(2-aminophenyl)benzamides. Bioorg Med Chem Lett 20:3142–3145

Buchwald M, Kramer OH, Heinzel T (2009) HDACi–targets beyond chromatin. Cancer Lett 280:160–167

Candelaria M, Herrera A, Labardini J, Gonzalez-Fierro A, Trejo-Becerril C, Taja-Chayeb L, Perez-Cardenas E, de la Cruz-Hernandez E, Arias-Bofill D, Vidal S, Cervera E, Duenas-Gonzalez A (2011) Hydralazine and magnesium valproate as epigenetic treatment for myelodysplastic syndrome. Preliminary results of a phase-II trial. Ann Hematol 90:379–387

Cashen A, Juckett M, Jumonville A, Litzow M, Flynn PJ, Eckardt J, LaPlant B, Laumann K, Erlichman C, DiPersio J (2012) Phase II study of the histone deacetylase inhibitor belinostat (PXD101) for the treatment of myelodysplastic syndrome (MDS). Ann Hematol 91:33–38

Cervera E, Candelaria M, Lopez-Navarro O, Labardini J, Gonzalez-Fierro A, Taja-Chayeb L, Cortes J, Gordillo-Bastidas D, Duenas-Gonzalez A (2012) Epigenetic therapy with hydralazine and magnesium valproate reverses imatinib resistance in patients with chronic myeloid leukemia. Clin Lymphoma Myeloma Leuk 12:207–212

Chinnaiyan P, Chowdhary S, Potthast L, Prabhu A, Tsai YY, Sarcar B, Kahali S, Brem S, Yu HM, Rojiani A, Murtagh R, Pan E (2012) Phase I trial of vorinostat combined with bevacizumab and CPT-11 in recurrent glioblastoma. Neuro Oncol 14:93–100

Choudhary C, Kumar C, Gnad F, Nielsen ML, Rehman M, Walther TC, Olsen JV, Mann M (2009) Lysine acetylation targets protein complexes and co-regulates major cellular functions. Science 325:834–840

Chung EJ, Lee MJ, Lee S, Trepel JB (2006) Assays for pharmacodynamic analysis of histone deacetylase inhibitors. Expert Opin Drug Metab Toxicol 2:213–230

Coiffier B, Pro B, Prince HM, Foss F, Sokol L, Greenwood M, Caballero D, Borchmann P, Morschhauser F, Wilhelm M, Pinter-Brown L, Padmanabhan S, Shustov A, Nichols J, Carroll S, Balser J, Balser B, Horwitz S (2012) Results from a pivotal, open-label, phase II study of romidepsin in relapsed or refractory peripheral T-cell lymphoma after prior systemic therapy. J Clin Oncol 30:631–636

Corsetti MT, Salvi F, Perticone S, Baraldi A, De Paoli L, Gatto S, Pietrasanta D, Pini M, Primon V, Zallio F, Tonso A, Alvaro MG, Ciravegna G, Levis A (2011) Hematologic improvement and response in elderly AML/RAEB patients treated with valproic acid and low-dose Ara-C. Leuk Res 35:991–997

David KA, Mongan NP, Smith C, Gudas LJ, Nanus DM (2010) Phase I trial of ATRA-IV and Depakote in patients with advanced solid tumor malignancies. Cancer Biol Ther 9:678–684

Dimicoli S, Jabbour E, Borthakur G, Kadia T, Estrov Z, Yang H, Kelly M, Pierce S, Kantarjian H, Garcia-Manero G (2012) Phase II study of the histone deacetylase inhibitor panobinostat (LBH589) in patients with low or intermediate-1 risk myelodysplastic syndrome. Am J Hematol 87:127–129

Dizon DS, Blessing JA, Penson RT, Drake RD, Walker JL, Johnston CM, Disilvestro PA, Fader AN (2012a) A phase II evaluation of belinostat and carboplatin in the treatment of recurrent or persistent platinum-resistant ovarian, fallopian tube, or primary peritoneal carcinoma: a Gynecologic Oncology Group study. Gynecol Oncol 125:367–371

Dizon DS, Damstrup L, Finkler NJ, Lassen U, Celano P, Glasspool R, Crowley E, Lichenstein HS, Knoblach P, Penson RT (2012b) Phase II activity of belinostat (PXD-101), carboplatin, and paclitaxel in women with previously treated ovarian cancer. Int J Gynecol Cancer 22:979–986

Doi T, Hamaguchi T, Shirao K, Chin K, Hatake K, Noguchi K, Otsuki T, Mehta A, Ohtsu A (2013) Evaluation of safety, pharmacokinetics, and efficacy of vorinostat, a histone deacetylase inhibitor, in the treatment of gastrointestinal (GI) cancer in a phase I clinical trial. Int J Clin Oncol 18(1):87–95

Dong M, Ning ZQ, Xing PY, Xu JL, Cao HX, Dou GF, Meng ZY, Shi YK, Lu XP, Feng FY (2012) Phase I study of chidamide (CS055/HBI-8000), a new histone deacetylase inhibitor, in patients with advanced solid tumors and lymphomas. Cancer Chemother Pharmacol 69:1413–1422

Drappatz J, Lee EQ, Hammond S, Grimm SA, Norden AD, Beroukhim R, Gerard M, Schiff D, Chi AS, Batchelor TT, Doherty LM, Ciampa AS, Lafrankie DC, Ruland S, Snodgrass SM, Raizer JJ, Wen PY (2012) Phase I study of panobinostat in combination with bevacizumab for recurrent high-grade glioma. J Neurooncol 107:133–138

Dummer R, Beyer M, Hymes K, Epping MT, Bernards R, Steinhoff M, Sterry W, Kerl H, Heath K, Ahern JD, Hardwick JS, Garcia-Vargas J, Baumann K, Rizvi S, Frankel SR, Whittaker SJ, Assaf C (2012) Vorinostat combined with bexarotene for treatment of cutaneous T-cell lymphoma: in vitro and phase I clinical evidence supporting augmentation of retinoic acid receptor/retinoid X receptor activation by histone deacetylase inhibition. Leuk Lymphoma 53(8):1501–1508

Duvic M, Talpur R, Ni X, Zhang C, Hazarika P, Kelly C, Chiao JH, Reilly JF, Ricker JL, Richon VM, Frankel SR (2007) Phase 2 trial of oral vorinostat (suberoylanilide hydroxamic acid, SAHA) for refractory cutaneous T-cell lymphoma (CTCL). Blood 109:31–39

Duvic M, Dummer R, Becker JC, Poulalhon N, Ortiz Romero P, Grazia Bernengo M (2013) Panobinostat activity in both bexarotene-exposed and -naïve patients with refractory cutaneous T-cell lymphoma: results of a phase II trial. Eur J Cancer 49:386–394

Fakih MG, Fetterly G, Egorin MJ, Muindi JR, Espinoza-Delgado I, Zwiebel JA, Litwin A, Holleran JL, Wang K, Diasio RB (2010) A phase I, pharmacokinetic, and pharmacodynamic study of two schedules of vorinostat in combination with 5-fluorouracil and leucovorin in patients with refractory solid tumors. Clin Cancer Res 16:3786–3794

Fakih MG, Groman A, McMahon J, Wilding G, Muindi JR (2012) A randomized phase II study of two doses of vorinostat in combination with 5-FU/LV in patients with refractory colorectal cancer. Cancer Chemother Pharmacol 69:743–751

Fischer A, Sananbenesi F, Mungenast A, Tsai LH (2010) Targeting the correct HDAC(s) to treat cognitive disorders. Trends Pharmacol Sci 31:605–617

Fournel M, Bonfils C, Hou Y, Yan PT, Trachy-Bourget MC, Kalita A, Liu J, Lu AH, Zhou NZ, Robert MF, Gillespie J, Wang JJ, Ste-Croix H, Rahil J, Lefebvre S, Moradei O, Delorme D, Macleod AR, Besterman JM, Li Z (2008) MGCD0103, a novel isotype-selective histone deacetylase inhibitor, has broad spectrum antitumor activity in vitro and in vivo. Mol Cancer Ther 7:759–768

Friday BB, Anderson SK, Buckner J, Yu C, Giannini C, Geoffroy F, Schwerkoske J, Mazurczak M, Gross H, Pajon E, Jaeckle K, Galanis E (2012) Phase II trial of vorinostat in combination with bortezomib in recurrent glioblastoma: a north central cancer treatment group study. Neuro Oncol 14:215–221

Fukutomi A, Hatake K, Matsui K, Sakajiri S, Hirashima T, Tanii H, Kobayashi K, Yamamoto N (2012) A phase I study of oral panobinostat (LBH589) in Japanese patients with advanced solid tumors. Invest New Drugs 30:1096–1106

Furumai R, Matsuyama A, Kobashi N, Lee KH, Nishiyama M, Nakajima H, Tanaka A, Komatsu Y, Nishino N, Yoshida M, Horinouchi S (2002) FK228 (depsipeptide) as a natural prodrug that inhibits class I histone deacetylases. Cancer Res 62:4916–4921

Gandia P, Arellano C, Chalret du Rieu Q, Lochon I, Campone M, Pierga JY, Poublanc M, Hennebelle I, Filleron T, Chatelut E, Delord JP (2011) Unexpected high levels of vorinostat when combined with vinorelbine in patients with advanced cancer. Curr Clin Pharmacol 6:274–279

Giaccone G, Rajan A, Berman A, Kelly RJ, Szabo E, Lopez-Chavez A, Trepel J, Lee MJ, Cao L, Espinoza-Delgado I, Spittler J, Loehrer PJ Sr (2011) Phase II study of belinostat in patients with recurrent or refractory advanced thymic epithelial tumors. J Clin Oncol 29:2052–2059

Glozak MA, Sengupta N, Zhang X, Seto E (2005) Acetylation and deacetylation of non-histone proteins. Gene 363:15–23

Gong K, Xie J, Yi H, Li W (2012) CS055 (Chidamide/HBI-8000), a novel histone deacetylase inhibitor, induces G1 arrest, ROS-dependent apoptosis and differentiation in human leukaemia cells. Biochem J 443:735–746

Gottesfeld JM, Pandolfo M (2009) Development of histone deacetylase inhibitors as therapeutics for neurological disease. Future Neurol 4:775–784

Göttlicher M, Minucci S, Zhu P, Krämer OH, Schimpf A, Giavara S, Sleeman JP, Lo Coco F, Nervi C, Pelicci PG, Heinzel T (2001) Valproic acid defines a novel class of HDAC inhibitors inducing differentiation of transformed cells. EMBO J 20:6969–6978

Haberland M, Montgomery RL, Olson EN (2009) The many roles of histone deacetylases in development and physiology: implications for disease and therapy. Nat Rev Genet 10:32–42

Haigentz M Jr, Kim M, Sarta C, Lin J, Keresztes RS, Culliney B, Gaba AG, Smith RV, Shapiro GI, Chirieac LR, Mariadason JM, Belbin TJ, Greally JM, Wright JJ, Haddad RI (2012) Phase II trial of the histone deacetylase inhibitor romidepsin in patients with recurrent/metastatic head and neck cancer. Oral Oncol 48(12):1281–1288

Hainsworth JD, Infante JR, Spigel DR, Arrowsmith ER, Boccia RV, Burris HA (2011) A phase II trial of panobinostat, a histone deacetylase inhibitor, in the treatment of patients with refractory metastatic renal cell carcinoma. Cancer Invest 29:451–455

Hideshima T, Bradner JE, Wong J, Chauhan D, Richardson P, Schreiber SL, Anderson KC (2005) Small-molecule inhibition of proteasome and aggresome function induces synergistic antitumor activity in multiple myeloma. Proc Natl Acad Sci USA 102:8567–8572

Hoffmann K, Brosch G, Loidl P, Jung M (1999) A non-isotopic assay for histone deacetylase activity. Nucleic Acids Res 27:2057–2058

Iwamoto FM, Lamborn KR, Kuhn JG, Wen PY, Yung WK, Gilbert MR, Chang SM, Lieberman FS, Prados MD, Fine HA (2011) A phase I/II trial of the histone deacetylase inhibitor romidepsin for adults with recurrent malignant glioma: North American Brain Tumor Consortium Study 03-03. Neuro Oncol 13:509–516

Jagannath S, Dimopoulos MA, Lonial S (2010) Combined proteasome and histone deacetylase inhibition: a promising synergy for patients with relapsed/refractory multiple myeloma. Leuk Res 34:1111–1118

Jones P (2009) Histone deacetylase inhibitors. In: Sippl W, Jung M (eds) Epigenetic targets in drug discovery. Wiley VCH, New York, pp 185–223

Jones SF, Bendell JC, Infante JR, Spigel DR, Thompson DS, Yardley DA, Greco FA, Murphy PB, Burris HA 3rd (2011) A phase I study of panobinostat in combination with gemcitabine in the treatment of solid tumors. Clin Adv Hematol Oncol 9:225–230

Jones SF, Infante JR, Spigel DR, Peacock NW, Thompson DS, Greco FA, McCulloch W, Burris Iii HA (2012) Phase 1 results from a study of romidepsin in combination with gemcitabine in patients with advanced solid tumors. Cancer Invest 30:481–486

Khan O, La Thangue NB (2012) HDAC inhibitors in cancer biology: emerging mechanisms and clinical applications. Immunol Cell Biol 90:85–94

Kim GD, Choi YH, Dimtchev A, Jeong SJ, Dritschilo A, Jung M (1999) Sensing of ionizing radiation-induced DNA damage by ATM through interaction with histone deacetylase. J Biol Chem 274:31127–31130

Kirschbaum M, Frankel P, Popplewell L, Zain J, Delioukina M, Pullarkat V, Matsuoka D, Pulone B, Rotter AJ, Espinoza-Delgado I, Nademanee A, Forman SJ, Gandara D, Newman E (2011) Phase II study of vorinostat for treatment of relapsed or refractory indolent non-Hodgkin's lymphoma and mantle cell lymphoma. J Clin Oncol 29:1198–1203

Kirschbaum MH, Goldman BH, Zain JM, Cook JR, Rimsza LM, Forman SJ, Fisher RI (2012) A phase 2 study of vorinostat for treatment of relapsed or refractory Hodgkin lymphoma: Southwest Oncology Group Study S0517. Leuk Lymphoma 53:259–262

Lane S, Gill D, McMillan NA, Saunders N, Murphy R, Spurr T, Keane C, Fan HM, Mollee P (2012) Valproic acid combined with cytosine arabinoside in elderly patients with acute myeloid leukemia has in vitro but limited clinical activity. Leuk Lymphoma 53:1077–1083

Lassen U, Molife LR, Sorensen M, Engelholm SA, Vidal L, Sinha R, Penson RT, Buhl-Jensen P, Crowley E, Tjornelund J, Knoblauch P, de Bono JS (2010) A phase I study of the safety and pharmacokinetics of the histone deacetylase inhibitor belinostat administered in combination with carboplatin and/or paclitaxel in patients with solid tumours. Br J Cancer 103:12–17

Latham JA, Dent SY (2007) Cross-regulation of histone modifications. Nat Struct Mol Biol 14:1017–1024

Leder A, Orkin S, Leder P (1975) Differentiation of erythroleukemic cells in the presence of inhibitors of DNA synthesis. Science 190:893–894

Lin RJ, Sternsdorf T, Tini M, Evans RM (2001) Transcriptional regulation in acute promyelocytic leukemia. Oncogene 20:7204–7215

Luo J, Su F, Chen D, Shiloh A, Gu W (2000) Deacetylation of p53 modulates its effect on cell growth and apoptosis. Nature 408:377–381

Ma X, Ezzeldin HH, Diasio RB (2009) Histone deacetylase inhibitors: current status and overview of recent clinical trials. Drugs 69:1911–1934

Mateos M, Spencer A, Taylor K, Lonial S, De La Rubia J, Facon T, Bengoudifa B, Hazell K, Bourquelot PM, San-Miguel JF (2010) Phase Ib study of oral panobinostat (LBH589) plus lenalidomide (LEN) plus dexamethasone (DEX) in patients (Pts) with relapsed (Rel) or Rel and refractory (Ref) multiple myeloma (MM). J Clin Oncol (Meeting Abstracts) 28(Suppl):8030

McKinsey TA (2012) Therapeutic potential for HDAC inhibitors in the heart. Annu Rev Pharmacol Toxicol 52:303–319

Millward M, Price T, Townsend A, Sweeney C, Spencer A, Sukumaran S, Longenecker A, Lee L, Lay A, Sharma G, Gemmill RM, Drabkin HA, Lloyd GK, Neuteboom ST, McConkey DJ, Palladino MA, Spear MA (2012) Phase 1 clinical trial of the novel proteasome inhibitor marizomib with the histone deacetylase inhibitor vorinostat in patients with melanoma, pancreatic and lung cancer based on in vitro assessments of the combination. Invest New Drugs 30(6):2303–2317

Moffat D, Patel S, Day F, Belfield A, Donald A, Rowlands M, Wibawa J, Brotherton D, Stimson L, Clark V, Owen J, Bawden L, Box G, Bone E, Mortenson P, Hardcastle A, van Meurs S, Eccles S, Raynaud F, Aherne W (2010) Discovery of 2-(6-{[(6-fluoroquinolin-2-yl)methyl] amino}bicyclo[3.1.0]hex-3-yl)-N-hydroxypyrim idine-5-carboxamide (CHR-3996), a class I selective orally active histone deacetylase inhibitor. J Med Chem 53:8663–8678

Mohammed TA, Holen KD, Jaskula-Sztul R, Mulkerin D, Lubner SJ, Schelman WR, Eickhoff J, Chen H, Loconte NK (2011) A pilot phase II study of valproic acid for treatment of low-grade neuroendocrine carcinoma. Oncologist 16:835–843

Morita S, Oizumi S, Minami H, Kitagawa K, Komatsu Y, Fujiwara Y, Inada M, Yuki S, Kiyota N, Mitsuma A, Sawaki M, Tanii H, Kimura J, Ando Y (2012) Phase I dose-escalating study of panobinostat (LBH589) Administered intravenously to Japanese patients with advanced solid tumors. Invest New Drugs 30(5):1950–1957

Munster PN, Thurn KT, Thomas S, Raha P, Lacevic M, Miller A, Melisko M, Ismail-Khan R, Rugo H, Moasser M, Minton SE (2011) A phase II study of the histone deacetylase inhibitor vorinostat combined with tamoxifen for the treatment of patients with hormone therapy-resistant breast cancer. Br J Cancer 104:1828–1835

Niesvizky R, Ely S, Mark T, Aggarwal S, Gabrilove JL, Wright JJ, Chen-Kiang S, Sparano JA (2011) Phase 2 trial of the histone deacetylase inhibitor romidepsin for the treatment of refractory multiple myeloma. Cancer 117:336–342

Novotny-Diermayr V, Sangthongpitag K, Hu CY, Wu X, Sausgruber N, Yeo P, Greicius G, Pettersson S, Liang AL, Loh YK, Bonday Z, Goh KC, Hentze H, Hart S, Wang H, Ethirajulu K, Wood JM (2010) SB939, a novel potent and orally active histone deacetylase inhibitor with high tumor exposure and efficacy in mouse models of colorectal cancer. Mol Cancer Ther 9:642–652

Offidani M, Polloni C, Cavallo F, Marina Liberati A, Ballanti S, Pulini S, Catarini M, Alesiani F, Corvatta L, Gentili S, Caraffa P, Boccadoro M, Leoni P, Palumbo A (2012) Phase II study of melphalan, thalidomide and prednisone combined with oral panobinostat in patients with relapsed/refractory multiple myeloma. Leuk Lymphoma 53(9):1722–1727

Ohtani K, Dimmeler S (2011) Epigenetic regulation of cardiovascular differentiation. Cardiovasc Res 90:404–412

Olsen EA, Kim YH, Kuzel TM, Pacheco TR, Foss FM, Parker S (2007) Phase IIb multicenter trial of vorinostat in patients with persistent, progressive, or treatment refractory cutaneous T-cell lymphoma. J Clin Oncol 25:3109–3115

Otterson GA, Hodgson L, Pang H, Vokes EE (2010) Phase II study of the histone deacetylase inhibitor Romidepsin in relapsed small cell lung cancer (Cancer and Leukemia Group B 30304). J Thorac Oncol 5:1644–1648

Pandolfi PP (2001) Histone deacetylases and transcriptional therapy with their inhibitors. Cancer Chemother Pharmacol 48(Suppl 1):S17–S19

Parsons PG, Hansen C, Fairlie DP, West ML, Danoy PA, Sturm RA, Dunn IS, Pedley J, Ablett EM (1997) Tumor selectivity and transcriptional activation by azelaic bishydroxamic acid in human melanocytic cells. Biochem Pharmacol 53:1719–1724

Pasqualucci L, Migliazza A, Basso K, Houldsworth J, Chaganti RS, Dalla-Favera R (2003) Mutations of the BCL6 proto-oncogene disrupt its negative autoregulation in diffuse large B-cell lymphoma. Blood 101:2914–2923

Piekarz RL, Frye R, Turner M, Wright JJ, Allen SL, Kirschbaum MH (2009) Phase II multi-institutional trial of the histone deacetylase inhibitor romidepsin as monotherapy for patients with cutaneous T-cell lymphoma. J Clin Oncol 27:5410–5417

Piekarz RL, Frye R, Prince HM, Kirschbaum MH, Zain J, Allen SL, Jaffe ES, Ling A, Turner M, Peer CJ, Figg WD, Steinberg SM, Smith S, Joske D, Lewis I, Hutchins L, Craig M, Fojo AT, Wright JJ, Bates SE (2011) Phase 2 trial of romidepsin in patients with peripheral T-cell lymphoma. Blood 117:5827–5834

Pili R, Salumbides B, Zhao M, Altiok S, Qian D, Zwiebel J, Carducci MA, Rudek MA (2012) Phase I study of the histone deacetylase inhibitor entinostat in combination with 13-cis retinoic acid in patients with solid tumours. Br J Cancer 106:77–84

Plumb JA, Finn PW, Williams RJ, Bandara MJ, Romero MR, Watkins CJ, La Thangue NB, Brown R (2003) Pharmacodynamic response and inhibition of growth of human tumor xenografts by the novel histone deacetylase inhibitor PXD101. Mol Cancer Ther 2:721–728

Ramalingam SS, Kummar S, Sarantopoulos J, Shibata S, LoRusso P, Yerk M, Holleran J, Lin Y, Beumer JH, Harvey RD, Ivy SP, Belani CP, Egorin MJ (2010) Phase I study of vorinostat in patients with advanced solid tumors and hepatic dysfunction: a National Cancer Institute Organ Dysfunction Working Group study. J Clin Oncol 28:4507–4512

Rambaldi A, Dellacasa CM, Finazzi G, Carobbio A, Ferrari ML, Guglielmelli P, Gattoni E, Salmoiraghi S, Finazzi MC, Di Tollo S, D'Urzo C, Vannucchi AM, Barosi G, Barbui T (2010) A pilot study of the Histone-Deacetylase inhibitor Givinostat in patients with JAK2V617F positive chronic myeloproliferative neoplasms. Br J Haematol 150:446–455

Rathkopf D, Wong BY, Ross RW, Anand A, Tanaka E, Woo MM, Hu J, Dzik-Jurasz A, Yang W, Scher HI (2010) A phase I study of oral panobinostat alone and in combination with docetaxel in patients with castration-resistant prostate cancer. Cancer Chemother Pharmacol 66:181–189

Razak AR, Hotte SJ, Siu LL, Chen EX, Hirte HW, Powers J, Walsh W, Stayner LA, Laughlin A, Novotny-Diermayr V, Zhu J, Eisenhauer EA (2011) Phase I clinical, pharmacokinetic and pharmacodynamic study of SB939, an oral histone deacetylase (HDAC) inhibitor, in patients with advanced solid tumours. Br J Cancer 104:756–762

Ree AH, Dueland S, Folkvord S, Hole KH, Seierstad T, Johansen M, Abrahamsen TW, Flatmark K (2010) Vorinostat, a histone deacetylase inhibitor, combined with pelvic palliative radiotherapy for gastrointestinal carcinoma: the Pelvic Radiation and Vorinostat (PRAVO) phase 1 study. Lancet Oncol 11:459–464

Riggs MG, Whittaker RG, Neumann JR, Ingram VM (1977) n-Butyrate causes histone modification in HeLa and Friend erythroleukaemia cells. Nature 268:462–464

Saito A, Yamashita T, Mariko Y, Nosaka Y, Tsuchiya K, Ando T, Suzuki T, Tsuruo T, Nakanishi O (1999) A synthetic inhibitor of histone deacetylase, MS-27-275, with marked in vivo antitumor activity against human tumors. Proc Natl Acad Sci USA 96:4592–4597

Sauve AA, Wolberger C, Schramm VL, Boeke JD (2006) The biochemistry of sirtuins. Annu Rev Biochem 75:435–465

Scherpereel A, Berghmans T, Lafitte JJ, Colinet B, Richez M, Bonduelle Y, Meert AP, Dhalluin X, Leclercq N, Paesmans M, Willems L, Sculier JP (2011) Valproate-doxorubicin: promising therapy for progressing mesothelioma. A phase II study. Eur Respir J 37:129–135

Stathis A, Hotte SJ, Chen EX, Hirte HW, Oza AM, Moretto P, Webster S, Laughlin A, Stayner LA, McGill S, Wang L, Zhang WJ, Espinoza-Delgado I, Holleran JL, Egorin MJ, Siu LL (2011) Phase I study of decitabine in combination with vorinostat in patients with advanced solid tumors and non-Hodgkin's lymphomas. Clin Cancer Res 17:1582–1590

Strickler JH, Starodub AN, Jia J, Meadows KL, Nixon AB, Dellinger A, Morse MA, Uronis HE, Marcom PK, Zafar SY, Haley ST, Hurwitz HI (2012) Phase I study of bevacizumab, everolimus, and panobinostat (LBH-589) in advanced solid tumors. Cancer Chemother Pharmacol 70(2):251–258

Ueda H, Manda T, Matsumoto S, Mukumoto S, Nishigaki F, Kawamura I, Shimomura K (1994) FR901228, a novel antitumor bicyclic depsipeptide produced by Chromobacterium violaceum No. 968. III. Antitumor activities on experimental tumors in mice. J Antibiot (Tokyo) 47:315–323

Verdin E, Dequiedt F, Kasler HG (2003) Class II histone deacetylases: versatile regulators. Trends Genet 19:286–293

Verdin E, Dequiedt F, Fischle W, Frye R, Marshall B, North B (2004) Measurement of mammalian histone deacetylase activity. Methods Enzymol 377:180–196

Wagner JM, Hackanson B, Lubbert M, Jung M (2010) Histone deacetylase (HDAC) inhibitors in recent clinical trials for cancer therapy. Clin Epigenetics 1:117–136

Walter RB, Medeiros BC, Powell BL, Schiffer CA, Appelbaum FR, Estey EH (2012) Phase II trial of vorinostat and gemtuzumab ozogamicin as induction and post-remission therapy in older adults with previously untreated acute myeloid leukemia. Haematologica 97:739–742

Wang Z, Zang C, Cui K, Schones DE, Barski A, Peng W, Zhao K (2009) Genome-wide mapping of HATs and HDACs reveals distinct functions in active and inactive genes. Cell 138:1019–1031

Wang H, Cao Q, Dudek AZ (2012) Phase II study of panobinostat and bortezomib in patients with pancreatic cancer progressing on gemcitabine-based therapy. Anticancer Res 32:1027–1031

Weichert W (2009) HDAC expression and clinical prognosis in human malignancies. Cancer Lett 280:168–176

Whittaker SJ, Demierre MF, Kim EJ, Rook AH, Lerner A, Duvic M, Scarisbrick J, Reddy S, Robak T, Becker JC, Samtsov A, McCulloch W, Kim YH (2010) Final results from a multicenter, international, pivotal study of romidepsin in refractory cutaneous T-cell lymphoma. J Clin Oncol 28:4485–4491

Wightman F, Ellenberg P, Churchill M, Lewin SR (2012) HDAC inhibitors in HIV. Immunol Cell Biol 90:47–54

Wong NS, Seah E, Wang LZ, Yeo WL, Yap HL, Chuah B, Lim YW, Ang PC, Tai BC, Lim R, Goh BC, Lee SC (2011) Impact of UDP-gluconoryltransferase 2B17 genotype on vorinostat metabolism and clinical outcomes in Asian women with breast cancer. Pharmacogenet Genomics 21:760–768

Yong WP, Goh BC, Soo RA, Toh HC, Ethirajulu K, Wood J, Novotny-Diermayr V, Lee SC, Yeo WL, Chan D, Lim D, Seah E, Lim R, Zhu J (2011) Phase I and pharmacodynamic study of an orally administered novel inhibitor of histone deacetylases, SB939, in patients with refractory solid malignancies. Ann Oncol 22:2516–2522

Yoo CB, Jones PA (2006) Epigenetic therapy of cancer: past, present and future. Nat Rev Drug Discov 5:37–50

Yoshida M, Kijima M, Akita M, Beppu T (1990) Potent and specific inhibition of mammalian histone deacetylase both in vivo and in vitro by trichostatin A. J Biol Chem 265:17174–17179

Younes A, Oki Y, Bociek RG, Kuruvilla J, Fanale M, Neelapu S, Copeland A, Buglio D, Galal A, Besterman J, Li Z, Drouin M, Patterson T, Ward MR, Paulus JK, Ji Y, Medeiros LJ, Martell RE (2011) Mocetinostat for relapsed classical Hodgkin's lymphoma: an open-label, single-arm, phase 2 trial. Lancet Oncol 12:1222–1228

Younes A, Sureda A, Ben-Yehuda D, Zinzani PL, Ong TC, Prince HM, Harrison SJ, Kirschbaum M, Johnston P, Gallagher J, Le Corre C, Shen A, Engert A (2012) Panobinostat in patients with relapsed/refractory Hodgkin's lymphoma after autologous stem-cell transplantation: results of a phase II study. J Clin Oncol 30:2197–2203

Zhang Y, Gilquin B, Khochbin S, Matthias P (2006) Two catalytic domains are required for protein deacetylation. J Biol Chem 281:2401–2404

Zou H, Wu Y, Navre M, Sang BC (2006) Characterization of the two catalytic domains in histone deacetylase 6. Biochem Biophys Res Commun 341:45–50

11 Clinical Implications of Epigenetic Alterations in Lung Cancer

David S. Schrump

11.1 Introduction

Lung cancer ranks among the most lethal malignancies worldwide, with an incidence exceeding 1,000,000 cases per year. Approximately 80 % of pulmonary carcinomas are non-small cell lung cancers (NSCLC) comprised primarily of squamous cell cancers, adenocarcinomas, bronchoalveolar carcinomas, and large cell (anaplastic) cancers with or without neuroendocrine features. The remaining 20 % are primarily small cell lung cancers (SCLC), which exhibit unique molecular genetic, biologic, and clinical features (Coe et al. 2006; Du et al. 2010a).

The vast majority of lung cancers are directly attributable to cigarette smoking, and gene expression profiles in tobacco-associated lung cancers are markedly different than those observed in tumors arising in nonsmokers (Lam et al. 2007; Brambilla and Gazdar 2009). During recent years considerable information has accumulated regarding irreversible genetic alterations involving proto-oncogenes and tumor suppressor genes, which contribute to malignant transformation in tobacco-exposed respiratory epithelia (Sato et al. 2007; Soh et al. 2009; Weir et al. 2007; Sos et al. 2009). However, less information is available pertaining to the frequency and clinical relevance of potentially reversible, epigenetic events involving DNA methylation and posttranslational modifications of core histone proteins that alter chromatin structure and perturb gene expression during pulmonary carcinogenesis (Brambilla and Gazdar 2009; Schrump et al. 2007; Bowman et al. 2009). The following presentation will focus on epigenetic regulators of gene expression in tobacco-induced lung cancers (Table 11.1) and ongoing efforts to develop epigenetic regimens for the treatment and prevention of these malignancies.

D.S. Schrump, MD
Thoracic Oncology Section, Surgery Branch, Center for Cancer Research, National Cancer Institute, Rm. 4-3940, 10 Center Drive, MSC 1201, Bethesda, MD 20892-1201, USA
e-mail: david_schrump@nih.gov

M. Lübbert, P.A. Jones (eds.), *Epigenetic Therapy of Cancer*,
DOI 10.1007/978-3-642-38404-2_11,

Table 11.1 Epigenetic regulators of gene expression implicated in lung cancer

DNMT1	SUV39H1
DNMT3b	SUV39H2
MBD2	G9a
HDAC1	KDM1
HDAC3	KDM5B
HDAC5	BMI1
HDAC10	EZH2

11.2 DNA Methyltransferases and Methylated DNA-Binding Proteins in Lung Cancer

DNA methylation is the major epigenetic mechanism mediating dynamic patterns of gene expression during differentiation and normal cellular homeostasis (Hernandez et al. 2011), as well as long-term repression of gene expression associated with imprinting and X-chromosome inactivation (Hirasawa and Feil 2010; Berdasco and Esteller 2010; De Carvalho et al. 2010). To date, three major DNMTs (DNMT1, 3a, and 3b), with numerous isoforms, have been characterized in somatic cells, all of which mediate transfer of a methyl group from S-adenosylmethionine to the 5′ position of cytosine in the context of CpG. Whereas the specificities of various isoforms have not been fully elucidated and considerable overlap exists (Choi et al. 2010), DNMT1 binds preferentially to hemimethylated DNA and functions primarily as a maintenance methyltransferase; DNMT3a and 3b, which exhibit distinct flanking sequence preferences (Wienholz et al. 2010), interact primarily with unmethylated or hemimethylated DNA to mediate de novo DNA methylation. An additional isoform-designated DNMT3L, which is normally expressed only in germ cells (Goll and Bestor 2005), lacks methyltransferase activity and functions to enhance targeting of DNMT3a and 3b to DNA (Wienholz et al. 2010).

Increasing evidence indicates that altered expression/activity of DNMTs contributes to the pathogenesis of tobacco-induced lung cancers and prognosis of patients with these malignancies. For example, increased DNMT expression/activity coincides with progression to lung cancer in mice exposed to the tobacco carcinogen, NNK (Belinsky et al. 1996). Whereas the mechanisms contributing to DNMT overexpression in human lung cancers have not been fully defined, recent studies suggest that wt p53 suppresses DNMT1 expression via formation of a complex with SP-1 and several chromatin modifiers within the DNMT1 promoter (Lin et al. 2010a); overexpression of SP-1 enhances MDM-2-mediated degradation of p53, resulting in upregulation of DNMT1; consistent with these findings, increased DNMT1 levels correlate significantly with p53 mutations and enhanced SP-1 expression in primary lung cancers.

Damiani et al. (2008) reported that hypermethylation of several tumor suppressor genes, including CDH1, CDH13, GATA5, and PAX5 in immortalized human bronchial epithelial cells (HBEC) exposed to the tobacco carcinogens methyl-nitrosourea (MNU) or benzo-a-pyrene diolepoxide (BPDE) was dependent on DNMT1. Consistent with these findings, Lin et al. (2010b) observed that NNK induces nuclear accumulation of DNMT1 and subsequent hypermethylation of p16, RAR-β, and FHIT in human lung fibroblasts. In contrast, Liu et al. (2010) reported that hypermethylation of RASSF1A and RAR-β coincides with decreased DNMT1/DNMT3b expression ratios in HBEC exposed to cigarette smoke condensate. These findings suggest differential silencing of tumor suppressors by DNMTs during pulmonary carcinogenesis.

Kim et al. (2006) observed increased expression of DNMT1 and DNMT3b in approximately 50 % of lung cancer specimens, which coincided with hypermethylation of a variety of tumor suppressor genes; overexpression of DNMT1 correlated with p16 promoter hypermethylation and diminished patient survival. Lin et al. (2007) reported that coordinate expression of DNMT1, 3a, and 3b coincided with increased methylation of a variety of tumor suppressor genes including p16, FHIT, and RAR-β in lung cancers and diminished survival of patients with these neoplasms; this phenomenon was especially pronounced in smokers with squamous cell carcinomas. In an additional study, Lin et al. (2010b) examined DNMT1 expression in 124 lung cancers and observed that high-level intranuclear DNMT1 levels correlated significantly with smoking status and diminished patient survival. Vallbohmer et al. (2006) examined DNMT1, 3a, and 3b expression levels relative to methylation status of APC, DAPK, GSTP1, and MGMT in 91 lung cancer specimens and adjacent normal lung samples. Expression of the three DNMTs was higher in tumors compared to normal lung. Whereas no correlation was observed between DNMT expression and DNA methylation, hypermethylation status was an independent adverse prognostic factor.

Xing et al. (2008) used quantitative RT-PCR techniques to examine DMNT1 and DNMT3b, as well as methylated DNA-binding protein 2 (MBD2) expression in 148 resected NSCLCs. High-level DNMT1 expression correlated significantly with increased risk of cancer-related death in all patients, whereas increased DNMT3b expression was associated with poor outcome in patients less than 65 years of age. High-level expression of MBD2 correlated with poor survival in male patients and those with squamous cell carcinomas. Combinatorial effects of DNMT1 and 3b, DMNT1 and MBD2, and DNMT3b and MBD2 were evident in male patients and those with squamous cell carcinomas. Collectively, aforementioned clinical data as well as laboratory experiments indicating that knockdown of DNMT1 and/or 3b induces genotoxic stress and apoptosis (Kassis et al. 2006), whereas knockdown of MBD2 inhibits growth and tumorigenicity of cultured lung cancer cells (Campbell et al. 2004), attest to the relevance of aberrant expression of these modulators of DNA methylation during pulmonary carcinogenesis.

Shen et al. (2002) observed that a novel polymorphism, which enhances DNMT3b expression, increases lung cancer risk. More recently, Paliwal et al. (2010) observed DNA methylation-mediated silencing of CHRNalpha3, encoding the nicotinic acetylcholine receptor alpha 3 subunit (nAChRalpha3) within the 15q25.1 lung cancer susceptibility locus. DNA-demethylating agents restored nAChRalpha3 expression, and ectopic expression of this gene induced apoptosis in cultured lung cancer cells. Conversely, knockdown of CHRNalpha3 activated AKT signaling and rendered lung cancer cells resistant to apoptosis-inducing compounds. Collectively, these observations provide potential mechanistic links between aberrant DNA methylation and susceptibility to lung cancer.

11.3 Histone Acetylases/Deacetylases and Histone Methyltransferases/Demethylases in Lung Cancer

Lysine-rich tails of core histone proteins (H2A, H2B, H3, and H4), which protrude from the nucleosome, provide sites for highly diverse, reversible, covalent modifications such as acetylation, methylation, phosphorylation, and ubiquitination that alter chromatin structure and modulate gene expression (Barth and Imhof 2010; Scharf and Imhof 2010; Lee et al. 2010). To date, acetylation/deacetylation and methylation/demethylation have been the most extensively characterized histone modifications in cancer cells (Sawan and Herceg 2010). Acetylation of core histones is governed by opposing actions of a variety histone acetyl transferases (HAT) such as GNAT, p300(KAT3B), P/CAF(KAT2B), CBP(KAT3A), as well as MYST family proteins, which exhibit highly restricted substrate specificities, and histone deacetylases (HDACs), 18 of which comprise four classes based on structural homologies, substrates, and cellular localization (Sawan and Herceg 2010; Schrump 2009). Methylation of core histones is mediated by the opposing actions of a variety of histone methyltransferases (HMTs), such as SUV39H, Ga9(KMT1C), MLL(KMT2), EZH2 (KMT6), and RIZ1(KMT8), and histone demethylases (HDMTs) including LSD1(KDM1), GASC1(KDM4C), UTX(KDM6A), JHDM3(KDM4), and JARID1(KDM5), all of which are components of multi-protein chromatin remodeling complexes and exhibit unique as well as overlapping substrate specificities (Scharf and Imhof 2010; Sawan and Herceg 2010; Albert and Helin 2010; Pedersen and Helin 2010).

Relatively limited information is available concerning the direct clinical implications of aberrant expression of HATs and HDACs, as well as HMTs and HDMTs in lung cancers. Park et al. (2005) observed no correlation between a variety of polymorphisms involving HDACs 1–8 and lung cancer risk. Sasaki et al. (2004) reported that increased HDAC1 mRNA levels coincided with advanced stage of disease in lung cancer patients. Interestingly, although no published studies have simultaneously examined DNMTs and HDACs in lung cancer specimens, recent data indicate that HDAC1 deacetylates DNMT1, thereby protecting it from proteosomal degradation in colon cancer cells, providing a potential mechanistic link between HDAC1 overexpression and aberrant DNA methylation during malignant transformation (Du et al. 2010b).

In a recent study involving nearly 100 lung cancer patients, Minamiya et al. (2010) observed that individuals with tumors exhibiting high-level HDAC3 expression had significantly shorter disease-free survivals than patients whose tumors had low HDAC3 expression. Multivariate analysis revealed that HDAC3 overexpression was an independent prognosticator of poor survival in patients with adenocarcinomas, but not those with squamous cell carcinomas. In an additional study, Osada et al. (2004) observed that reduced expression of several class II HDACs (particularly HDACs 5 and 10) correlated with adverse outcome in lung cancer patients.

Less information is available regarding roles of specific HMTs or HDMTs in the pathogenesis of lung cancer. Yoon et al. (2006) observed that a polymorphism within the 3′ UTR of SUV39H2 was associated with increased risk of squamous cell carcinomas, whereas several polymorphisms involving RIZ-1 correlated with diminished lung cancer risk (Yoon et al. 2007). Chen et al. (2006) reported that hypoxia increases Ga9 methyltransferase activity resulting in increased levels of H3K9me2 within promoter regions of DHFR and MLH1 and diminished expression of these tumor suppressor genes in lung cancer cells. More recent studies by these investigators have demonstrated that G9a expression enhances invasion and metastatic potential of lung cancer cells via epigenetic silencing of the cell adhesion molecule, EP-CAM (Chen et al. 2010).

Hayami et al. (2010) observed overexpression of KDM5B, which demethylates H3K4Me3/Me2, in a large panel of small cell as well as non-small cell lung cancers. Subsequent analysis revealed significant correlation between KDM5B overexpression and increased expression of E2F1 and E2F2. Knockdown of KDM5B diminished expression of E2F1and E2F2 and inhibited expression of a variety of genes mediating cell cycle progression. In subsequent studies, Hayami et al. (2011) observed upregulation of KDM1, which catalyzes demethylation of H3K4Me2/Me1 and possibly H3K9Me2/Me1, in small cell lung cancers relative to normal lung tissues; knockdown of KDM1 induced G1 arrest without apoptosis in cultured lung cancer cells. Consistent with these findings, Watanabe et al. (2008) observed that knockdown of KMT6 (which mediates trimethylation of H3K27), KMT1C, SETB1, or SUV39H1 inhibited proliferation and soft agar colony formation of immortalized or fully transformed respiratory epithelial cells, implicating these modifiers of histone methylation in the pathogenesis of lung cancer.

Several recent studies suggest that the cumulative effects of perturbed acetylation and methylation of core histones observed in lung cancers may be clinically relevant. Seligson et al. (2009) reported that decreased levels of H3K4Me2 and H3K18Ac correlated significantly with reduced survival of patients with early stage lung cancers undergoing potentially curative resections. Van Den Broeck (2008) observed hyperacetylation of H4K5 and H4K8, hypoacetylation of H4K12/H4K16, and decreased H4K20Me3 levels in lung cancer cells relative to adjacent normal respiratory epithelia. Whereas loss of H4K20Me3 was more common in squamous cell carcinomas, this histone alteration, which coincided with diminished expression of SUV4-20h2, was not associated with patient outcome. In contrast, loss of H4K20Me3 in early stage adenocarcinomas correlated significantly with decreased patient survival.

Barlési et al. (2007) used recursive partitioning analysis (RPA) to classify 138 lung cancer patients into seven groups based on histology, TNM stage, and global expression levels of H3K4Me2, H2AK5Ac, and H3K9Ac; the groups exhibited significant differences in disease free, as well as overall survivals. Interestingly, the four groups comprising stage I patients displayed dramatic differences, with a median survival of 10 months for adenocarcinoma patients with high-level intratumoral H3K9Ac, compared to 147 months for non-adenocarcinoma patients with high-level intratumoral H3K4Me2 expression. Cox regression confirmed that RPA was an independent prognosticator of survival. Collectively, these data suggest that histone alterations mediated by aberrant expression of HATs, HDACs, HMTs and HDMTs contribute to the pathogenesis and clinical evolution of lung cancers – particularly early stage neoplasms.

11.4 Polycomb Group Proteins in Lung Cancer

During recent years the polycomb group proteins (PcG), which mediate pluripotency in stem cells, have emerged as critical determinants of long-term gene repression in normal cells, as well as aberrant gene silencing in cancer cells (Sawarkar and Paro 2010; Christophersen and Helin 2010; Surface et al. 2010; Sauvageau and Sauvageau 2010; Mills 2010). Two major polycomb repressive complexes (PRC) have been identified in mammals. The maintenance complex, PRC1, consists of core subunits of various paralogs of PCGF, PHC, RING1, CBX, and SCML, as well as SFMBT and L3MBTL proteins. The initiation complex, PRC2, consists of EZH2, SUZ12, PCL, and EED (Sauvageau and Sauvageau 2010; Mills 2010). More than 1,000 genes, many of which contain homeobox domains and mediate cellular differentiation, are potential PcG targets (Bracken et al. 2006).

Whereas the mechanisms by which PcG proteins mediate transcriptional repression have not been fully elucidated (Morey and Helin 2010), several recent studies highlight the potential relevance of aberrant polycomb expression/activity during pulmonary carcinogenesis. For example, stem cell polycomb group targets are significantly more likely to have cancer-specific promoter hypermethylation than non-polycomb targets, and H3K27Me3 is a mark associated with promoters of all tumor suppressor genes that are hypermethylated in cancer cells (Jones and Baylin 2007; Widschwendter et al. 2007). Consistent with these findings, Liu et al. (2010) observed that polycomb target genes were sevenfold more likely to undergo DNA hypermethylation in cultured HBEC exposed to cigarette smoke condensate. Predilection for DNA hypermethylation appears to be related to DNA sequence as well as binding of polycomb repressive complexes (McCabe et al. 2009).

Presently, the mechanisms contributing to aberrant expression of PcG genes during pulmonary carcinogenesis have not been fully defined; however, the vast majority of lung cancers exhibit disruption of Rb-mediated regulation of E2F, and a number of PcG genes including EZH2, EED, and SUZ12 are potential E2F targets (Coe et al. 2006; Bracken et al. 2003). Inactivation of p16, which is observed in 30–40 % of NSCLCs (Brambilla and Gazdar 2009; Sato et al. 2007), results in upregulation of EZH2 and SUZ12 and targeting of these PcG proteins as well as DNMTs to HOXA9 in cultured cancer cells (Reynolds et al. 2006). Downregulation of several micro-RNAs such as miR-101 and miR-26a that normally target the 3′ UTR of EZH2 increases EZH2 expression during malignant transformation (Friedman et al. 2009; Lu et al. 2011), and recent data indicate that downregulation of miR-101 directly contributes to overexpression of EZH2 in lung cancer cells (Zhang et al. 2011).

Increased expression of BMI1(PCGF4) and EZH2 in primary lung cancers and their precursor lesions indicates that dysregulation of PcG complexes occurs early during multi-step pulmonary carcinogenesis (Breuer et al. 2004). Recent laboratory as well as translational studies suggests that BMI1 and EZH2 directly contribute to initiation and progression of lung cancers. For example, Dovey et al. (2008) observed that BMI1-deficient mice develop significantly fewer and smaller k-ras-induced lung tumors due to diminished capacity of BMI1-deficient bronchoalveolar stem cells (BASCs) to exhibit self-renewal and proliferate in response to oncogenic stimulation. Using a different murine model, Becker et al. (2009) observed that knockout of BMI1 did not diminish initiation, but significantly inhibited progression of lung tumors induced by oncogenic RAF. In both of these models, reduced lung tumor development was attributable to upregulation of p16 and/or p19/ARF. Consistent with these findings, increased expression of BMI1 correlates significantly with diminished expression of p16 and p14/ARF in primary human lung cancers (Vonlanthen et al. 2001).

Several recent studies have examined the prognostic significance of BMI1 and EZH2 expression in lung cancer patients. Vrzalikova et al. (2008) used immunohistochemistry (IHC) techniques to examine BMI1 expression in 179 NSCLCs including 106 squamous cell, 58 adeno-, and 15 large cell carcinomas. Nearly 70 % of samples exhibited moderate or strong nuclear immunoreactivity for BMI1. Subsequent analysis revealed that BMI1 expression correlated significantly with advanced stage of disease (stages III or IV), as well as decreased disease free survival for patients with stage I or II neoplasms. An additional study pertaining to IHC analysis of 134 resected pulmonary adenocarcinomas demonstrated that BMI1 expression was higher in stage III tumors relative to stage I or II cancers; multivariate analysis revealed that BMI1 expression was an independent prognosticator of poor survival of adenocarcinoma patients (Zhang et al. 2010).

Kikuchi et al. (2010) used IHC techniques to examine BMI1 and EZH2 expression in 157 resected NSCLC specimens, including 65 squamous cell carcinomas, 82 adenocarcinomas, 7 adenosquamous carcinomas, and 2 large cell carcinomas. In contrast to aforementioned results, BMI1 expression did not appear to be associated with any clinicopathologic features. However, high intratumoral EZH2 expression correlated significantly with non-adenocarcinoma histology, increased proliferation index, moderate to poor differentiation, and significantly decreased patient survival in all stages; the adverse impact of EZH2 expression was particularly apparent in stage I neoplasms.

A recent series of laboratory experiments further highlights the relevance of polycomb-mediated gene repression in the pathogenesis of tobacco-induced lung cancers. Hussain et al. (2009) cultured human lung cancer cells in normal media with or without cigarette smoke condensate (CSC) under clinically relevant exposure conditions. Ten-day CSC exposure diminished expression of Dickkopf-1(Dkk-1), encoding a secreted antagonist of Wnt signaling, and dramatically increased tumorigenicity of lung cancer cells in nude mice. Repression of Dkk-1 coincided with decreased H4K16Ac, increased H3K27Me3, and recruitment of SirT1, EZH2, SUZ12, and BMI1 without DNA hypermethylation within the Dkk-1 promoter; these results were consistent with recent studies demonstrating gene silencing by polycomb repressive complexes in the absence of DNA methylation (Kondo et al. 2008). Removal of CSC from culture media resulted in loss of promoter-associated polycomb repressive complexes and re-expression of Dkk-1. Knockdown of EZH2 abrogated CSC-mediated inhibition of Dkk-1 expression. CSC exposure or knockdown of Dkk-1 activated Wnt signaling in lung cancer cells, as well as normal small airway epithelial cells (SAEC). Furthermore, knockdown of

Dkk-1 recapitulated the protumorigenic effects of CSC exposure in lung cancer cells. Collectively, these data provided the first direct evidence that cigarette smoke engages polycomb machinery to activate cancer stem cell signaling networks (Konigshoff and Eickelberg 2010; Espada et al. 2009; Vermeulen et al. 2010) in normal as well as malignantly transformed respiratory epithelia cells.

11.5 Clinical Relevance of Epigenomic Reprogramming in Lung Cancer Cells

As with other neoplasms (Berdasco and Esteller 2010), epigenomic events during pulmonary carcinogenesis are manifested simultaneously as genomic hypomethylation, primarily involving repetitive DNA sequences (Ehrlich 2009; Ting et al. 2011), and site-specific DNA hypermethylation silencing numerous homeobox and tumor suppressor genes (Schrump and Nguyen 2005). Although recent studies suggest that global DNA demethylation may be linked to aberrant DNA repair (Schar and Fritsch 2011; Ha et al. 2011), decreased DNMT1 expression (Liu et al. 2010; Yamada et al. 2005), or replication independent DNA demethylases (Ehrlich 2009; Rai et al. 2010), the mechanisms mediating genomic demethylation during malignant transformation remain elusive. Irrespective of the mechanisms, global DNA demethylation results in derepression of endogenous retroviruses, pseudogenes, and imprinted alleles, thereby enhancing genomic instability (Ehrlich 2009; Howard et al. 2008; Holm et al. 2005) (Table 11.2). For example, several human endogenous retroviruses (HER) including HER-E are activated in lung cancers (Yi and Kim 2007); furthermore, 40–80 % of lung cancers exhibit loss of imprinting (LOI) involving the H19/IgF2, p57, or paternally expressed imprinted gene 1/mesoderm-specific transcript (PEG1/MEST) loci (Kohda et al. 2001; Kondo et al. 1996, 1995).

Global DNA demethylation also results in derepression of a variety of genes that are silent in normal somatic cells, yet exhibit stage-specific expression during germ cell development in testes or ovaries (Table 11.2). To date, more than 100 of these "cancer-testis (CT)" genes have been identified, approximately half of which map to the X chromosome (Stevenson et al. 2007). Relative to autosomal CT genes, CT-X-chromosome (CT-X) genes are more frequently activated in cancer cells, and particular gene families appear to be simultaneously derepressed in a tumor-specific manner.

Coordinate activation of CT genes during malignant transformation suggests direct or functional interactions of their respective gene products, and several recent studies indicate that proteins encoded by CT genes may contribute to the malignant phenotype of lung cancer cells. For example, MAGE-C1 directly binds to NY-ESO-1 (Cho et al. 2006). BORIS enhances activation of NY-ESO-1 and MAGE-A1 (Hong et al. 2005; Vatolin et al. 2005) and increases telomerase expression in cancer cells (Renaud et al. 2011). Multiple MAGE family members including MAGE-A3 and MAGE-A2 complex with and inactivate Kap-1, a corepressor of p53 (Yang et al. 2007; Monte et al. 2006). CAGE enhances cell cycle progression and chemoresistance in cancer cells via upregulation of cyclin D, cyclin E, and AP-1, and

Table 11.2 Genes frequently derepressed in lung cancer cells

Imprinted genes	Chromosome
H19	11p15.5
IGF2	11p15.5
MEST	7q32
Cancer testis genes	Chromosome
BORIS	20q13.2
MAGE-A	Xq28
MAGE-B	Xp21
MAGE-C	Xq26
MAGE-D	Xp21
MAGE-E	Xq13
MAGE-F	3q26
MAGE-G	15q11
MAGE-H	Xp11
MAGE-I	Xp11
MAGE-J	Xp11
MAGE-K	Xq24
MAGE-L	15q11
NY-ESO-1	Xq28
LAGE-1	Xq28
SSX	Xp11.2
GAGE	Xp11.4
PAGE	Xp11.23
XAGE	Xp11.22
TRAG-3	Xq28
L-SAGE	Xq28
SCP-1	1p13
SAGE	Xq28
HAGE	6q12
BRDT	1p31
MMA-1	21q22
OY-TES-1	12p13
NY-BR-3	18
HOM-TES-85	Xq24
CAGE	Xp22
CT-17	21q11
C-TAGE-1	18–11
HCA-661	Xq2
KK-LC-1	Xq22
CT-45	Xq26-3

suppression of p53 function (Por et al. 2010; Kim et al. 2010). Furthermore, MAGE-C1, MAGE-A3, and GAGE-7C confer resistance to apoptosis mediated by Fas ligand, IFN-γ, chemotherapeutic agents, or radiation (Atanackovic et al. 2010; Cilensek et al. 2002).

Despite aforementioned data suggesting that CT gene expression enhances the malignant phenotype of cancer cells, limited evidence indicates that CT gene activation during pulmonary carcinogenesis directly impacts diagnosis or prognosis of lung cancer patients. In general, lung cancers exhibit heterogeneous patterns of CT gene activation, the magnitude of which coincides with advanced stage of disease (Konishi et al. 2004). Grunwald et al. (2006) reported that 80 % of NSCLCs expressed one of seven CT genes (MAGE-A3, NY-ESO-1, LAGE-1, BRDT, Hom-TES-85, TPX-1, and LDHC), and nearly one half of tumors expressed at least two of these genes; CT gene expression appeared to be more frequent in squamous cell carcinomas. Melloni et al. (2004) detected MAGE-A1, -2, -3, GAGE-1, -2, -8, and MAGE-B2 expression in 25–40 % of 46 resected lung cancers, and observed that GAGE expression correlated with diminished patient survival. Gure et al. (2005) examined CT-X gene expression in tumors from over 500 lung cancer patients undergoing potentially curative resections. Approximately 90 % of squamous cell carcinomas and 70 % of adenocarcinomas or bronchoalveolar cancers expressed one or more of nine CT-X genes (MAGE-A1, MAGE-A3, MAGE-A4, MAGE-A10, MAGE-C1, NY-ESO-1, LAGE-1, SSX2, and SSX4). Derepression of CT-X genes coincided with tobacco use and advanced stage of disease; expression of NY-ESO-1 and/or MAGE-A3 correlated with poor survival.

As previously mentioned, a variety of tumor suppressor genes appear to be targeted by polycomb as well as DNA methylation-mediated repression mechanisms during pulmonary carcinogenesis (Schrump and Nguyen 2005; Pfeifer and Rauch 2009) (Table 11.3). Several recent studies analyzing large numbers of resected NSCLCs suggest that complex genetic and environmental interactions contribute to aberrant DNA hypermethylation in lung cancers (Vaissiere et al. 2009) and that tobacco-associated lung cancers exhibit considerably different DNA methylation profiles relative to tumors arising in nonsmokers (Toyooka et al. 2006). Unlike the effects of DNA hypomethylation, the clinical ramifications of hypermethylation of tumor suppressor genes in tobacco-induced lung cancers are more evident.

Toyooka et al. (2003) examined methylation status of a variety of tumor suppressor genes including p16, RASSF1A, APC, RAR-β, and CDH13 (E-cadherin) in approximately 350 lung cancer patients and observed that methylation of p16 correlated significantly with poor outcome in patients with adenocarcinomas. Additional studies have indicated that methylation-mediated silencing of RASSF1A correlates significantly with tobacco exposure commencing during adolescence (Marsit et al. 2005; Endoh et al. 2003). Methylation of the FHIT promoter correlates with advanced stage of disease and diminished survival of lung cancer patients (Maruyama et al. 2004); RECK promoter methylation correlates with k-ras mutations and lymph node metastases in these patients (Chang et al. 2006). Furthermore, methylation of the TSLC1/IGSF4 promoter correlates with tobacco exposure and poor outcome in lung cancer patients (Kikuchi et al. 2006), and methylation of oligodendrocyte transcription factor 1 (OLIG1) correlates with diminished survival of these patients (Brena et al. 2007). In contrast, methylation of 14-3-3σ, which encodes a protein involved in nuclear translocation of class II HDACs, enhances chemosensitivity and overall survival in lung cancer patients (Ramirez et al. 2005).

Gu et al. (2006) examined methylation status of nine genes (p16, CDH1, TIMP3, RASSF1A, FHIT, APC, DAPK, MGMT, and GSTP1) in approximately 150 resected lung cancers. The overall methylation index was higher in adenocarcinomas

Table 11.3 Genes frequently hypermethylated in lung cancer cells

ALDH1A3	
APC	XRCC5
CTSZ	CCNA1
DAPK	p15INK4b
Dkk-1	TSLC1/IGSF4
FHIT	p16/p14ARF
GATA-4/5	RAR-β
GST-π	RASSF1A
HIC-1	TFPI-2
IRF7	FABP3
LOX	CDH-13
MDR-1	TIMP-3
MGMT	TMS-1
MLH-1	THBS-1
MSX1	BCN1
NRCAM	
OLIG-1	
RECK	
RIPK3	PAX3
SFRP	ASC
WIF-1	BRCA1/2

compared to squamous cell carcinomas, tumors from heavy vs. light smokers, and tumors from older vs. younger patients. Individuals with tumors exhibiting p16 promoter methylation had significantly worse survival (median = 21.7 months) than patients with cancers expressing this tumor suppressor gene (median = 62.5 months). Brock et al. (Brock et al. 2008) examined DNA methylation status of seven tumor suppressor genes in 51 patients with resected stage I NSCLC who recurred within 40 months following surgery compared to 166 control patients who did not recur during this observation period; promoter methylation of p16, CDH13, RASSF1A, and APC correlated significantly with early tumor recurrence.

In an additional study, Castro et al. (2010) used a methylation-specific multiplex ligation-dependent probe amplification assay (MS-MLPA) to examine the DNA methylation status of 18 tumor suppressors in 54 lung cancer specimens. DNA methylation profiles distinguished squamous cell carcinomas from adenocarcinomas. Methylation of RUNX3, SFRP4, DLC1, and SCGB3A1 was associated with disease recurrence, whereas methylation of HTLF, SFRP5, and TIMP3 correlated significantly with decreased patient survival.

11.6 Targeting Epigenetic Regulators for Lung Cancer Therapy

Identification of epigenetic regulators of gene expression during pulmonary carcinogenesis provides a rationale for the use of chromatin remodeling agents for lung cancer therapy. To date, most epigenetic therapies for lung cancers have focused on the evaluation of pharmacologic inhibitors of DNMT and HDAC activity (Schrump 2009; Brueckner et al. 2007). Specifically these trials have evaluated the nucleoside analogues, 5-azacytidine (5-AC) and 5-aza-2′-deoxycytidine (DAC), as well as HDAC inhibitors (HDACi) such as depsipeptide (DP; romidepsin), sodium butyrate, and SAHA (vorinostat) either alone or in combination with other chromatin remodeling agents or conventional chemotherapy regimens. When interpreting results of these trials, it is important to recognize that the antitumor effects of DNA-demethylating agents and HDACi are not solely attributable to reactivation of tumor suppressor genes aberrantly silenced by epigenetic mechanisms (Xiong and Epstein 2009). For instance, cytotoxicity mediated by DAC is attributable in part to formation of DNMT-DNA adducts (particularly those involving DNMT 3a and 3b) (Oka et al. 2005) as well as DNA damage (Palii et al. 2008). HDACi promote acetylation of a variety of nonhistone proteins such as p53 and Hsp90, thereby modulating cell cycle progression and apoptosis in cancer cells (Schrump 2009; Yu et al. 2002; Lundqvist et al. 2006; Yu et al. 2007). DNA-demethylating agents in combination with HDACi induce DNA damage (Luszczek et al. 2010) and inhibit removal of incorporated abases (Chai et al. 2008) in lung cancer cells.

In a phase I/II study, Momparler et al. (1997) treated 15 lung cancer patients with DAC administered at various doses over 8 h and observed prolonged survival (>5 years) in one of nine evaluable patients. In a more recent phase I trial, Schrump et al. (2006) treated 18 lung cancer patients with escalating doses of DAC administered via continuous 72 h infusions. The maximum tolerated dose of DAC was 75 mg/m^2; myelosuppression was dose limiting. Although no objective responses were observed, two patients exhibited prolonged stabilization of disease (>1 year). Nearly one quarter of all patients exhibited induction of p16, MAGE-3, or NY-ESO-1 in posttreatment tumor biopsies. Quantitative RT-PCR analysis of sequential tumor biopsies from one of the two patients with prolonged stabilization of disease revealed a steady increase in MAGE-3 and NY-ESO-1 mRNA copy numbers, coinciding with increased NY-ESO-1 antibody titers following 6 months of therapy.

In a phase II trial, Schrump et al. (2008) treated 18 lung cancer patients with DP (~18 mg/m^2) administered as a 4 h infusion on days 1 and 7 of a 21-day cycle. Transient stabilization of disease (2–6 months) was observed in nine patients. Steady state DP levels during infusion ranged from 384 to 1,114 ng/ml (median: 667 ng/ml), decreasing to ~10 ng/ml within 4 h following the infusion. Intratumoral levels of H3Ac and p21 were increased in approximately 50 % of patients following DP therapy. In addition, several patients exhibited enhanced expression of NY-ESO-1 and MAGE-A3 in tumor biopsies following DP infusions.

In a more recent trial, Otterson et al. (2010) treated 16 SCLC patients with DP (13 mg/m^2) administered as 4-h infusions on days 1, 8, and 16 of a 29-day cycle. No objective responses were observed; transient stabilization of disease was observed in three patients. Median progression free survival was less than 2 months, and median overall survival approximated 6 months. In an additional phase II trial, Traynor et al. (2009) treated 16 patients with relapsed NSCLC with vorinostat 400 mg PO daily. No objective responses were observed in 14 evaluable patients. Median time to progression was 2.3 months, which was similar to that observed for lung cancer patients receiving other targeted agents. Collectively, results of these lung cancer trials are consistent with broader experience demonstrating minimal activity of HDACi as single agents in solid tumors (Schrump 2009).

Numerous preclinical studies have demonstrated either additive or synergistic proapoptotic effects of HDACi in combination with standard cytotoxic chemotherapeutics or targeted agents in lung cancer cells (Yu et al. 2007; Bruzzese et al. 2009; Yeow et al. 2006; Zhang et al. 2009). The mechanisms underlying this phenomenon appear to be related to HDACi-mediated induction of reactive oxygen species, depletion of oncoprotein expression, and inhibition of survival signaling (Schrump 2009; Yu et al. 2002, 2007). Ramalingam et al. (2010) randomly assigned 94 chemo-naive patients with stage IV NSCLC to receive carboplatin and paclitaxel with either vorinostat (400 mg) on days 1–14 of a 21-day cycle or placebo. The median number of treatment cycles was four in both arms. Median response rate was significantly improved in patients receiving vorinostat vs. placebo (34 % vs. 12.5 %). Whereas progression free and overall survival in patients receiving vorinostat increased by 2–3 months, this survival benefit was not statistically significant.

Several investigators have demonstrated that HDACi potentiate tumor suppressor as well as CT-X gene induction in cancer cells mediated by DNA-demethylating agents (Schrump et al. 2007; Cameron et al. 1999; Weiser et al. 2001). In a recent phase I trial at the NCI, 31 patients with thoracic neoplasms (15 of whom had lung cancer) were treated with sequential DAC/DP infusions. DAC was administered as a continuous 72 h infusion commencing on day 1 of a 35-day treatment cycle; DP was administered as a 4 h infusion immediately following DAC and on day 10. Median steady state DAC and DP levels were 13.4 ng/ml (range 4.7–78 ng/ml) and 323 ng/ml (range 136–923 ng/ml), respectively. Whereas no objective tumor regressions were observed, several patients exhibited stabilization of disease lasting 4–6 months.

Gene expression profiles in laser-captured tumor cells from pre- and posttreatment biopsies from 8 lung cancer patients receiving DAC/DP infusions were analyzed relative to profiles in laser-captured lung cancer cells and normal respiratory epithelia from 20 patients undergoing potentially curative resections. Interestingly, those genes that were induced or repressed by sequential DAC/DP were repressed or induced, respectively, in lung cancers relative to normal cells. A similar phenomenon was observed following analysis of biopsy specimens from patients receiving DAC or DP as single agents (Fig. 11.1). Collectively, these findings raise the possibility that DAC, DP, and sequential DAC/DP regimens partially reverse aberrant lung cancer gene expression in vivo (Schrump DS, manuscript in preparation). The fact that these molecular responses did not translate into more prolonged disease stabilization or tumor regressions strongly suggests suboptimal durations of drug exposure.

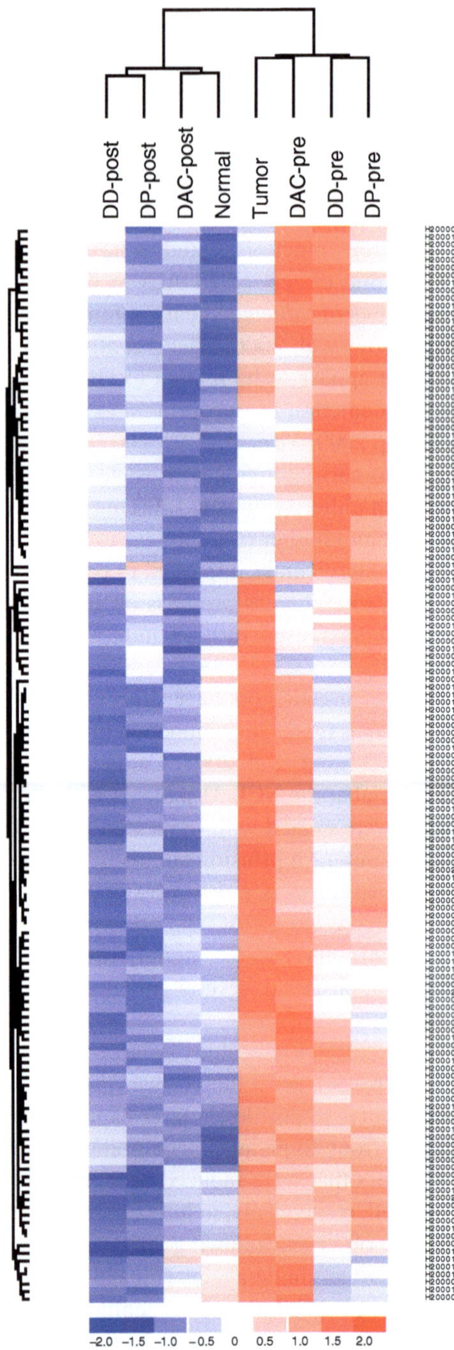

Fig. 11.1 Representative heat map corresponding to gene expression profiles in laser-captured lung cancer cells from pre- and posttreatment biopsies from patients receiving decitabine (*DAC*), depsipeptide (*DP*), or sequential decitabine/depsipeptide (*DD*) infusions, as well as tumor and histologically normal respiratory epithelia from patients undergoing potentially curative lung cancer resections. Epigenetic therapy appears to shift lung cancer gene expression profiles toward those observed in normal respiratory epithelia

11.7 Ongoing Clinical Efforts at the National Cancer Institute

An alternative to combining cytotoxic chemotherapeutics with DNA-demethylating agents and HDACi involves the development of gene induction regimens in conjunction with immunotherapy protocols for lung cancer therapy. Derepression of CT genes during pulmonary carcinogenesis results in expression of highly restricted antigens that are potential targets for lung cancer immunotherapy. Of particular interest in this regard are NY-ESO-1, MAGE-A3, and MAGE-A1, which are expressed in 25–40 % of NSCLC and >75 % of SCLC (Schrump and Nguyen 2005). Interestingly, immune responses to these cancer testis antigens (CTAs) are exceedingly uncommon in lung cancer patients (Groeper et al. 2007; Stockert et al. 1998) due in part to low level, heterogeneous CTA expression, deficiencies regarding antigen processing and presentation – particularly in SCLC (Delp et al. 2000) – and intratumoral or circulating immunosuppressive regulatory T cells (Tregs) (Li et al. 2007; Ju et al. 2009; Elkord et al. 2010).

Because CT genes are derepressed via epigenetic mechanisms during pulmonary carcinogenesis, it is conceivable that chromatin remodeling agents can be used to enhance immunogenicity of lung cancer cells, facilitating their eradication by endogenous immune mechanisms or adoptively transferred T cells. Our previous studies have demonstrated synergistic activation of CT gene expression in cultured lung cancer cells, but not normal epithelia or lymphoid cells following exposure to DNA-demethylating agents and HDACi such as DAC and DP (Schrump et al. 2007; Hong et al. 2005). Furthermore, we have demonstrated that DAC and DP can upregulate NY-ESO-1 as well as MAGE-A3 expression in primary lung cancers (Schrump et al. 2006; Schrump et al. 2008). Following DAC or sequential DAC/DP exposure, lung cancer cells can be recognized by T cells expressing native or genetically engineered T-cell receptors (TCR) specific for peptide epitopes of NY-ESO-1 or MAGE-A3 (Weiser et al. 2001; Chinnasamy et al. 2011; Wargo et al. 2009). Lastly, using an immunocompetent murine model, we have demonstrated that a CTA-induced in vivo by DAC can be targeted by adoptively transferred CTL (Guo et al. 2006). Collectively, these studies established proof of principle for the use of chromatin remodeling agents in conjunction with immunotherapy regimens in lung cancer patients.

Whereas several FDA-approved HDACi augment DAC-mediated induction of NY-ESO-1 and MAGE-A3 in lung cancer cells, these agents may not be optimal for clinical use in lung cancer patients due to their ability to potentiate immunosuppression by Tregs (Akimova et al. 2010). As such our recent efforts have focused on the identification of novel strategies to augment CT gene expression in lung cancer cells. Our analysis has revealed that knockdown of KDM1, KDM5B, or KMT6 markedly enhances DAC-mediated activation of CT-X genes in lung cancer cells. DZNep, a pharmacologic inhibitor of KMT6 expression, significantly augments DAC-mediated induction of CT-X genes in lung cancer – but not normal cells.

Table 11.4 Quantitative RT-PCR analysis of CT gene expression in primary cancer lines exposed to normal media (NM) with or without DAC (1 μM × 6 day)

		MAGE-A3	NY-ESO-1	BORIS	MAGE-A1	CT45	SSX1	SSX2
Pt. L	NM	42	1	0	3	243	1	1722
DAC	664	12158	41	0	8027	1039	2400	
Pt. B	NM	8	0	0	0	0	5	0
DAC	10693	7870	645	0	2762	4088	1063	
Pt. J	NM	416	2	3	31	96	1	0
DAC	1449	768	44	712	4863	603	42	
Pt. K	NM	52035	7	30	0	27889	8	1
DAC	97486	2514	2518	0	55214	715	1510	
Pt. T	NM	168	9	6	384	951544	32	8
DAC	3133	1866	398	3811	918361	3162	4184	
Testis		10185	9252	11304	10812	9633	9747	10860

mRNA copy #/β-actin e4

Following DAC-DZNep exposure, lung cancer cells can be lysed by T cells genetically engineered to recognize NY-ESO-1 or MAGE-A3. In additional studies we have observed that knockdown of KDM1, KDM5B or KMT6, or DZNep exposure markedly enhances DAC-mediated activation of a variety of tumor suppressor genes aberrantly silenced in lung cancer cells (Rao et al., manuscript in preparation). These findings are consistent with recent experiments by Huang et al. (2009) demonstrating that oligoamine analogues that inhibit KDM1 potentiate DAC-mediated derepression of SFRP-2 in cultured colon cancer cells and suggest that combining DNA-demethylating agents with compounds that modulate histone lysine methylation may represent novel epigenetic strategies for lung cancer therapy.

An additional strategy to treat micrometastatic disease involves the use of autologous epigenetically modified tumor cell vaccines to induce immunity to a variety of CTAs that potentially can be upregulated in lung cancer cells in vivo by systemic gene induction regimens (Schrump et al. 2006, 2008). In recent experiments, we successfully established tumor lines from 18 of 50 patients (36 %) with primary thoracic malignancies. Eight of these lines were treated with DAC ± DP under a variety of exposure conditions. Quantitative RT-PCR analysis revealed dose-dependent induction of CT genes including BORIS, MAGE-1, MAGE-3, NY-ESO-1, CT-45, and SSX. Representative results pertaining to 6-day DAC exposure are depicted in Table 11.4. Variable patterns of CT gene expression have been observed in untreated as well as DAC-treated cells. Cytokine release assays confirmed recognition of epigenetically modified tumor cells by allogeneic T cells encoding receptors for NY-ESO-1 and MAGE-A3 (Fig. 11.2).

The aforementioned data have provided the preclinical rationale for a recently initiated protocol utilizing epigenetically modified autologous tumor cell vaccines as a means to induce immunity to CT-X antigens in lung cancer patients. The cell-based vaccines will be administered with ISCOMATRIX™, a proprietary adjuvant that accelerates and potentiates immune responses to a variety of antigens including NY-ESO-1(Maraskovsky et al. 2009; Schnurr et al. 2009). The vaccines will be

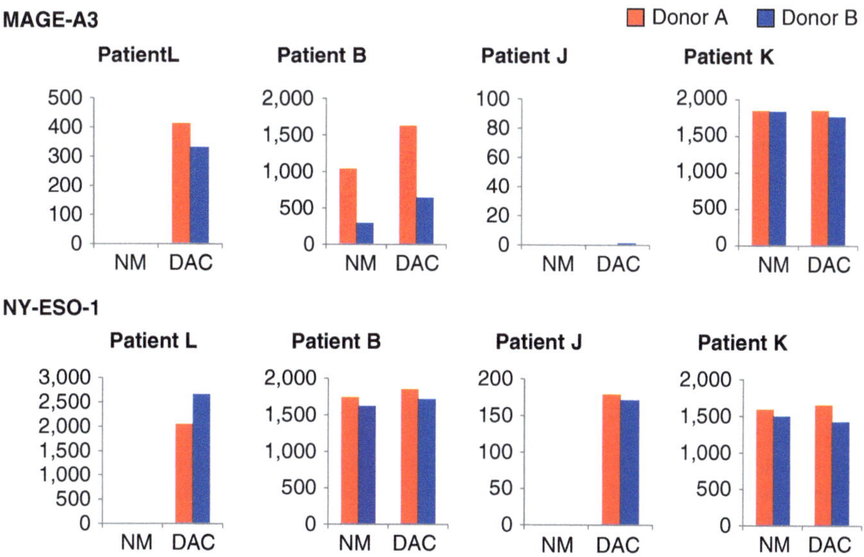

Fig. 11.2 Interferon-γ release assays demonstrating recognition of DAC-treated primary lung cancer cells by allogeneic T cells engineered to express receptors against HLA-*A0201 restricted epitopes of NY-ESO-1 and MAGE-A3

administered in conjunction with celecoxib at doses that potentially inhibit function of immunosuppressive T-regulatory cells, which are abnormally increased in lung cancer patients (Shimizu et al. 2010; Karagoz et al. 2010; Lee et al. 2009; Ruter et al. 2009) and have been shown to markedly attenuate immune responses to NY-ESO-1 vaccines in these individuals (Gnjatic et al. 2009).

Conclusions

Although considerable data suggest that epigenetic regulators of gene expression contribute to initiation and progression of lung cancers, none of the aforementioned aberrations observed during pulmonary carcinogenesis have been sufficiently validated as diagnostic or prognostic variables in lung cancer patients. Nevertheless, recent insights pertaining to lung cancer epigenetics provide new opportunities for intervention in this disease. Of particular concern regarding the use of chromatin remodeling agents for lung cancer therapy are observations that genes aberrantly hypermethylated in cancer cells do not revert to a fully euchromatin state (McGarvey et al. 2006) and that genes, which have been derepressed by DNA-demethylating agents, cannot be maintained in an active state by HDACi (Egger et al. 2007). These laboratory data, together with results of recent clinical trials, suggest that epigenetic therapies may need to be administered for prolonged periods to be efficacious and that additional regimens utilizing histone methyltransferase inhibitors, conventional chemotherapeutic regimens, molecularly targeted agents, or immunotherapies may be necessary in order for chromatin remodeling agents to mediate differentiation/senescence/death of lung cancer cells in vivo. Further analysis of epigenetic mechanisms associated with pulmonary carcinogenesis, as well as the identification of novel compounds that specifically target components of the epigenetic machinery that are dysregulated during malignant transformation, will inevitably hasten the development of more efficacious epigenetic regimens for the treatment and possible prevention of lung cancer.

References

Akimova T, Ge G, Golovina T, Mikheeva T, Wang L, Riley JL et al (2010) Histone/protein deacetylase inhibitors increase suppressive functions of human FOXP3+ Tregs. Clin Immunol 136:348–363

Albert M, Helin K (2010) Histone methyltransferases in cancer. Semin Cell Dev Biol 21:209–220

Atanackovic D, Hildebrandt Y, Jadczak A, Cao Y, Luetkens T, Meyer S et al (2010) Cancer-testis antigens MAGE-C1/CT7 and MAGE-A3 promote the survival of multiple myeloma cells. Haematologica 95:785–793

Barlesi F, Giaccone G, Gallegos-Ruiz MI, Loundou A, Span SW, Lefesvre P et al (2007) Global histone modifications predict prognosis of resected non small-cell lung cancer. J Clin Oncol 25:4358–4364

Barth TK, Imhof A (2010) Fast signals and slow marks: the dynamics of histone modifications. Trends Biochem Sci 35:618–626

Becker M, Korn C, Sienerth AR, Voswinckel R, Luetkenhaus K, Ceteci F et al (2009) Polycomb group protein Bmi1 is required for growth of RAF driven non-small-cell lung cancer. PLoS One 4:e4230

Belinsky SA, Nikula KJ, Baylin SB, Issa JP (1996) Increased cytosine DNA-methyltransferase activity is target-cell-specific and an early event in lung cancer. Proc Natl Acad Sci U S A 93:4045–4050

Berdasco M, Esteller M (2010) Aberrant epigenetic landscape in cancer: how cellular identity goes awry. Dev Cell 19:698–711

Bowman RV, Wright CM, Davidson MR, Francis SM, Yang IA, Fong KM (2009) Epigenomic targets for the treatment of respiratory disease. Expert Opin Ther Targets 13:625–640

Bracken AP, Pasini D, Capra M, Prosperini E, Colli E, Helin K (2003) EZH2 is downstream of the pRB-E2F pathway, essential for proliferation and amplified in cancer. EMBO J 22:5323–5335

Bracken AP, Dietrich N, Pasini D, Hansen KH, Helin K (2006) Genome-wide mapping of Polycomb target genes unravels their roles in cell fate transitions. Genes Dev 20:1123–1136

Brambilla E, Gazdar A (2009) Pathogenesis of lung cancer signalling pathways: roadmap for therapies. Eur Respir J 33:1485–1497

Brena RM, Morrison C, Liyanarachchi S, Jarjoura D, Davuluri RV, Otterson GA et al (2007) Aberrant DNA methylation of OLIG1, a novel prognostic factor in non-small cell lung cancer. PLoS Med 4:e108

Breuer RH, Snijders PJ, Smit EF, Sutedja TG, Sewalt RG, Otte AP et al (2004) Increased expression of the EZH2 polycomb group gene in BMI-1-positive neoplastic cells during bronchial carcinogenesis. Neoplasia 6:736–743

Brock MV, Hooker CM, Ota-Machida E, Han Y, Guo M, Ames S et al (2008) DNA methylation markers and early recurrence in stage I lung cancer. N Engl J Med 358:1118–1128

Brueckner B, Kuck D, Lyko F (2007) DNA methyltransferase inhibitors for cancer therapy. Cancer J 13:17–22

Bruzzese F, Rocco M, Castelli S, Di GE, Desideri A, Budillon A (2009) Synergistic antitumor effect between vorinostat and topotecan in small cell lung cancer cells is mediated by generation of reactive oxygen species and DNA damage-induced apoptosis. Mol Cancer Ther 8:3075–3087

Cameron EE, Bachman KE, Myohanen S, Herman JG, Baylin SB (1999) Synergy of demethylation and histone deacetylase inhibition in the re-expression of genes silenced in cancer. Nat Genet 21:103–107

Campbell PM, Bovenzi V, Szyf M (2004) Methylated DNA-binding protein 2 antisense inhibitors suppress tumourigenesis of human cancer cell lines in vitro and in vivo. Carcinogenesis 25:499–507

Castro M, Grau L, Puerta P, Gimenez L, Venditti J, Quadrelli S et al (2010) Multiplexed methylation profiles of tumor suppressor genes and clinical outcome in lung cancer. J Transl Med 8:86

Chai G, Li L, Zhou W, Wu L, Zhao Y, Wang D et al (2008) HDAC inhibitors act with 5-aza-2′-deoxycytidine to inhibit cell proliferation by suppressing removal of incorporated abases in lung cancer cells. PLoS One 3:e2445

Chang HC, Cho CY, Hung WC (2006) Silencing of the metastasis suppressor RECK by RAS oncogene is mediated by DNA methyltransferase 3b-induced promoter methylation. Cancer Res 66:8413–8420

Chen H, Yan Y, Davidson TL, Shinkai Y, Costa M (2006) Hypoxic stress induces dimethylated histone H3 lysine 9 through histone methyltransferase G9a in mammalian cells. Cancer Res 66:9009–9016

Chen MW, Hua KT, Kao HJ, Chi CC, Wei LH, Johansson G et al (2010) H3K9 histone methyltransferase G9a promotes lung cancer invasion and metastasis by silencing the cell adhesion molecule Ep-CAM. Cancer Res 70:7830–7840

Chinnasamy N, Wargo JA, Yu Z, Rao M, Frankel TL, Riley JP et al (2011) A TCR targeting the HLA-A*0201-restricted epitope of MAGE-A3 recognizes multiple epitopes of the MAGE-A antigen superfamily in several types of cancer. J Immunol 186:685–696

Cho HJ, Caballero OL, Gnjatic S, Andrade VC, Colleoni GW, Vettore AL et al (2006) Physical interaction of two cancer-testis antigens, MAGE-C1 (CT7) and NY-ESO-1 (CT6). Cancer Immun 6:12

Choi SH, Heo K, Byun HM, An W, Lu W, Yang AS (2011) Identification of preferential target sites for human DNA methyltransferases. Nucleic Acids Res 39(1):104–118. doi: doi: 10.1093/nar/gkq774

Christophersen NS, Helin K (2010) Epigenetic control of embryonic stem cell fate. J Exp Med 207:2287–2295

Cilensek ZM, Yehiely F, Kular RK, Deiss LP (2002) A member of the GAGE family of tumor antigens is an anti-apoptotic gene that confers resistance to Fas/CD95/APO-1, Interferon-gamma, taxol and gamma-irradiation. Cancer Biol Ther 1:380–387

Coe BP, Lockwood WW, Girard L, Chari R, Macaulay C, Lam S et al (2006) Differential disruption of cell cycle pathways in small cell and non-small cell lung cancer. Br J Cancer 94: 1927–1935

Damiani LA, Yingling CM, Leng S, Romo PE, Nakamura J, Belinsky SA (2008) Carcinogen-induced gene promoter hypermethylation is mediated by DNMT1 and causal for transformation of immortalized bronchial epithelial cells. Cancer Res 68:9005–9014

De Carvalho DD, You JS, Jones PA (2010) DNA methylation and cellular reprogramming. Trends Cell Biol 20:609–617

Delp K, Momburg F, Hilmes C, Huber C, Seliger B (2000) Functional deficiencies of components of the MHC class I antigen pathway in human tumors of epithelial origin. Bone Marrow Transplant 25(Suppl 2):S88–S95

Dovey JS, Zacharek SJ, Kim CF, Lees JA (2008) Bmi1 is critical for lung tumorigenesis and bronchioalveolar stem cell expansion. Proc Natl Acad Sci U S A 105:11857–11862

Du L, Schageman JJ, Irnov, Girard L, Hammond SM, Minna JD et al (2010a) MicroRNA expression distinguishes SCLC from NSCLC lung tumor cells and suggests a possible pathological relationship between SCLCs and NSCLCs. J Exp Clin Cancer Res 29:75

Du Z, Song J, Wang Y, Zhao Y, Guda K, Yang S et al (2010b) DNMT1 stability is regulated by proteins coordinating deubiquitination and acetylation-driven ubiquitination. Sci Signal 3:ra80

Egger G, Aparicio AM, Escobar SG, Jones PA (2007) Inhibition of histone deacetylation does not block resilencing of p16 after 5-aza-2'-deoxycytidine treatment. Cancer Res 67:346–353
Ehrlich M (2009) DNA hypomethylation in cancer cells. Epigenomics 1:239–259
Elkord E, Alcantar-Orozco EM, Dovedi SJ, Tran DQ, Hawkins RE, Gilham DE (2010) T regulatory cells in cancer: recent advances and therapeutic potential. Expert Opin Biol Ther 10:1573–1586
Endoh H, Yatabe Y, Shimizu S, Tajima K, Kuwano H, Takahashi T et al (2003) RASSF1A gene inactivation in non-small cell lung cancer and its clinical implication. Int J Cancer 106:45–51
Espada J, Calvo MB, Diaz-Prado S, Medina V (2009) Wnt signalling and cancer stem cells. Clin Transl Oncol 11:411–427
Friedman JM, Liang G, Liu CC, Wolff EM, Tsai YC, Ye W et al (2009) The putative tumor suppressor microRNA-101 modulates the cancer epigenome by repressing the polycomb group protein EZH2. Cancer Res 69(6):2623–2629
Gnjatic S, Altorki NK, Tang DN, Tu SM, Kundra V, Ritter G et al (2009) NY-ESO-1 DNA vaccine induces T-cell responses that are suppressed by regulatory T cells. Clin Cancer Res 15:2130–2139
Goll MG, Bestor TH (2005) Eukaryotic cytosine methyltransferases. Annu Rev Biochem 74:481–514
Groeper C, Gambazzi F, Zajac P, Bubendorf L, Adamina M, Rosenthal R et al (2007) Cancer/testis antigen expression and specific cytotoxic T lymphocyte responses in non small cell lung cancer. Int J Cancer 120:337–343
Grunwald C, Koslowski M, Arsiray T, Dhaene K, Praet M, Victor A et al (2006) Expression of multiple epigenetically regulated cancer/germline genes in nonsmall cell lung cancer. Int J Cancer 118:2522–2528
Gu J, Berman D, Lu C, Wistuba II, Roth JA, Frazier M et al (2006) Aberrant promoter methylation profile and association with survival in patients with non-small cell lung cancer. Clin Cancer Res 12:7329–7338
Guo ZS, Hong JA, Irvine KR, Chen GA, Spiess PJ, Liu Y et al (2006) De novo induction of a cancer/testis antigen by 5-aza-2′-deoxycytidine augments adoptive immunotherapy in a murine tumor model. Cancer Res 66:1105–1113
Gure AO, Chua R, Williamson B, Gonen M, Ferrera CA, Gnjatic S et al (2005) Cancer-testis genes are coordinately expressed and are markers of poor outcome in non-small cell lung cancer. Clin Cancer Res 11:8055–8062
Ha K, Lee GE, Palii SS, Brown KD, Takeda Y, Liu K et al (2011) Rapid and transient recruitment of DNMT1 to DNA double-strand breaks is mediated by its interaction with multiple components of the DNA damage response machinery. Hum Mol Genet 20:126–140
Hayami S, Yoshimatsu M, Veerakumarasivam A, Unoki M, Iwai Y, Tsunoda T et al (2010) Overexpression of the JmjC histone demethylase KDM5B in human carcinogenesis: involvement in the proliferation of cancer cells through the E2F/RB pathway. Mol Cancer 9:59
Hayami S, Kelly JD, Cho HS, Yoshimatsu M, Unoki M, Tsunoda T et al (2011) Overexpression of LSD1 contributes to human carcinogenesis through chromatin regulation in various cancers. Int J Cancer 128:574–586
Hernandez DG, Nalls MA, Gibbs JR, Arepalli S, van der Brug M, Chong S et al (2011) Distinct DNA methylation changes highly correlated with chronological age in the human brain. Hum Mol Genet 20:1164–1172
Hirasawa R, Feil R (2010) Genomic imprinting and human disease. Essays Biochem 48:187–200
Holm TM, Jackson-Grusby L, Brambrink T, Yamada Y, Rideout WM III, Jaenisch R (2005) Global loss of imprinting leads to widespread tumorigenesis in adult mice. Cancer Cell 8:275–285
Hong JA, Kang Y, Abdullaev Z, Flanagan PT, Pack SD, Fischette MR et al (2005) Reciprocal binding of CTCF and BORIS to the NY-ESO-1 promoter coincides with derepression of this cancer-testis gene in lung cancer cells. Cancer Res 65:7763–7774
Howard G, Eiges R, Gaudet F, Jaenisch R, Eden A (2008) Activation and transposition of endogenous retroviral elements in hypomethylation induced tumors in mice. Oncogene 27: 404–408

Huang Y, Stewart TM, Wu Y, Baylin SB, Marton LJ, Perkins B et al (2009) Novel oligoamine analogues inhibit lysine-specific demethylase 1 and induce reexpression of epigenetically silenced genes. Clin Cancer Res 15:7217–7228

Hussain M, Rao M, Humphries AE, Hong JA, Liu F, Yang M et al (2009) Tobacco smoke induces polycomb-mediated repression of Dickkopf-1 in lung cancer cells. Cancer Res 69:3570–3578

Jones PA, Baylin SB (2007) The epigenomics of cancer. Cell 128:683–692

Ju S, Qiu H, Zhou X, Zhu B, Lv X, Huang X et al (2009) CD13+CD4+CD25hi regulatory T cells exhibit higher suppressive function and increase with tumor stage in non-small cell lung cancer patients. Cell Cycle 8:2578–2585

Karagoz B, Bilgi O, Gumus M, Erikci AA, Sayan O, Turken O et al (2010) CD8+. Med Oncol 27:29–33

Kassis ES, Zhao M, Hong JA, Chen GA, Nguyen DM, Schrump DS (2006) Depletion of DNA methyltransferase 1 and/or DNA methyltransferase 3b mediates growth arrest and apoptosis in lung and esophageal cancer and malignant pleural mesothelioma cells. J Thorac Cardiovasc Surg 131:298–306

Kikuchi S, Yamada D, Fukami T, Maruyama T, Ito A, Asamura H et al (2006) Hypermethylation of the TSLC1/IGSF4 promoter is associated with tobacco smoking and a poor prognosis in primary nonsmall cell lung carcinoma. Cancer 106:1751–1758

Kikuchi J, Kinoshita I, Shimizu Y, Kikuchi E, Konishi J, Oizumi S et al (2010) Distinctive expression of the polycomb group proteins Bmi1 polycomb ring finger oncogene and enhancer of zeste homolog 2 in nonsmall cell lung cancers and their clinical and clinicopathologic significance. Cancer 116:3015–3024

Kim H, Kwon YM, Kim JS, Han J, Shim YM, Park J et al (2006) Elevated mRNA levels of DNA methyltransferase-1 as an independent prognostic factor in primary nonsmall cell lung cancer. Cancer 107:1042–1049

Kim Y, Park H, Park D, Lee YS, Choe J, Hahn JH et al (2010) Cancer/testis antigen CAGE exerts negative regulation on p53 expression through HDAC2 and confers resistance to anti-cancer drugs. J Biol Chem 285:25957–25968

Kohda M, Hoshiya H, Katoh M, Tanaka I, Masuda R, Takemura T et al (2001) Frequent loss of imprinting of IGF2 and MEST in lung adenocarcinoma. Mol Carcinog 31:184–191

Kondo M, Suzuki H, Ueda R, Osada H, Takagi K, Takahashi T et al (1995) Frequent loss of imprinting of the H19 gene is often associated with its overexpression in human lung cancers. Oncogene 10:1193–1198

Kondo M, Matsuoka S, Uchida K, Osada H, Nagatake M, Takagi K et al (1996) Selective maternal-allele loss in human lung cancers of the maternally expressed p57KIP2 gene at 11p15.5. Oncogene 12:1365–1368

Kondo Y, Shen L, Cheng AS, Ahmed S, Boumber Y, Charo C et al (2008) Gene silencing in cancer by histone H3 lysine 27 trimethylation independent of promoter DNA methylation. Nat Genet 40:741–750

Konigshoff M, Eickelberg O (2010) WNT signaling in lung disease: a failure or a regeneration signal? Am J Respir Cell Mol Biol 42:21–31

Konishi J, Toyooka S, Aoe M, Omura Y, Washio K, Tsukuda K et al (2004) The relationship between NY-ESO-1 mRNA expression and clinicopathological features in non-small cell lung cancer. Oncol Rep 11:1063–1067

Lam DC, Girard L, Ramirez R, Chau WS, Suen WS, Sheridan S et al (2007) Expression of nicotinic acetylcholine receptor subunit genes in non-small-cell lung cancer reveals differences between smokers and nonsmokers. Cancer Res 67:4638–4647

Lee SY, Choi HK, Lee KJ, Jung JY, Hur GY, Jung KH et al (2009) The immune tolerance of cancer is mediated by IDO that is inhibited by COX-2 inhibitors through regulatory T cells. J Immunother 32:22–28

Lee JS, Smith E, Shilatifard A (2010) The language of histone crosstalk. Cell 142:682–685

Li H, Yu JP, Cao S, Wei F, Zhang P, An XM et al (2007) CD4 +CD25 + regulatory T cells decreased the antitumor activity of cytokine-induced killer (CIK) cells of lung cancer patients. J Clin Immunol 27:317–326

Lin RK, Hsu HS, Chang JW, Chen CY, Chen JT, Wang YC (2007) Alteration of DNA methyltransferases contributes to 5′CpG methylation and poor prognosis in lung cancer. Lung Cancer 55:205–213

Lin RK, Wu CY, Chang JW, Juan LJ, Hsu HS, Chen CY et al (2010a) Dysregulation of p53/Sp1 control leads to DNA methyltransferase-1 overexpression in lung cancer. Cancer Res 70:5807–5817

Lin RK, Hsieh YS, Lin P, Hsu HS, Chen CY, Tang YA et al (2010b) The tobacco-specific carcinogen NNK induces DNA methyltransferase 1 accumulation and tumor suppressor gene hypermethylation in mice and lung cancer patients. J Clin Invest 120:521–532

Liu F, Killian JK, Yang M, Walker RL, Hong JA, Zhang M et al (2010) Epigenomic alterations and gene expression profiles in respiratory epithelia exposed to cigarette smoke condensate. Oncogene 29:3650–3664

Lu J, He ML, Wang L, Chen Y, Liu X, Dong Q et al (2011) MiR-26a inhibits cell growth and tumorigenesis of nasopharyngeal carcinoma through repression of EZH2. Cancer Res 71(1):225–233

Lundqvist A, Abrams SI, Schrump DS, Alvarez G, Suffredini D, Berg M et al (2006) Bortezomib and depsipeptide sensitize tumors to tumor necrosis factor-related apoptosis-inducing ligand: a novel method to potentiate natural killer cell tumor cytotoxicity. Cancer Res 66:7317–7325

Luszczek W, Cheriyath V, Mekhail TM, Borden EC (2010) Combinations of DNA methyltransferase and histone deacetylase inhibitors induce DNA damage in small cell lung cancer cells: correlation of resistance with IFN-stimulated gene expression. Mol Cancer Ther 9:2309–2321

Maraskovsky E, Schnurr M, Wilson NS, Robson NC, Boyle J, Drane D (2009) Development of prophylactic and therapeutic vaccines using the ISCOMATRIX adjuvant. Immunol Cell Biol 87:371–376

Marsit CJ, Kim DH, Liu M, Hinds PW, Wiencke JK, Nelson HH et al (2005) Hypermethylation of RASSF1A and BLU tumor suppressor genes in non-small cell lung cancer: implications for tobacco smoking during adolescence. Int J Cancer 114:219–223

Maruyama R, Sugio K, Yoshino I, Maehara Y, Gazdar AF (2004) Hypermethylation of FHIT as a prognostic marker in nonsmall cell lung carcinoma. Cancer 100:1472–1477

McCabe MT, Lee EK, Vertino PM (2009) A multifactorial signature of DNA sequence and polycomb binding predicts aberrant CpG island methylation. Cancer Res 69:282–291

McGarvey KM, Fahrner JA, Greene E, Martens J, Jenuwein T, Baylin SB (2006) Silenced tumor suppressor genes reactivated by DNA demethylation do not return to a fully euchromatic chromatin state. Cancer Res 66:3541–3549

Melloni G, Ferreri AJ, Russo V, Gattinoni L, Arrigoni G, Ceresoli GL et al (2004) Prognostic significance of cancer-testis gene expression in resected non-small cell lung cancer patients. Oncol Rep 12:145–151

Mills AA (2010) Throwing the cancer switch: reciprocal roles of polycomb and trithorax proteins. Nat Rev Cancer 10:669–682

Minamiya Y, Ono T, Saito H, Takahashi N, Ito M, Motoyama S et al (2010) Strong expression of HDAC3 correlates with a poor prognosis in patients with adenocarcinoma of the lung. Tumour Biol 31:533–539

Momparler RL, Bouffard DY, Momparler LF, Dionne J, Belanger K, Ayoub J (1997) Pilot phase I-II study on 5-aza-2′-deoxycytidine (Decitabine) in patients with metastatic lung cancer. Anticancer Drugs 8:358–368

Monte M, Simonatto M, Peche LY, Bublik DR, Gobessi S, Pierotti MA et al (2006) MAGE-A tumor antigens target p53 transactivation function through histone deacetylase recruitment and confer resistance to chemotherapeutic agents. Proc Natl Acad Sci U S A 103:11160–11165

Morey L, Helin K (2010) Polycomb group protein-mediated repression of transcription. Trends Biochem Sci 35:323–332

Oka M, Meacham AM, Hamazaki T, Rodic N, Chang LJ, Terada N (2005) De novo DNA methyltransferases Dnmt3a and Dnmt3b primarily mediate the cytotoxic effect of 5-aza-2′-deoxycytidine. Oncogene 24:3091–3099

Osada H, Tatematsu Y, Saito H, Yatabe Y, Mitsudomi T, Takahashi T (2004) Reduced expression of class II histone deacetylase genes is associated with poor prognosis in lung cancer patients. Int J Cancer 112:26–32

Otterson GA, Hodgson L, Pang H, Vokes EE (2010) Phase II study of the histone deacetylase inhibitor Romidepsin in relapsed small cell lung cancer (Cancer and Leukemia Group B 30304). J Thorac Oncol 5:1644–1648

Palii SS, Van Emburgh BO, Sankpal UT, Brown KD, Robertson KD (2008) DNA methylation inhibitor 5-Aza-2′-deoxycytidine induces reversible genome-wide DNA damage that is distinctly influenced by DNA methyltransferases 1 and 3B. Mol Cell Biol 28:752–771

Paliwal A, Vaissiere T, Krais A, Cuenin C, Cros MP, Zaridze D et al (2010) Aberrant DNA methylation links cancer susceptibility locus 15q25.1 to apoptotic regulation and lung cancer. Cancer Res 70:2779–2788

Park JM, Lee GY, Choi JE, Kang HG, Jang JS, Cha SI et al (2005) No association between polymorphisms in the histone deacetylase genes and the risk of lung cancer. Cancer Epidemiol Biomarkers Prev 14:1841–1843

Pedersen MT, Helin K (2010) Histone demethylases in development and disease. Trends Cell Biol 20:662–671

Pfeifer GP, Rauch TA (2009) DNA methylation patterns in lung carcinomas. Semin Cancer Biol 19:181–187

Por E, Byun HJ, Lee EJ, Lim JH, Jung SY, Park I et al (2010) The cancer/testis antigen CAGE with oncogenic potential stimulates cell proliferation by up-regulating cyclins D1 and E in an AP-1- and E2F-dependent manner. J Biol Chem 285:14475–14485

Rai K, Sarkar S, Broadbent TJ, Voas M, Grossmann KF, Nadauld LD et al (2010) DNA demethylase activity maintains intestinal cells in an undifferentiated state following loss of APC. Cell 142:930–942

Rao M, Chinnasamy N, Hong JA, Zhang Y, Zhang M, Xi S, et al. Inhibition of histone lysine methylation enhances cancer-testis antigen expression in lung cancer cells: implications for adoptive immunotherapy of cancer. Cancer Res 2011;71:4192–204.

Ramalingam SS, Maitland ML, Frankel P, Argiris AE, Koczywas M, Gitlitz B et al (2010) Carboplatin and Paclitaxel in combination with either vorinostat or placebo for first-line therapy of advanced non-small-cell lung cancer. J Clin Oncol 28:56–62

Ramirez JL, Rosell R, Taron M, Sanchez-Ronco M, Alberola V, de Las PR et al (2005) 14-3-3sigma methylation in pretreatment serum circulating DNA of cisplatin-plus-gemcitabine-treated advanced non-small-cell lung cancer patients predicts survival: The Spanish Lung Cancer Group. J Clin Oncol 23:9105–9112

Renaud S, Loukinov D, Alberti L, Vostrov A, Kwon YW, Bosman FT et al (2011) BORIS/CTCFL-mediated transcriptional regulation of the hTERT telomerase gene in testicular and ovarian tumor cells. Nucleic Acids Res 39:862–873

Reynolds PA, Sigaroudinia M, Zardo G, Wilson MB, Benton GM, Miller CJ et al (2006) Tumor suppressor p16INK4A regulates polycomb-mediated DNA hypermethylation in human mammary epithelial cells. J Biol Chem 281:24790–24802

Ruter J, Barnett BG, Kryczek I, Brumlik MJ, Daniel BJ, Coukos G et al (2009) Altering regulatory T cell function in cancer immunotherapy: a novel means to boost the efficacy of cancer vaccines. Front Biosci 14:1761–1770

Sasaki H, Moriyama S, Nakashima Y, Kobayashi Y, Kiriyama M, Fukai I et al (2004) Histone deacetylase 1 mRNA expression in lung cancer. Lung Cancer 46:171–178

Sato M, Shames DS, Gazdar AF, Minna JD (2007) A translational view of the molecular pathogenesis of lung cancer. J Thorac Oncol 2:327–343

Sauvageau M, Sauvageau G (2010) Polycomb group proteins: multi-faceted regulators of somatic stem cells and cancer. Cell Stem Cell 7:299–313

Sawan C, Herceg Z (2010) Histone modifications and cancer. Adv Genet 70:57–85

Sawarkar R, Paro R (2010) Interpretation of developmental signaling at chromatin: the Polycomb perspective. Dev Cell 19:651–661

Schar P, Fritsch O (2011) DNA repair and the control of DNA methylation. Prog Drug Res 67:51–68

Scharf AN, Imhof A (2011) Every methyl counts – epigenetic calculus. FEBS Lett 585(13):2001–2007. doi: 10.1016/j.febslet.2010.11.029

Schnurr M, Orban M, Robson NC, Shin A, Braley H, Airey D et al (2009) ISCOMATRIX adjuvant induces efficient cross-presentation of tumor antigen by dendritic cells via rapid cytosolic antigen delivery and processing via tripeptidyl peptidase II. J Immunol 182:1253–1259
Schrump DS (2009) Cytotoxicity mediated by histone deacetylase inhibitors in cancer cells: mechanisms and potential clinical implications. Clin Cancer Res 15:3947–3957
Schrump DS, Nguyen DM (2005) Targeting the epigenome for the treatment and prevention of lung cancer. Semin Oncol 32:488–502
Schrump DS, Fischette MR, Nguyen DM, Zhao M, Li X, Kunst TF et al (2006) Phase I study of decitabine-mediated gene expression in patients with cancers involving the lungs, esophagus, or pleura. Clin Cancer Res 12:5777–5785
Schrump DS, Hong JA, Nguyen DM (2007) Utilization of chromatin remodeling agents for lung cancer therapy. Cancer J 13:56–64
Schrump DS, Fischette MR, Nguyen DM, Zhao M, Li X, Kunst TF et al (2008) Clinical and molecular responses in lung cancer patients receiving Romidepsin. Clin Cancer Res 14:188–198
Seligson DB, Horvath S, McBrian MA, Mah V, Yu H, Tze S et al (2009) Global levels of histone modifications predict prognosis in different cancers. Am J Pathol 174:1619–1628
Shen H, Wang L, Spitz MR, Hong WK, Mao L, Wei Q (2002) A novel polymorphism in human cytosine DNA-methyltransferase-3B promoter is associated with an increased risk of lung cancer. Cancer Res 62:4992–4995
Shimizu K, Nakata M, Hirami Y, Yukawa T, Maeda A, Tanemoto K (2010) Tumor-infiltrating Foxp3+ regulatory T cells are correlated with cyclooxygenase-2 expression and are associated with recurrence in resected non-small cell lung cancer. J Thorac Oncol 5:585–590
Soh J, Okumura N, Lockwood WW, Yamamoto H, Shigematsu H, Zhang W et al (2009) Oncogene mutations, copy number gains and mutant allele specific imbalance (MASI) frequently occur together in tumor cells. PLoS One 4:e7464
Sos ML, Michel K, Zander T, Weiss J, Frommolt P, Peifer M et al (2009) Predicting drug susceptibility of non-small cell lung cancers based on genetic lesions. J Clin Invest 119:1727–1740
Stevenson BJ, Iseli C, Panji S, Zahn-Zabal M, Hide W, Old LJ et al (2007) Rapid evolution of cancer/testis genes on the X chromosome. BMC Genomics 8:129
Stockert E, Jäger E, Chen YT, Scanlan MJ, Gout I, Karbach J et al (1998) A survey of the humoral immune response of cancer patients to a panel of human tumor antigens. J Exp Med 187:1349–1354
Surface LE, Thornton SR, Boyer LA (2010) Polycomb group proteins set the stage for early lineage commitment. Cell Stem Cell 7:288–298
Ting DT, Lipson D, Paul S, Brannigan BW, Akhavanfard S, Coffman EJ et al (2011) Aberrant overexpression of satellite repeats in pancreatic and other epithelial cancers. Science 331:593–596
Toyooka S, Maruyama R, Toyooka KO, McLerran D, Feng Z, Fukuyama Y et al (2003) Smoke exposure, histologic type and geography-related differences in the methylation profiles of non-small cell lung cancer. Int J Cancer 103:153–160
Toyooka S, Tokumo M, Shigematsu H, Matsuo K, Asano H, Tomii K et al (2006) Mutational and epigenetic evidence for independent pathways for lung adenocarcinomas arising in smokers and never smokers. Cancer Res 66:1371–1375
Traynor AM, Dubey S, Eickhoff JC, Kolesar JM, Schell K, Huie MS et al (2009) Vorinostat (NSC# 701852) in patients with relapsed non-small cell lung cancer: a Wisconsin Oncology Network phase II study. J Thorac Oncol 4:522–526
Vaissiere T, Hung RJ, Zaridze D, Moukeria A, Cuenin C, Fasolo V et al (2009) Quantitative analysis of DNA methylation profiles in lung cancer identifies aberrant DNA methylation of specific genes and its association with gender and cancer risk factors. Cancer Res 69:243–252
Vallbohmer D, Brabender J, Yang D, Schneider PM, Metzger R, Danenberg KD et al (2006) DNA methyltransferases messenger RNA expression and aberrant methylation of CpG islands in non-small-cell lung cancer: association and prognostic value. Clin Lung Cancer 8:39–44
Van Den Broeck A, Brambilla E, Moro-Sibilot D, Lantuejoul S, Brambilla C, Eymin B et al (2008) Loss of histone H4K20 trimethylation occurs in preneoplasia and influences prognosis of non-small cell lung cancer. Clin Cancer Res 14:7237–7245
Vatolin S, Abdullaev Z, Pack SD, Flanagan PT, Custer M, Loukinov DI et al (2005) Conditional expression of the CTCF-paralogous transcriptional factor BORIS in normal cells results in

demethylation and derepression of MAGE-A1 and reactivation of other cancer-testis genes. Cancer Res 65:7751–7762

Vermeulen L, De Sousa E, Melo F, van der Heijden M, Cameron K, de Jong JH, Borovski T et al (2010) Wnt activity defines colon cancer stem cells and is regulated by the microenvironment. Nat Cell Biol 12:468–476

Vonlanthen S, Heighway J, Altermatt HJ, Gugger M, Kappeler A, Borner MM et al (2001) The bmi-1 oncoprotein is differentially expressed in non-small cell lung cancer and correlates with INK4A-ARF locus expression. Br J Cancer 84:1372–1376

Vrzalikova K, Skarda J, Ehrmann J, Murray PG, Fridman E, Kopolovic J et al (2008) Prognostic value of Bmi-1 oncoprotein expression in NSCLC patients: a tissue microarray study. J Cancer Res Clin Oncol 134:1037–1042

Wargo JA, Robbins PF, Li Y, Zhao Y, El-Gamil M, Caragacianu D et al (2009) Recognition of NY-ESO-1+ tumor cells by engineered lymphocytes is enhanced by improved vector design and epigenetic modulation of tumor antigen expression. Cancer Immunol Immunother 58:383–394

Watanabe H, Soejima K, Yasuda H, Kawada I, Nakachi I, Yoda S et al (2008) Deregulation of histone lysine methyltransferases contributes to oncogenic transformation of human broncho-epithelial cells. Cancer Cell Int 8:15

Weir BA, Woo MS, Getz G, Perner S, Ding L, Beroukhim R et al (2007) Characterizing the cancer genome in lung adenocarcinoma. Nature 450:893–898

Weiser TS, Guo ZS, Ohnmacht GA, Parkhurst ML, Tong-On P, Marincola FM et al (2001) Sequential 5-Aza-2 deoxycytidine-depsipeptide FR901228 treatment induces apoptosis preferentially in cancer cells and facilitates their recognition by cytolytic T lymphocytes specific for NY-ESO-1. J Immunother 24:151–161

Widschwendter M, Fiegl H, Egle D, Mueller-Holzner E, Spizzo G, Marth C et al (2007) Epigenetic stem cell signature in cancer. Nat Genet 39:157–158

Wienholz BL, Kareta MS, Moarefi AH, Gordon CA, Ginno PA, Chedin F (2010) DNMT3L modulates significant and distinct flanking sequence preference for DNA methylation by DNMT3A and DNMT3B in vivo. PLoS Genet 6:e1001106. doi: 10.1371/journal.pgen.1001106

Xing J, Stewart DJ, Gu J, Lu C, Spitz MR, Wu X (2008) Expression of methylation-related genes is associated with overall survival in patients with non-small cell lung cancer. Br J Cancer 98:1716–1722

Xiong J, Epstein RJ (2009) Growth inhibition of human cancer cells by 5-aza-2′-deoxycytidine does not correlate with its effects on INK4a/ARF expression or initial promoter methylation status. Mol Cancer Ther 8:779–785

Yamada Y, Jackson-Grusby L, Linhart H, Meissner A, Eden A, Lin H et al (2005) Opposing effects of DNA hypomethylation on intestinal and liver carcinogenesis. Proc Natl Acad Sci U S A 102:13580–13585

Yang B, O'Herrin SM, Wu J, Reagan-Shaw S, Ma Y, Bhat KM et al (2007) MAGE-A, mMage-b, and MAGE-C proteins form complexes with KAP1 and suppress p53-dependent apoptosis in MAGE-positive cell lines. Cancer Res 67:9954–9962

Yeow WS, Ziauddin MF, Maxhimer JB, Shamimi-Noori S, Baras A, Chua A et al (2006) Potentiation of the anticancer effect of valproic acid, an antiepileptic agent with histone deacetylase inhibitory activity, by the kinase inhibitor Staurosporine or its clinically relevant analogue UCN-01. Br J Cancer 94:1436–1445

Yi JM, Kim HS (2007) Molecular phylogenetic analysis of the human endogenous retrovirus E (HERV-E) family in human tissues and human cancers. Genes Genet Syst 82:89–98

Yoon KA, Hwangbo B, Kim IJ, Park S, Kim HS, Kee HJ et al (2006) Novel polymorphisms in the SUV39H2 histone methyltransferase and the risk of lung cancer. Carcinogenesis 27:2217–2222

Yoon KA, Park S, Hwangbo B, Shin HD, Cheong HS, Shin HR et al (2007) Genetic polymorphisms in the Rb-binding zinc finger gene RIZ and the risk of lung cancer. Carcinogenesis 28:1971–1977

Yu X, Guo ZS, Marcu MG, Neckers L, Nguyen DM, Chen GA et al (2002) Modulation of p53, ErbB1, ErbB2, and Raf-1 expression in lung cancer cells by depsipeptide FR901228. J Natl Cancer Inst 94:504–513

Yu XD, Wang SY, Chen GA, Hou CM, Zhao M, Hong JA et al (2007) Apoptosis induced by depsipeptide FK228 coincides with inhibition of survival signaling in lung cancer cells. Cancer J 13:105–113

Zhang W, Peyton M, Xie Y, Soh J, Minna JD, Gazdar AF et al (2009) Histone deacetylase inhibitor romidepsin enhances anti-tumor effect of erlotinib in non-small cell lung cancer (NSCLC) cell lines. J Thorac Oncol 4:161–166

Zhang XY, Dong QG, Huang JS, Huang AM, Shi CL, Jin B et al (2010) The expression of stem cell-related indicators as a prognostic factor in human lung adenocarcinoma. J Surg Oncol 102:856–862

Zhang JG, Guo JF, Liu DL, Liu Q, Wang JJ (2011) MicroRNA-101 exerts tumor-suppressive functions in Non-small cell lung cancer through directly targeting enhancer of zeste homolog 2. J Thorac Oncol 6:671–678

Epigenetic Disturbances in Colorectal Cancer

12

Sarah Derks and Manon van Engeland

12.1 Introduction

Colorectal cancer is a major contributor to cancer-related death with over one million new patients diagnosed each year in both the USA and Europe.

Most CRCs develop from premalignant adenomas that are thought to arise from pluripotent stem cells located in intestinal crypts. The exact cell of origin is unclear. There are models that postulate that every cell has malignant potential, while others suggest that only the cancer stem cell can initiate colorectal carcinogenesis. About 5 % of premalignant adenomas will develop into a carcinoma with invasive and metastatic potential. Which adenoma progresses into cancer is unknown. Much of the understanding of the histological progression of normal epithelium into adenomas and carcinomas is based on the model of Vogelstein and coworkers in the early 1990s. In this model, CRC development involves sequential genetic abnormalities such as *TP53*, *KRAS* (Bos et al. 1987), and *APC* (Nakamura et al. 1991) mutations and allelic deletions of chromosomes 5, 17, and 18 (Fearon and Vogelstein 1990). Later it became apparent that CRC is a heterogeneous disease. About 85 % of CRCs can be characterized by a condition of aneuploidy and an increased rate of loss of heterozygosity (LOH) (Douglas et al. 2004; Hermsen et al. 2002), also called the chromosomal instability phenotype (CIN), while the remaining 15 % of CRCs are characterized by microsatellite instability (MSI), which is caused by inactivation of the mismatch repair gene

S. Derks
Department of Medical Oncology, VU University Medical Center,
Amsterdam, The Netherlands

M. van Engeland (✉)
Department of Pathology, GROW – School for Oncology and Developmental Biology,
Maastricht University Medical Center, 616, Maastricht 6200 MD, The Netherlands
e-mail: manon.van.engeland@mumc.nl

M. Lübbert, P.A. Jones (eds.), *Epigenetic Therapy of Cancer*,
DOI 10.1007/978-3-642-38404-2_12, © Springer-Verlag Berlin Heidelberg 2014

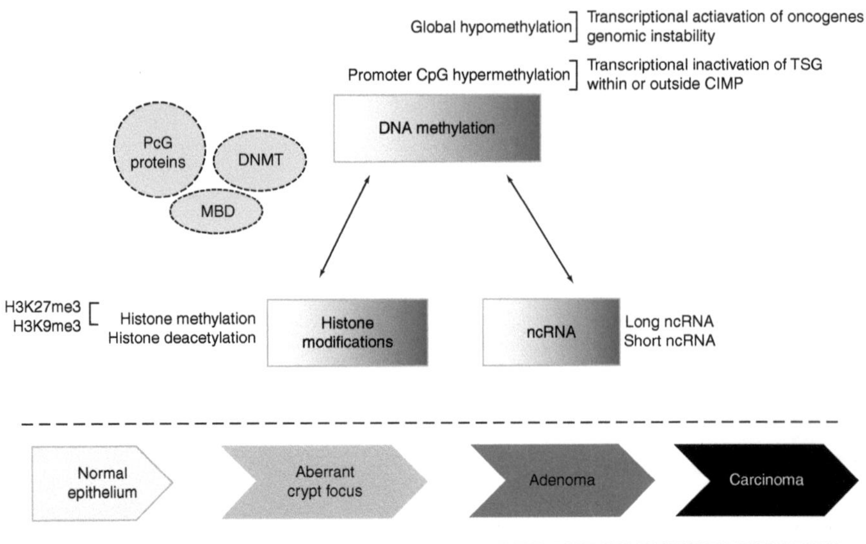

Fig. 12.1 Epigenetic modifications in colorectal cancer. Epigenetic disturbances that accompany the transition of normal epithelium to adenoma and carcinoma involve DNA methylation, histone modifications, and noncoding RNAs. CpG dinucleotides hypermethylation is catalyzed by DNA methyltransferases (*DNMTs*) and bound by methyl-binding (*MBD*) proteins. Some genes are targeted by Polycomb proteins that are able to catalyze H3K27 trimethylation. This process is accompanied by histone deacetylases to remove histone acetylation and histone methyltransferase to methylate H3K9 as well. These epigenetic modifications constitute a "closed" chromatin structure and a transcriptional silenced state

MHL1 (Cunningham et al. 1998; Herman et al. 1998) by mutation (Lynch syndrome) and DNA hypermethylation (sporadic CRCs).

The identification of epigenetic mechanisms contributing to the clinical presentation of a disease, i.e., promoter CpG island methylation in sporadic MSI CRCs, and other epigenetic alterations significantly added to the model for CRC carcinogenesis (Fig. 12.1). Promoter CpG island hypermethylation is the most extensively studied epigenetic modification in CRC and plays a pivotal role in carcinogenesis by transcriptional silencing of DNA repair and tumor suppressor genes (Herman and Baylin 2003). A rapid increase in advances in genome-wide approaches to map DNA methylation and histone modifications has yielded important insight into the extent of epigenetic disturbances in CRC. DNA methylation occurs in a network of other epigenetic alterations such as histone tail modifications, chromosome looping, and noncoding RNAs which interact and influence each other in a specific way (van Engeland et al. 2011). Nowadays, it has become increasingly apparent that epigenetic abnormalities are promising as biomarkers for early detection, prognosis, and response to therapy.

Here we provide an overview of the epigenetic alterations in CRC and discuss how they will contribute to CRC management in the future.

12.2 DNA Methylation: The CRC Methylome

In the last three decades, it has become clear that aberrant DNA methylation, DNA hypomethylation as well as hypermethylation, occurs at a genome-wide scale in CRC and is associated with altered gene expression and genomic instability.

DNA hypomethylation was one of the first recognized epigenetic alterations in CRC (Goelz et al. 1985). Global depletion of the 5-methylcytosine content occurs predominantly at CpG dinucleotides in repetitive sequences (satellite and LINE repeats, retrotransposons, and endogenous retroviral elements) (Ehrlich 2002; Feinberg and Tycko 2004; Irizarry et al. 2009). Originally, hypomethylation was hypothesized to be associated with widespread oncogene activation in CRC. Later it became clear that loss of methylation also causes altered chromosome replication and leads to genomic instability (Suzuki et al. 2006). A recent study of Berman et al. (2012) showed that hypomethylated regions cover almost half of the genome and demonstrate a specific spatial organization with hypermethylated areas (Berman et al. 2012). Regions of focal CpG island hypermethylation are located within regions of long-range (>100 kb) hypomethylation. Hypomethylated regions are associated with genes that gain expression in the tumor. These upregulated genes contain regions with an overrepresentation of AP-1-binding sequences of the Fos-Jun dimer, which is thought to be associated with chromatin remodeling (Aguilera et al. 2011).

DNA hypermethylation of CpG dinucleotides is one of the best studied epigenetic aberrations in CRC and occurs at CpG island containing promoter regions (Gardiner-Garden and Frommer 1987) as well as regions with less dense CpG dinucleotides situated in the proximity (~2 kb) of CpG islands called CpG shores (Irizarry et al. 2009). In normal cells, promoter CpG islands and CpG shores are not hypermethylated, with the exception of tissue-specific genes, which become hypermethylated early in development and differentiation (Irizarry et al. 2009; Straussman et al. 2009). In cancer cells, CpG hypermethylation at these sites results in transcriptional silencing of tumor suppressor genes, which is a gene- and tissue-specific process.

High-throughput epigenome-wide analyses have visualized the extent of DNA methylation in CRC and shown that in CRC about 400–600 genes are hypermethylated (Schuebel et al. 2007). A subset of these methylated genes are driver genes of which promoter CpG island methylation occurs exclusively in cancer. These genes have shown to function in regulating a diversity of functions such as proliferation, migration, angiogenesis, apoptosis, DNA stability, and repair (Schuebel et al. 2007; Weber et al. 2005). Disrupted key pathways driving colorectal carcinogenesis are WNT signaling, transforming growth factor-β (TGFβ) signaling, epidermal growth factor (EGFR) signaling, RAS/RAF/MAPK signaling, and phosphatidylinositol 3-kinase (PI3K) but also other pathways affecting DNA repair cell cycle control, p53 network, and apoptosis are affected. In these pathways, multiple genes are hypermethylated among which *APC*, *MLH1*, *MGMT*, *CHFR*, *RASSF1A*, *P14ARF*, and *P16INK4A* (Table 12.1).

Table 12.1 Genes and ncRNAs aberrantly expressed in CRC and potential role as biomarker

Signaling pathways	Hyper/hypomethylated genes/ ncRNAs	Early detection	Biomarker prognosis (good/poor)	Treatment response
WNT	*APC*, *SFRP1*, *SFRP2*, *SFRP4*, *SFRP5*, *SOX17*, *WNT5a*, *DKK1*, *DKK3*, *WIF1*, *AXIN2*, *LGR5*, *TFAP2*	*SFRP1* (Zhang et al. 2007) *SFRP2* (Muller et al. 2004), *APC* (Leung et al. 2005), *WIF1* (Lee et al. 2009)	*LGR5*, poor (de Sousa et al. 2011)	*TFAP2*, 5-FU resistance (Ebert et al. 2012)
RAS/RAF/MAPK	*RASSF1A*, *RASSF2A*, *EPHB2*, *RAB32*, *NORE1*	*RASSF2A* (Lee et al. 2009)		
TP53	*HIC1*, *miRNA34a*, *miRNA34b*, *miRNA34c*			
PI3K	*PIK3CA*			
IGF	*IGF2*		*IGF2*, poor (Baba et al. 2010)	
Cell cycle regulation	*CDKN2A*, *KLF4*		*CDKN2A*, poor (Esteller et al. 2001; Maeda et al. 2003; Shima et al. 2011)	
Cell signaling	*Vimentin*	*Vimentin* (Li et al. 2009; Easwaran et al. 2010)		
Transcription regulation	*GATA4*, *GATA5*, *RUNX3*, *CDX1*, *HLTF*, *FOXL2*, *ALX4*, *ASCL2*	*GATA4* (Hellebrekers et al. 2009) , *ALX4* (Ebert et al. 2006; Tanzer et al. 2010), *HLTF* (Leung et al. 2005)	*ASCL2*, poor (de Sousa et al. 2011) *HLTF*, poor (Herbst et al. 2009)	
DNA repair/stability	*MLH1*, *MGMT*, *WRN*, *CHFR*	*MLH1* (Leung et al. 2005), *MGMT* (Lee et al. 2009)	*CHFR*, poor (Tanaka et al. 2011)	*MLH1*, 5-FU (Ogino et al. 2007c) *WRN*, irinotecan resistance (Agrelo et al. 2006)
Apoptosis	*BNIP3*, *IRF8*, *DAPK*, *HRK*	*DAPK* (Yamaguchi et al. 2003)		
Cytokines	*OSMR*, *SEPT9*	*OSMR* (Kim et al. 2009), *SEPT9* (Lofton-Day et al. 2008)		

Tissue factor	*TFPI2*	*TFPI2* (Glockner et al. 2009)		
Other/unknown pathway	*NDRG4*, *LINE-1*, *UGT1A1*, *HOTAIR*	*NDRG4* (Melotte et al. 2009)	*LINE-1*, poor (Tanaka et al. 2011)	*UGT1A1*, irinotecan resistance (Gagnon et al. 2006) *LINE-1*, 5-FU sensitivity (Kawakami et al. 2011)
CIMP	*MINT1*, *MINT2*, *MINT31*,*CDKN2A*, *MLH1* *CACNA1G*, *IGF2*, *NEUROG1*, *RUNX3*, *SOCS1*		*Good* (Ogino et al. 2007c), poor (Ogino et al. 2007c)	5-FU sensitivity (Warusavitarne and Schnitzler 2007) 5-FU resistance (Ogino et al. 2007c)
Long ncRNA	*HOTAIR*, *MALAT-1*		*HOTAIR*, poor (Tsai et al. 2010) *MALAT-1*, poor (Xu et al. 2011)	

This table is not exhaustive and represents genes and noncoding RNAs, which are aberrantly expressed by epigenetic mechanisms in CRC and have a promising role as biomarker for early detection and prediction of prognosis and response to therapy

CIMP CpG island methylation phenotype, *5-FU* 5-fluorouracil

12.3 How Is CpG Methylation Mediated in CRC?

CpG hypermethylation is mediated by a family of DNA methyltransferases (DNMTs) that catalyze the transfer of a methyl group of S-adenosyl methionine to a cytosine. DNMT3a and 3b regulate de novo methylation and are responsible for the establishment of methylation, while DNMT1 is responsible for the maintenance of methylation (Clements et al. 2012). Besides its methyltransferase activity, DNMT1 can also repress transcription of specific genes by associating with histone deacetylases HDAC1, HDAC2, and LSD1. This process is independent of CpG methylation which explains why a subgroup of unmethylated genes is upregulated after treatment with DNA-demethylating drug 5-aza-2′-deoxycytidine.

Methylated CpG residues influence gene expression by recruitment of methyl-CpG-binding domain (MBD) proteins such as MBD1, MBD2, and MeCP2. These proteins prevent binding of other DNA-binding proteins such as CTCF (Hark et al. 2000) and transcription factors to their target sequences and thereby inhibit gene transcription. Furthermore, CpG methylation influences gene transcription by a close interaction with chromatin remodeling processes such as histone (de)acetylation and (de)methylation. Transcriptional inactive genes show a repressive chromatin state characterized by trimethylation of histone 3 lysine 9 (H3K9me3) and lysine 27 (H3K27me3) and deacetylation of H3 and H4 (Ohm et al. 2007). To the contrary, transcriptionally active genes are enriched with di- and trimethylation of histone H3 lysine 4 (H3K4me2/me3) and acetylation of key H3 and H4 amino acids near the transcription start site. The repressive chromatin mark is initiated by Polycomb group of proteins 2 (PRC2). The Polycomb group of proteins (PRC) control long-term transcriptional repression of genes and associate within two multimeric complexes: PRC1 and PRC2 (Sparmann and van Lohuizen 2006). PRC2 is involved in the initiation of silencing by forming H3K27me3 and H3K9me3. PRC2 contains EZH2 (among SUZ12 and EED), which functions as a histone methyltransferase that methylates H3K27, and to a lesser extent H3K9. This mark can attract PRC1 containing BMI1 that recognizes H3K27me3. PRC1 has a role in long-term silencing and includes besides BMI1 the CBX and HPH family of proteins, YY1, RING1/1a, and RING2/1b. Enrichment of EZH2 and the H3K27 mark has been shown to be a characteristic of DNA hypermethylated promoters and silenced genes (Ohm et al. 2007; Squazzo et al. 2006).

It has been shown that EZH2 expression increases during colorectal cancer progression (Wang et al. 2010). EZH2 overexpression and specific polymorphisms in particular are associated with poor prognosis (Crea et al. 2012; Wang et al. 2010). The same association has been described for BMI (Du et al. 2010).

12.4 Which Genes Become Methylated?

One of the key questions that remain to be answered is the mechanism behind the disrupted epigenome in CRC. Aberrant DNA methylation is a tissue-specific process, and the underlying mechanism determining gene specificity is not known.

One hypothesis proposes a role for local DNA sequence features in CRC. Feltus et al. showed by an DNMT1 overexpression experiment involving DNA pattern recognition that methylation-prone- and methylation-resistant CpG islands can be distinguished by an underlying sequence signature based on the frequency of 13 DNA motifs. These motifs might represent protein-binding sites involved in the promotion or prevention of DNA methylation. Methylation-prone motifs, however, do not obviously resemble a transcription factor consensus sequence or protein-binding site. On the other hand, transcription factors PML-RARA and c-MYC (Brenner et al. 2005) have shown to be able to initiate DNA methylation by the recruitment of DNMTs to specific loci. The opposite is observed for the presence of Alu elements and Sp1-binding sites as well as binding of the insulator protein CTCF which are all associated with resistance to DNA methylation (Berman et al. 2012).

Interestingly, genes that become methylated in CRC have shown to be premarked with PcG proteins EZH2 (Bracken et al. 2006; Ohm et al. 2007; Viré et al. 2006) and CBX7 in embryonic stem cell stage. A recent study demonstrated that genes with a methylation-prone sequence motif and genes characterized by Polycomb group protein occupancy in embryonic stem cells are strongly related. These data suggest that tumor-specific targeting of DNA methylation is preprogrammed by epigenetic marks that normally regulate the expression of embryonic genes.

12.5 CpG Island Core Regions

Recent studies have shown that transcriptional inactivation of a gene does not require methylation of the entire CpG island but that CpG methylation of a specific regions within a CpG island, the core region, determines gene silencing. For example, for *P16INK4A* (Gonzalgo et al. 1998) and *MLH1*, it has been reported that a small region in exon 1 and a region proximal of the transcription start site, designated as core regions, determine transcriptional activity. Also for *hTERT* (Zinn et al. 2007), *NDRG4*, and *WIF1* among others, core regions have been identified that were associated with gene silencing and specific clinic-pathologic characteristics. Core regions are often located close to the transcription start site within a CpG island but can theoretically also be present at distant loci such as enhancers.

Methylation outside these core regions is also frequently observed in CRC and has been described to be associated with ageing and inflammation without necessarily affecting gene transcription. DNA methylation at these sites can spread to neighboring regions and to core regions, which might explain the linkage between ageing, inflammation, and cancer.

Therefore, when studying promoter CpG island methylation, it is important to determine CpG methylation at an expression regulating core region of a gene and the association with gene silencing and clinic-pathologic characteristics.

12.6 Chromatin Looping and Long-Range Epigenetic Silencing

Besides epigenetic silencing of individual genes, multiple genes can be transcriptionally silenced coordinately. Due to higher-order chromatin structures and subsequent chromatin looping, it has been shown that different hypermethylated CpG islands can physically interact, cluster, and cooperate in attracting repressor proteins and ensure a transcriptional silenced state. This has been described for *GATA4* (Tiwari et al. 2008) in which DNA looping is crucial for complete gene silencing and affects an entire chromosomal region (Easwaran et al. 2010).

Furthermore, also genes located on large stretches on specific chromosomal regions can undergo simultaneous gene silencing; a phenomenon termed long-range epigenetic silencing. Frigola et al. were the first one to demonstrated epigenetic silencing of a 4 Mb region at chromosome 2q14.2 in CRC. Promoter CpG island methylation was observed in three distinct regions of up to 12 CpG islands (spanning 1 MB) harboring several candidate tumor suppressor genes. Neighboring genes in this 2q14.2 4 MB region were also transcriptionally suppressed and marked with inactive chromatin marks (H3K9me2), even in the absence of promoter CpG island hypermethylation.

Since then, LRES has been reported for more regions in CRC among which a 4-Mb chromosomal region on 3p22 which flanks the *MLH1* gene and chromosomal region 5q32.2. The mechanism underlying LRES is not known. It is not clear whether LRES is initiated by a critical target gene and that a silenced heterochromatin state is spread to innocent bystanders or that neighboring genes are coordinately suppressed due to a specific spatial organization in the nucleus. Whether LRES is a general mechanism involving more chromosomes needs to be unraveled.

12.7 The CpG Island Methylator Phenotype

A specific subset of CRCs displays an exceptionally high frequency of concordantly hypermethylated genes, a phenotype designated as the "CpG island methylation phenotype" (CIMP). CIMP-positive CRCs are well accepted as etiological and clinically distinct CRC subgroup as they are frequently MSI and show characteristics including older age, female sex, proximal tumor location, poor differentiation, *BRAF* mutation, and wild-type *TP53* (Hawkins et al. 2002; Ogino et al. 2007b; Samowitz et al. 2005, 2007; van Rijnsoever et al. 2002; Weisenberger et al. 2006).

Since the introduction of CIMP by Toyota in 1999 (Toyota et al. 1999), however, the concept is under debate (Hughes et al. 2012). The use of different CIMP markers and detection techniques throughout the years has caused confusion by reporting conflicting associations. Different attempts have been made to standardize the gene panel among which a study of Weisenberger et al. who screened 195 CpG islands in 295 CRCs, for a high specificity to a subclass with a high number of methylated genes and selected five gene promoters (*CACNA1G, IGF2, NEUROG1, RUNX3, and SOCS1*) as markers for CIMP (Weisenberger et al. 2006). Although Weisenbergers marker panel outperforms other definitions of CIMP in respect to an association with specific phenotypic characteristics, a bimodal distribution of methylation is only present in MSI CRC and not in MSS/CIMP CRCs (Lee et al. 2008; Nosho et al. 2008; Ogino et al. 2007b). To overcome this problem, Ferracin et al. identified a new panel of markers containing *CACNA1G*, *IGF2*, *RUNX3*, *HTR6*, *RIZ1*, *MINT31*, and *MAP1B* that allows a more distinct classification of CIMP tumors in MSS CRC.

Besides CIMP, a subgroup of CRCs with a lower number of hypermethylated genes, CIMP-low, has been described (Derks et al. 2008; Iacopetta et al. 2006). CIMP-low is associated with *MGMT* CpG island promoter methylation, mutant *KRAS* (Ogino et al. 2006, 2007a), and a poor prognosis (Barault et al. 2008).

Why some genes are methylated within the concept of CIMP(-high) and others in CIMP-low is not known. One of the biggest knowledge deficits remains that the biological cause of CIMP is unclear and that a universal definition is still under debate (Hughes et al. 2012).

12.8 Noncoding RNAs

An additional mechanism of epigenetic regulation involves the role of noncoding (nc) RNAs. ncRNAs are grouped into two major classes based on transcript size: small ncRNAs, microRNAs (miRNA) and short interference RNAs (siRNA),and long ncRNAs (Khalil et al. 2009; Ponjavic et al. 2009). miRNAs serve as regulators of gene expression by annealing to complementary mRNA and core promoter sequences which can lead to translational repression, accelerated mRNA turnover, and heterochromatin formation. miRNAs have important regulatory functions in many biological processes such as cellular proliferation, differentiation, angiogenesis, and apoptosis. Dysregulation of miRNA that is involved in the expression of oncogenes or tumor suppressor genes plays an important role in cancer initiation and cancer progression and metastasis. miRNAs described to be involved in CRC affect multiple processes such as epithelial differentiation (miRNA-141 and miRNA-200c), migration and invasion (miRNA-373 and miRNA-520c), WNT signaling (miRNA-145, miRNA-135a and miRNA-135b), TP53 pathway (miRNA-34b and miRNA-34c), and cell cycle regulation(miRNA-124a) among others frequently undergo promoter CpG island hypermethylation in CRC. Promoter CpG island methylation of miRNA-137 and miRNA-342 has been shown to occur in early stages of CRC (Grady et al. 2008), while silencing of miRNA-148a, miRNA-34b, miRNA-34c, and miRNA-9 has been associated with metastatic CRC. Emerging evidence indicates that every cancer has its own miRNA signature. The availability of miRNA analysis will map the extent of miRNA dysregulation in CRC.

Long ncRNAs, on the other hand, are able to regulate expression of multiple genes by an interaction with chromatin-modifying complexes (Khalil et al. 2009; Ponjavic et al. 2009). Recently, it was shown that long ncRNA Hox transcript antisense intergenic RNA (HOTAIR) is able to epigenetically suppress multiple genes by binding PRC2 subunits (SUZ12 and EZH2) to its 5′ side and thereby trimethylate H3K27 (Kogo et al. 2011). Furthermore, *HOTAIR* can bind histone-modifying complex LSD1/CoREST/REST to its 3′ side and demethylate H3K4 (Tsai et al. 2010). Recently, it has been shown that in CRC *HOTAIR* expression is increased and is associated with liver metastasis and a poor prognosis (Kogo et al. 2011). Another long ncRNA, metastasis associated lung adenocarcinoma transcript 1 (MALAT-1) has been described as well and associates with CRC metastasis (Xu et al. 2011).

12.9 Translational CRC Epigenetics

Due to the high incidence and central role of epigenetic changes in colorectal cancer development, many studies have focused on the development of epigenetic biomarkers in CRC. Furthermore, patients within the same disease stage can demonstrate considerable variation in survival. Biomarkers to assist in the selection of optimal treatment regimes are needed, and multiple methylation markers have shown proof of principle.

12.9.1 Early Detection: Diagnostic Biomarkers

It is known that a reduction in CRC incidence and mortality can be achieved by early detection and removal of premalignant lesions (Zauber et al. 2012). Multiple methods have been described of which colonoscopy is considered the gold standard. Screening compliance, however, is low because of the invasive character of the procedure (Gatto et al. 2003). The (immunological) fecal occult blood test (FOBT) has recently been shown to be a good alternative (Quintero et al. 2012). Subjects are more likely to participate in screening programs using fecal test, but these test do not detect premalignant lesions with the same sensitivity (Imperiale et al. 2004; Quintero et al. 2012). The use of biomarkers, specifically epigenetic biomarkers, in stool, blood, or other body fluids, is a promising alternative due to their noninvasive and potentially highly sensitive character. Several studies have shown proof of principle for the detection of methylation biomarkers in colorectal adenoma- or carcinoma-derived DNA in stool and blood (Ebert et al. 2006; Frattini et al. 2006).

The detection of biomarkers in stool is based on cellular shedding from colorectal neoplasms. Promoter CpG island methylation of exon 1 of Vimentin (VIM) (Itzkowitz et al. 2007) can be detected in stool with a sensitivity of 83 % and specificity of 82 % and is nowadays commercially available in the USA (Itzkowitz et al. 2008, 2007; Li et al. 2009). Due to the high sensitivity of PCR-based methods, different methylation blood markers have been shown proof of principle as well, among which promoter CpG island methylation of *SEPT9* (Lofton-Day et al. 2008) and *TFPI2* (Hibi et al. 2012).

Nowadays, a diversity of fecal and blood methylation markers, single or in panel, are described to detect CRCs with promising sensitivity and specificity (Table 12.1). Like many early studies of biomarkers, however, the numbers of cases and controls analyzed are limited. Results still have to be validated in large independent prospective screening studies, and the sensitivity, specificity, and cost-effectiveness have to be compared directly to colonoscopy and FOBT. Thus, although promising, these issues need to be addressed before epigenetic markers for early detection of CRC can be implemented into clinical practice.

12.9.2 Prognostic Markers

In addition to markers for early detection, methylation biomarkers to predict risk for disease recurrence or metastatic disease could enhance current CRC treatment, particularly in the intermediate stages of disease where treatment decisions are most difficult. Epigenetic changes are potentially useful in this setting. Several publications report a prognostic role for presence of CIMP and promoter methylation of individual genes such as *p16INK4A*, *p14ARF*, *HLTF*, *and CHFR*, among others (Table 12.1), but their effects seem to be dependent on the presence of other methylated markers or adjuvant treatment (Smits et al. 2008). Furthermore, also *LINE-1* hypomethylation (Ogino et al. 2008) and high *miRNA-21* expression are associated with poor prognosis which is independent of other clinical characteristics.

Interestingly, a recent study showed that elevated expression of WNT target genes was associated with good prognosis (de Sousa et al. 2011). This study showed that several WNT target genes among which *ASCL2* and *LGR5* become silenced by promoter CpG island methylation and that this was a strong predictor of disease recurrence.

These examples of potential prognostic use of alterations in DNA methylation highlight the need for validation of the clinical utility in observational, population-based studies to assess the natural course of disease.

12.9.3 Predictive Markers

Multiple anticancer agents are used in metastatic CRC among which the intravenous and oral fluoropyrimidines, 5-FU and capecitabine, the platinum derivative oxaliplatin, the camptothecin derivative and topoisomerase inhibitor irinotecan, and the monoclonal antibodies directed against epidermal growth factor receptor (EGFR) (cetuximab and panitumumab) and vascular endothelial growth factor (VEGF), bevacizumab.

These anticancer agents are used in a standardized treatment protocols. It is known, however, that treatment response can vary greatly among patients and that these differences can be explained by the differences in underlying molecular alterations.

Sensitivity to topoisomerase inhibitor irinotecan, for instance, is dependent upon CpG island methylation of *Werner syndrome gene* (*WRN*) *and UGT1A1* (Gagnon et al. 2006).

CpG island promoter methylation of the DNA repair gene *MGMT* has shown to be associated with resistance to alkylating agents. This association was first described in gliomas (Esteller et al. 2000), and also in CRC, decreased *MGMT* expression has been proposed as marker of sensitivity for oxaliplatin (Park et al. 2010). Furthermore, MSI- and CIMP-positive CRCs show a reduced sensitivity to 5-FU (Warusavitarne and Schnitzler 2007). Recently, Ebert et al. have shown that promoter CpG island methylation of *transcription factor AP-2 epsilon* (*TFAP2*) is associated with resistance to 5-FU-based chemotherapy as well. Although the underlying molecular mechanism is not clear yet, the probability of response was 6 times higher among patients without *TFAP2* promoter methylation.

On a broader level, truncating mutations in the human histone deacetylase gene *HDAC2* in MSI-H CRC are reported to be associated with resistance to the antiproliferative and proapoptotic effects of the HDAC inhibitor trichostatin A (TSA), although this could not be confirmed in an independent study.

Despite these examples and other studies of predictive epigenetic markers in CRC, none have yet been developed to the point of clinical utility. Research on molecular markers is susceptible to publication bias and false-positive results due to small population sizes, selection bias, and small effect sizes, emphasizing the need for confirmation studies to determine the reproducibility of the data. Validation of newly discovered and current markers in randomized clinical trials of colorectal cancer treatment using comparable techniques will be required to truly assess clinical utility.

Conclusions

Colorectal cancer has provided an excellent model for studying the epigenetic basis of cancer. A revolution in epigenetic cancer research has been successful in unraveling the CRC epigenome and shown that DNA methylation, chromatin modifications, and noncoding RNAs occur in a coordinate fashion. Epigenetic changes play an important role in the initiation and progression of colorectal cancer. Future studies should focus on the translation of this knowledge into patient care by the implementation of epigenetic biomarkers for early detection, risk stratification, and tailored cancer treatment but also by the development of therapies to target epigenetic changes.

References

Agrelo R, Cheng WH, Setien F et al (2006) Epigenetic inactivation of the premature aging Werner syndrome gene in human cancer. Proc Natl Acad Sci USA 23:8822–8827

Aguilera C, Nakagawa K, Sancho R et al (2011) c-Jun N-terminal phosphorylation antagonises recruitment of the Mbd3/NuRD repressor complex. Nature 7329:231–235

Baba Y, Nosho K, Shima K et al (2010) Hypomethylation of the IGF2 DMR in colorectal tumors, detected by bisulfite pyrosequencing, is associated with poor prognosis. Gastroenterology 6:1855–1864

Barault L, Charon-Barra C, Jooste V et al (2008) Hypermethylator phenotype in sporadic colon cancer: study on a population-based series of 582 cases. Cancer Res 20:8541–8546

Berman BP, Weisenberger DJ, Aman JF et al (2012) Regions of focal DNA hypermethylation and long-range hypomethylation in colorectal cancer coincide with nuclear lamina-associated domains. Nat Genet 1:40–46

Bos JL, Fearon ER, Hamilton SR et al (1987) Prevalence of ras gene mutations in human colorectal cancers. Nature 6120:293–297

Bracken AP, Dietrich N, Pasini D et al (2006) Genome-wide mapping of Polycomb target genes unravels their roles in cell fate transitions. Genes Dev 9:1123–1136

Brenner C, Deplus R, Didelot C et al (2005) Myc represses transcription through recruitment of DNA methyltransferase corepressor. EMBO J 2:336–346

Clements EG, Mohammad HP, Leadem BR et al (2012) DNMT1 modulates gene expression without its catalytic activity partially through its interactions with histone-modifying enzymes. Nucleic Acids Res 40(10):4334–4346

Crea F, Fornaro L, Paolicchi E et al (2012) An EZH2 polymorphism is associated with clinical outcome in metastatic colorectal cancer patients. Ann Oncol 23(5):1207–1213

Cunningham JM, Christensen ER, Tester DJ et al (1998) Hypermethylation of the hMLH1 promoter in colon cancer with microsatellite instability. Cancer Res 15:3455–3460
de Sousa EMF, Colak S, Buikhuisen J et al (2011) Methylation of cancer-stem-cell-associated Wnt target genes predicts poor prognosis in colorectal cancer patients. Cell Stem Cell 5:476–485
Derks S, Postma C, Carvalho B et al (2008) Integrated analysis of chromosomal, microsatellite and epigenetic instability in colorectal cancer identifies specific associations between promoter methylation of pivotal tumour suppressor and DNA repair genes and specific chromosomal alterations. Carcinogenesis 2:434–439
Douglas EJ, Fiegler H, Rowan A et al (2004) Array comparative genomic hybridization analysis of colorectal cancer cell lines and primary carcinomas. Cancer Res 14:4817–4825
Du J, Li Y, Li J et al (2010) Polycomb group protein Bmi1 expression in colon cancers predicts the survival. Med Oncol 4:1273–1276
Easwaran HP, Van Neste L, Cope L et al (2010) Aberrant silencing of cancer-related genes by CpG hypermethylation occurs independently of their spatial organization in the nucleus. Cancer Res 20:8015–8024
Ebert MP, Model F, Mooney S et al (2006) Aristaless-like homeobox-4 gene methylation is a potential marker for colorectal adenocarcinomas. Gastroenterology 5:1418–1430
Ebert MP, Tanzer M, Balluff B et al (2012) TFAP2E-DKK4 and chemoresistance in colorectal cancer. N Engl J Med 1:44–53
Ehrlich M (2002) DNA methylation in cancer: too much, but also too little. Oncogene 35:5400–5413
Esteller M, Garcia-Foncillas J, Andion E et al (2000) Inactivation of the DNA-repair gene MGMT and the clinical response of gliomas to alkylating agents. N Engl J Med 19:1350–1354
Esteller M, Gonzalez S, Risques RA et al (2001) K-ras and p16 aberrations confer poor prognosis in human colorectal cancer. J Clin Oncol 2:299–304
Fearon ER, Vogelstein B (1990) A genetic model for colorectal tumorigenesis. Cell 5:759–767
Feinberg AP, Tycko B (2004) The history of cancer epigenetics. Nat Rev Cancer 2:143–153
Frattini M, Gallino G, Signoroni S et al (2006) Quantitative analysis of plasma DNA in colorectal cancer patients: a novel prognostic tool. Ann N Y Acad Sci 1075:185–190
Gagnon JF, Bernard O, Villeneuve L et al (2006) Irinotecan inactivation is modulated by epigenetic silencing of UGT1A1 in colon cancer. Clin Cancer Res 6:1850–1858
Gardiner-Garden M, Frommer M (1987) CpG islands in vertebrate genomes. J Mol Biol 2:261–282
Gatto NM, Frucht H, Sundararajan V et al (2003) Risk of perforation after colonoscopy and sigmoidoscopy: a population-based study. J Natl Cancer Inst 3:230–236
Glockner SC, Dhir M, Yi JM et al (2009) Methylation of TFPI2 in stool DNA: a potential novel biomarker for the detection of colorectal cancer. Cancer Res 11:4691–4699
Goelz SE, Vogelstein B, Hamilton SR et al (1985) Hypomethylation of DNA from benign and malignant human colon neoplasms. Science 4696:187–190
Gonzalgo ML, Hayashida T, Bender CM et al (1998) The role of DNA methylation in expression of the p19/p16 locus in human bladder cancer cell lines. Cancer Res 6:1245–1252
Grady WM, Parkin RK, Mitchell PS et al (2008) Epigenetic silencing of the intronic microRNA hsa-miR-342 and its host gene EVL in colorectal cancer. Oncogene 27:3880–3888
Hark AT, Schoenherr CJ, Katz DJ et al (2000) CTCF mediates methylation-sensitive enhancer-blocking activity at the H19/Igf2 locus. Nature 6785:486–489
Hawkins N, Norrie M, Cheong K et al (2002) CpG island methylation in sporadic colorectal cancers and its relationship to microsatellite instability. Gastroenterology 5:1376–1387
Hellebrekers DM, Lentjes MH, van den Bosch SM et al (2009) GATA4 and GATA5 are potential tumor suppressors and biomarkers in colorectal cancer. Clin Cancer Res 12:3990–3997
Herbst A, Wallner M, Rahmig K et al (2009) Methylation of helicase-like transcription factor in serum of patients with colorectal cancer is an independent predictor of disease recurrence. Eur J Gastroenterol Hepatol 5:565–569
Herman JG, Baylin SB (2003) Gene silencing in cancer in association with promoter hypermethylation. N Engl J Med 21:2042–2054

Herman JG, Umar A, Polyak K et al (1998) Incidence and functional consequences of hMLH1 promoter hypermethylation in colorectal carcinoma. Proc Natl Acad Sci USA 12:6870–6875

Hermsen M, Postma C, Baak J et al (2002) Colorectal adenoma to carcinoma progression follows multiple pathways of chromosomal instability. Gastroenterology 4:1109–1119

Hibi K, Goto T, Shirahata A et al (2012) Methylation of TFPI2 no longer detected in the serum DNA of colorectal cancer patients after curative surgery. Anticancer Res 3:787–790

Hughes LA, Khalid-de Bakker CA, Smits KM et al (2012) The CpG island methylator phenotype in colorectal cancer: progress and problems. Biochim Biophys Acta 1:77–85

Iacopetta B, Grieu F, Li W et al (2006) APC gene methylation is inversely correlated with features of the CpG island methylator phenotype in colorectal cancer. Int J Cancer 10:2272–2278

Imperiale TF, Ransohoff DF, Itzkowitz SH et al (2004) Fecal DNA versus fecal occult blood for colorectal-cancer screening in an average-risk population. N Engl J Med 26:2704–2714

Irizarry RA, Ladd-Acosta C, Wen B et al (2009) The human colon cancer methylome shows similar hypo- and hypermethylation at conserved tissue-specific CpG island shores. Nat Genet 2:178–186

Itzkowitz SH, Jandorf L, Brand R et al (2007) Improved fecal DNA test for colorectal cancer screening. Clin Gastroenterol Hepatol 1:111–117

Itzkowitz S, Brand R, Jandorf L et al (2008) A simplified, noninvasive stool DNA test for colorectal cancer detection. Am J Gastroenterol 11:2862–2870

Kawakami K, Matsunoki A, Kaneko M et al (2011) Long interspersed nuclear element-1 hypomethylation is a potential biomarker for the prediction of response to oral fluoropyrimidines in microsatellite stable and CpG island methylator phenotype-negative colorectal cancer. Cancer Sci 1:166–174

Khalil AM, Guttman M, Huarte M et al (2009) Many human large intergenic noncoding RNAs associate with chromatin-modifying complexes and affect gene expression. Proc Natl Acad Sci USA 28:11667–11672

Kim MS, Louwagie J, Carvalho B et al (2009) Promoter DNA methylation of oncostatin m receptor-beta as a novel diagnostic and therapeutic marker in colon cancer. PLoS One 8:e6555

Kogo R, Shimamura T, Mimori K et al (2011) Long noncoding RNA HOTAIR regulates polycomb-dependent chromatin modification and is associated with poor prognosis in colorectal cancers. Cancer Res 20:6320–6326

Lee S, Cho NY, Yoo EJ et al (2008) CpG island methylator phenotype in colorectal cancers: comparison of the new and classic CpG island methylator phenotype marker panels. Arch Pathol Lab Med 10:1657–1665

Lee BB, Lee EJ, Jung EH et al (2009) Aberrant methylation of APC, MGMT, RASSF2A, and Wif-1 genes in plasma as a biomarker for early detection of colorectal cancer. Clin Cancer Res 19:6185–6191

Leung WK, To KF, Man EP et al (2005) Quantitative detection of promoter hypermethylation in multiple genes in the serum of patients with colorectal cancer. Am J Gastroenterol 10:2274–2279

Li M, Chen WD, Papadopoulos N et al (2009) Sensitive digital quantification of DNA methylation in clinical samples. Nat Biotechnol 9:858–863

Lofton-Day C, Model F, Devos T et al (2008) DNA methylation biomarkers for blood-based colorectal cancer screening. Clin Chem 2:414–423

Maeda K, Kawakami K, Ishida Y et al (2003) Hypermethylation of the CDKN2A gene in colorectal cancer is associated with shorter survival. Oncol Rep 4:935–938

Melotte V, Lentjes MH, van den Bosch SM et al (2009) N-Myc downstream-regulated gene 4 (NDRG4): a candidate tumor suppressor gene and potential biomarker for colorectal cancer. J Natl Cancer Inst 13:916–927

Muller HM, Oberwalder M, Fiegl H et al (2004) Methylation changes in faecal DNA: a marker for colorectal cancer screening? Lancet 9417:1283–1285

Nakamura Y, Nishisho I, Kinzler KW et al (1991) Mutations of the adenomatous polyposis coli gene in familial polyposis coli patients and sporadic colorectal tumors. Princess Takamatsu Symp 22:285–292

Nosho K, Irahara N, Shima K et al (2008) Comprehensive biostatistical analysis of CpG island methylator phenotype in colorectal cancer using a large population-based sample. PLoS One 11:e3698

Ogino S, Kawasaki T, Kirkner GJ et al (2006) CpG island methylator phenotype-low (CIMP-low) in colorectal cancer: possible associations with male sex and KRAS mutations. J Mol Diagn 5:582–588

Ogino S, Kawasaki T, Kirkner GJ et al (2007a) Molecular correlates with MGMT promoter methylation and silencing support CpG island methylator phenotype-low (CIMP-low) in colorectal cancer. Gut 11:1564–1571

Ogino S, Kawasaki T, Kirkner GJ et al (2007b) Evaluation of markers for CpG island methylator phenotype (CIMP) in colorectal cancer by a large population-based sample. J Mol Diagn 3:305–314

Ogino S, Meyerhardt JA, Kawasaki T et al (2007c) CpG island methylation, response to combination chemotherapy, and patient survival in advanced microsatellite stable colorectal carcinoma. Virchows Arch 5:529–537

Ogino S, Nosho K, Kirkner GJ et al (2008) A cohort study of tumoral LINE-1 hypomethylation and prognosis in colon cancer. J Natl Cancer Inst 23:1734–1738

Ohm JE, McGarvey KM, Yu X et al (2007) A stem cell-like chromatin pattern may predispose tumor suppressor genes to DNA hypermethylation and heritable silencing. Nat Genet 2:237–242

Park JH, Kim NS, Park JY et al (2010) MGMT -535G>T polymorphism is associated with prognosis for patients with metastatic colorectal cancer treated with oxaliplatin-based chemotherapy. J Cancer Res Clin Oncol 8:1135–1142

Ponjavic J, Oliver PL, Lunter G et al (2009) Genomic and transcriptional co-localization of protein-coding and long non-coding RNA pairs in the developing brain. PLoS Genet 8:e1000617

Quintero E, Castells A, Bujanda L et al (2012) Colonoscopy versus fecal immunochemical testing in colorectal-cancer screening. N Engl J Med 8:697–706

Samowitz WS, Albertsen H, Herrick J et al (2005) Evaluation of a large, population-based sample supports a CpG island methylator phenotype in colon cancer. Gastroenterology 3:837–845

Samowitz WS, Slattery ML, Sweeney C et al (2007) APC mutations and other genetic and epigenetic changes in colon cancer. Mol Cancer Res 2:165–170

Schuebel KE, Chen W, Cope L et al (2007) Comparing the DNA hypermethylome with gene mutations in human colorectal cancer. PLoS Genet 9:1709–1723

Shima K, Nosho K, Baba Y et al (2011) Prognostic significance of CDKN2A (p16) promoter methylation and loss of expression in 902 colorectal cancers: cohort study and literature review. Int J Cancer 5:1080–1094

Smits KM, Cleven AH, Weijenberg MP et al (2008) Pharmacoepigenomics in colorectal cancer: a step forward in predicting prognosis and treatment response. Pharmacogenomics 12: 1903–1916

Sparmann A, van Lohuizen M (2006) Polycomb silencers control cell fate, development and cancer. Nat Rev Cancer 11:846–856

Squazzo SL, O'Geen H, Komashko VM et al (2006) Suz12 binds to silenced regions of the genome in a cell-type-specific manner. Genome Res 7:890–900

Straussman R, Nejman D, Roberts D et al (2009) Developmental programming of CpG island methylation profiles in the human genome. Nat Struct Mol Biol 5:564–571

Suzuki K, Suzuki I, Leodolter A et al (2006) Global DNA demethylation in gastrointestinal cancer is age dependent and precedes genomic damage. Cancer Cell 3:199–207

Tanaka M, Chang P, Li Y et al (2011) Association of CHFR promoter methylation with disease recurrence in locally advanced colon cancer. Clin Cancer Res 13:4531–4540

Tanzer M, Balluff B, Distler J et al (2010) Performance of epigenetic markers SEPT9 and ALX4 in plasma for detection of colorectal precancerous lesions. PLoS One 2:e9061

Tiwari VK, McGarvey KM, Licchesi JD et al (2008) PcG proteins, DNA methylation, and gene repression by chromatin looping. PLoS Biol 12:2911–2927

Toyota M, Ahuja N, Ohe-Toyota M et al (1999) CpG island methylator phenotype in colorectal cancer. Proc Natl Acad Sci USA 15:8681–8686

Tsai MC, Manor O, Wan Y et al (2010) Long noncoding RNA as modular scaffold of histone modification complexes. Science 5992:689–693

van Engeland M, Derks S, Smits KM et al (2011) Colorectal cancer epigenetics: complex simplicity. J Clin Oncol 29(10):1382–1391

van Rijnsoever M, Grieu F, Elsaleh H et al (2002) Characterisation of colorectal cancers showing hypermethylation at multiple CpG islands. Gut 6:797–802

Viré E, Brenner C, Deplus R et al (2006) The Polycomb group protein EZH2 directly controls DNA methylation. Nature 7078:871–874

Wang CG, Ye YJ, Yuan J et al (2010) EZH2 and STAT6 expression profiles are correlated with colorectal cancer stage and prognosis. World J Gastroenterol 19:2421–2427

Warusavitarne J, Schnitzler M (2007) The role of chemotherapy in microsatellite unstable (MSI-H) colorectal cancer. Int J Colorectal Dis 7:739–748

Weber M, Davies JJ, Wittig D et al (2005) Chromosome-wide and promoter-specific analyses identify sites of differential DNA methylation in normal and transformed human cells. Nat Genet 8:853–862

Weisenberger DJ, Siegmund KD, Campan M et al (2006) CpG island methylator phenotype underlies sporadic microsatellite instability and is tightly associated with BRAF mutation in colorectal cancer. Nat Genet 7:787–793

Xu C, Yang M, Tian J et al (2011) MALAT-1: a long non-coding RNA and its important 3' end functional motif in colorectal cancer metastasis. Int J Oncol 1:169–175

Yamaguchi S, Asao T, Nakamura J et al (2003) High frequency of DAP-kinase gene promoter methylation in colorectal cancer specimens and its identification in serum. Cancer Lett 1:99–105

Zauber AG, Winawer SJ, O'Brien MJ et al (2012) Colonoscopic polypectomy and long-term prevention of colorectal-cancer deaths. N Engl J Med 8:687–696

Zhang W, Bauer M, Croner RS et al (2007) DNA stool test for colorectal cancer: hypermethylation of the secreted frizzled-related protein-1 gene. Dis Colon Rectum 10:1618–1626; discussion 1626–1617

Zinn RL, Pruitt K, Eguchi S et al (2007) hTERT is expressed in cancer cell lines despite promoter DNA methylation by preservation of unmethylated DNA and active chromatin around the transcription start site. Cancer Res 1:194–201

Epigenetic Therapies in Solid Tumours: From Preclinical Models to Clinical Trial Results

13

Robert Brown, Juliane Steinmann, Janet Graham, and Ros Glasspool

13.1 Introduction

Since epigenetic marks are reversible, their maintenance enzymes are attractive targets for the development of epigenetic therapies (Kristensen et al. 2009; Lyko and Brown 2005). The DNMT inhibitors 5-azacytidine (Vidaza) and 5-aza-2′-deoxycytidine (Dacogen) show activity against haematological malignancies, whilst HDAC inhibitors, such as vorinostat (SAHA), have clinical activity in the treatment of cutaneous T cell lymphoma. However, the activity of these epigenetic therapies in solid tumours remains uncertain (Kristensen et al. 2009; Graham et al. 2009). Lack of specificity, poor delivery and nontarget-related toxicities have limited the clinical utility of DNMT and HDAC inhibitors to date in solid tumours, and better more targeted agents are required (Graham et al. 2009). Although pharmacodynamic markers have been used to optimise the treatment schedule and identify the biologically active dose of epigenetic therapies, especially when given in combination with chemotherapy, more specific and less toxic drugs are required. Tailoring epigenetic therapies to specific patient populations and specific tumour cell populations may also be important in maximising the clinical activity of these agents.

R. Brown (✉) • J. Graham
Epigenetics Unit, Department Surgery and Cancer, Imperial College London, IRDB 4th Floor, Hammersmith Hospital Campus, London W12 0NN, UK
e-mail: b.brown@imperial.ac.uk

J. Steinmann
Division of Hematology/Oncology, Department of Medicine, University of Freiburg Medical Center, Freiburg, Germany

R. Glasspool
Department of Medical Oncology, The Beatson West of Scotland Cancer Centre, Glasgow, UK

M. Lübbert, P.A. Jones (eds.), *Epigenetic Therapy of Cancer*,
DOI 10.1007/978-3-642-38404-2_13, © Springer-Verlag Berlin Heidelberg 2014

13.2 Demethylating Agents

Over 40 years ago, 5-azacytidine (Vidaza), a cytidine ribose nucleoside analogue, was identified as a potential anticancer therapy and subsequently shown to be a DNMT inhibitor (Jones 1985). It was hoped that the analogue 5-aza-2′-deoxycytidine (decitabine or Dacogen), which is already in the deoxy form, might reduce unwanted toxicity as it can only be incorporated into DNA (Oki et al. 2007). However, although decitabine does show greater DNA methylation inhibition and antitumour activity at equivalent doses to 5-azacytidine in experimental models (Momparler et al. 1984), myelosuppression does remain a significant problem. Zebularine (Zhou et al. 2002), another derivative of 5-azacytidine, has also been developed as a potentially less toxic analogue. Although zebularine was designed as an oral formulation, oral bioavailability is variable in different animal models raising concerns about its bioavailability in humans (Holleran et al. 2005; Cheng et al. 2003).

Initially, demethylating agents were examined clinically in solid tumours as single agents (Schwartsmann et al. 2000). They were given at their maximally tolerated doses where neutropenia was the dose-limiting toxicity. Few responses were seen at these relatively high doses. Issa and colleagues have argued that demethylating agents may be more biologically effective in haematological malignancies at lower, less toxic doses (Kantarjian and Issa 2005; Issa et al. 2004), suggesting that higher doses may inhibit demethylation due to cell cycle arrest preventing incorporation of the 5-azacytidine nucleotides into DNA and hence reducing subsequent demethylation. More recent clinical studies have used lower doses of drug and pharmacodynamic biomarkers of demethylation, such as levels of DNA methylation in surrogate and tumour tissue, to identify maximal biological effect rather than maximum tolerated dose (Appleton et al. 2007).

The original concept behind using epigenetic therapies such as demethylating agents as single agents was based largely on the hypothesis that many tumour suppressor genes are inactivated by epigenetic mechanisms and that reversal of epigenetic silencing at these genes would lead to suppression of tumour growth (Issa and Kantarjian 2009; Glasspool et al. 2006). One of the problems with this concept is that reversal of epigenetic silencing by demethylating agents is transitory and without continued inhibition of maintenance of the repressed epigenetic state, then genes will rapidly become re-silenced. However, the transitory reexpression of genes may provide a window of opportunity to combine such epigenetic therapies with other agents. For instance, DNA methylation and silencing of drug sensitivity genes has been implicated in mechanisms of acquired resistance to cytotoxic chemotherapy and reversal of this silencing may provide a window of opportunity to combine a demethylating agent with cytotoxic chemotherapy and hence overcome acquired drug resistance (Glasspool et al. 2006; Teodoridis et al. 2004).

In animal studies, demethylating agents sensitised tumours to cytotoxic chemotherapies such as carboplatin, suggesting that decitabine may indeed reverse clinical acquired drug resistance (Plumb et al. 2000). Appleton et al. (2007) have reported the results of a phase I trial of carboplatin and decitabine in patients with solid tumours. In the phase I study, patients received escalating doses of decitabine administered as a 6-h infusion on day 1 followed by carboplatin on day 8. The major toxicity was myelosuppression. Decitabine induced dose-dependent, reversible demethylation in peripheral blood cells (PBCs) maximally at day 10. Furthermore, decitabine induced demethylation of CpG island at gene promoters in PBCs, buccal cells and tumour biopsies, as well as elevation of epigenetically regulated gene expression. They concluded that decitabine could be combined safely with carboplatin at a dose and schedule that caused epigenetic changes equivalent to or greater than that observed in mice with carboplatin-sensitised xenografts. They recommended a dose/schedule for the phase II trial of decitabine 90 mg/m^2 (day 1) followed by carboplatin AUC 6 (day 8) every 28 days.

Two other phase I studies have investigated the combination of a demethylating agent and carboplatin in ovarian cancer patients (Fang et al. 2010; Fu et al. 2011). Both included patients with disease relapsing within 6 months of their last carboplatin and both used 5-day schedules for the demethylating agent. Fang et al. gave decitabine days 1–5 with carboplatin (AUC 5) on day 8, with a recommended dose of 10 mg/m^2 of decitabine. Fu et al. used azacytidine (75 mg/m^2 sc) days 1–5 with carboplatin (AUC 4 or 5) on day 2. Despite the relatively low-dose intensity of carboplatin- and platinum-resistant population, both studies saw responses (11 and 13.8 %). In the Fu study, the majority of patients with platinum-resistant disease had received other therapy prior to entry on to azacytidine plus carboplatin, with platinum-free intervals ranging from 6 to 31 months. Hence, some response to carboplatin alone could be expected; nevertheless, the results are interesting. It is of note that in both studies the responses occurred after several cycles suggesting that prolonged treatment with a demethylating agent may be required.

Following on from the recommended dose and schedule recommended by Appleton et al. of decitabine 90 mg/m^2 (day 1) followed by carboplatin AUC 6 (day 8) every 28 days, a randomised phase II trial was started in patients with recurrent ovarian cancer that had progressed within 6–12 months following the first round of platinum therapy (Glasspool et al. 2009). Based on previous studies showing acquired methylation of *hMLH1* following platinum treatment (Gifford et al. 2004), it was hypothesised that patients with methylation of specific genes within their tumours would have a greater chance of benefiting from the combined decitabine/carboplatin treatment. Therefore, the study was powered to contain a sufficient number of patients to allow the primary endpoint to be a comparison of response to carboplatin, with and without decitabine, in patients with methylated *hMLH1*.

However, the study was closed early, after a planned interim analysis, due to poor feasibility and lack of efficacy of the combination. The starting dose of decitabine was reduced from 90 to 45 mg/m^2 as the frequency of dose delays of carboplatin due to prolonged neutropenia were considered unacceptable. Also, none of the 11 patients on the combination arm, treated with 45 mg/m^2, completed 6 cycles, compared to 7 of 14 patients completing on carboplatin alone. In women that received more than one cycle of the combination, there were no objective radiological (RECIST) responses on the combination arm, and whilst two women had short-lived CA125 responses (59 and 63 days), these were not considered clinically relevant. In contrast 6 of 14 patients on carboplatin alone had responses consistent with the expected efficacy of carboplatin in this population. Also, grade 2/3 hypersensitivity reactions were more common with the combination treatment than with carboplatin alone (64 % vs. 21 %), as were prolonged treatment delays due to neutropenia (36 % (for 45 mg/m^2) vs. 14 %). Consequently decitabine was not considered to be effective or feasible for reversing platinum resistance with this dose and schedule (Glasspool et al. 2009).

The additional myelosuppression meant that less than half the patients in the combination arm received more than 2 cycles of treatment and so one possibility for the lack of efficacy seen in this phase II trial may have been the short duration of demethylation. In order for these agents to progress within the solid tumour setting, it will be important to develop agents that are less myelosuppressive or optimise schedules that are less toxic whilst retaining demethylating activity. Another feasible explanation may have been that the demethylation of certain genes, for instance *BRCA1*, led to an adverse affect counteracting the carboplatin sensitising effect of demethylated *MLH1* (Teodoridis et al. 2005). This again highlights the importance of patient selection based on their tumour methylation profile for treatments and future studies.

Matei et al. (2012) examined the combination of decitabine days 1–5 with carboplatin (AUC 5) on day 8, with a recommended dose of 10 mg/m^2 of decitabine in a nonrandomised phase II of ovarian cancer patients relapsing less than 6 months following last treatment. In contrast to the study of carboplatin and decitabine described above, they observed a response rate of 35 % and median PFS of 10.2 months, which is certainly higher than would be expected in a platinum-resistant population treated with carboplatin alone. Interestingly, despite the lower dose of carboplatin (AUC 5 q 28 days), Matei et al. had to give pegfilgastim to avoid prolonged neutropenia, and they also saw a high rate of hypersensitivity reactions (35 %).

The reasons for the difference between these two trials of decitabine and carboplatin in relapsed ovarian cancer are not clear (Glasspool et al. 2009; Matei et al. 2012). The low response rate in the study of Glasspool et al. (2009) was not explained by significant differences in carboplatin dose intensity. It is also possible that the 5-day schedule used by Matei et al. induced more prolonged demethylation during each cycle which was more effective in reversing resistance. Alternatively, the inclusion of patients with <6 months PFS may have selected a group of patients more responsive to demethylating agents than the 6–12-month group.

A phase I study of decitabine with doxorubicin and cyclophosphamide in children with neuroblastoma and other solid tumours has been reported (George et al. 2010). Patients received a 1-h decitabine infusion for 7 days, followed by doxorubicin (45 mg/m^2) and cyclophosphamide (1 g/m^2) on day 7. Biological studies included methylation and gene expression analyses of caspase-8, MAGE-1 and foetal haemoglobin (HbF) and expression profiling of pre- and post-treatment peripheral blood and bone marrow cells. The authors concluded that low-dose decitabine when combined with doxorubicin/cyclophosphamide has tolerable toxicity in children. However, doses of decitabine capable of producing clinically relevant biologic effects were not well tolerated with this combination.

A disadvantage of cytidine ribose nucleoside analogues is their incorporation into the entire genome and their lack of gene specificity, which leads to DNA damage throughout the genome. This unwanted toxicity could be avoided by inhibiting the DNMT catalytic site directly, without requiring incorporation into DNA. An increasing number of putative non-nucleoside DNMT inhibitors are now being examined for demethylating activity (Lyko and Brown 2005). However, the demethylating activity and ability to induce gene reexpression of some of these remains controversial, and benchmarking studies have shown substantially lower activity of the non-nucleoside inhibitors compared to nucleoside inhibitors (Brueckner et al. 2007; Yoo et al. 2007). One example of an alternative to nucleoside DNMT inhibitor is the oligonucleotide (20mer) antisense inhibitor of DNMT1 MG98 (Reid et al. 2002). MG98 downregulates DNMT1 in vitro and there is evidence of suppression of DNMT1 expression in some patients, but the downstream effects of DNA demethylation were not detectable in tumour or surrogate tissues in a comparable way to that observed for nucleoside DNMT inhibitors (Plummer et al. 2009; Klisovic et al. 2008). In a phase II clinical trial, MG98 failed to show efficacy in patients with renal cancer (Winquist et al. 2006).

Variation in drug metabolism in patients could influence the patients' response to DNMT inhibitors and thereby limit antitumour activity. For instance, deamination of 5-azacytidine and 5-aza-2′-deoxycytidine leads to their rapid inactivation, converting each of them into the respective 5-azauridine compound. The compound SGI110 (a 5-AzapG-3 dinucleotide) is protected from deamination by cytidine deaminase when given systemically but released 5-aza-2′-deoxycytidine in tumour cells (Yoo et al. 2007). Resistance to cytosine deamination may allow lower doses of DNMT inhibitor to be given with the same effect on demethylation in tumour cells but less systemic toxicity which could ameliorate some of the myelotoxicity associated with nucleoside DNMT inhibitors.

13.3 Histone Acetylation and HDAC Inhibitors

There have been a large number of studies examining the potential of targeting HDACs as anticancer targets, leading to a variety of types of HDAC inhibitor entering clinical trials (Bolden et al. 2006). Encouragement for the development of HDAC inhibitors in cancer came from reports of aberrant HDAC expression patterns in tumours and the suppression of tumour growth following knockdown of overexpressed HDACs (Bandyopadhyay et al. 2004). The hydroxamic acid moiety of HDAC inhibitors, such as vorinostat (SAHA), directly interacts with the zinc ion at the base of the catalytic pocket (Xu et al. 2007). However, it is worth emphasising that important regulatory proteins, such as hormone receptors, chaperon proteins and cytoskeleton proteins, regulating cell proliferation, immune response and cell death, are nonhistone substrates of HDACs (Bi and Jiang 2006). Thus, the effect of HDAC inhibitor treatment may be due to changes in these nonhistone proteins (Pediconi et al. 2003). Also, HDAC inhibitors are known to elevate reactive oxygen species (ROS) levels. This can induce cell death in a manner independent of caspase activation (Bolden et al. 2006).

Impressive results in clinical trials of the HDAC inhibitor vorinostat have been seen in cutaneous T cell lymphoma with partial responses of around 30 % in patients with advanced disease, many of whom have had multiple lines of previous chemotherapy (Duvic et al. 2007, 2009). However, the efficacy of these agents in solid tumours remains uncertain (Graham et al. 2009). Pooled clinical trial data from patients with solid or haematological malignancies show that vorinostat is well tolerated (Siegel et al. 2009). The most commonly reported drug-related adverse events are fatigue, nausea, diarrhoea, anorexia and vomiting, with the majority of adverse events being Grade 2 or less. Clinical trials of HDAC inhibitors in solid tumours have shown that pharmacodynamic responses in surrogate tissues (such as histone acetylation changes in lymphocytes) can be achieved at well-tolerated doses (Galanis et al. 2009; Steele et al. 2008). However, single agent efficacy has been limited in early clinical trials. For instance, in recurrent ovarian cancer patients, 2 out of 27 enrolled patients were progression-free over 6 months, with one having a partial response (Modesitt et al. 2008). Similarly, in advanced prostate cancer, the best objective response was stable disease in two (7 %) patients (Bradley et al. 2009). In recurrent and/or metastatic head and neck cancer, there were no confirmed responses in 12 patients (Blumenschein et al. 2008), and no responses were seen in 12 patients with breast cancer (although four patients did show stable disease) (Luu et al. 2008).

Many investigators feel that HDAC inhibitors are more likely to be effective in solid tumours if used in combination with cytotoxics or other biological therapy (Graham et al. 2009). Additive or synergistic activity with conventional anticancer agents has been shown in various models (Takai and Narahara 2010). One explanation for synergistic activity is that an increase in histone acetylation produces a more open DNA conformation which makes chromatin more permissive for gene transcription and hence reexpression of silenced genes. This could lead to increased expression of genes involved in apoptosis, including reexpression of pro-apoptotic genes and hence chemosensitisation. However, pretreatment of tumour cells with HDAC inhibitors may also increase initial damage and cause an increased DNA damage response. This could be as a result of a more open chromatin state resulting in greater DNA damage being induced following treatment with DNA damaging therapies, such as ionising radiation and platinum-based chemotherapy.

There are preclinical data in ovarian cancer models supporting the idea that the efficacy of carboplatin and paclitaxel might be improved by pretreating patients with HDAC inhibitors. A combination study of belinostat with carboplatin and paclitaxel showed enhanced growth inhibitory activity in ovarian tumour models (Qian et al. 2006). Furthermore, the HDAC inhibitor belinostat potentiates the chemosensitisation of decitabine in platinum-resistant ovarian xenografts in vivo (Steele et al. 2009). Pretreatment with vorinostat increases the cytotoxicity of a variety of DNA damaging agents, including platinum compounds, in cell line models (Kim et al. 2003). A novel HDAC inhibitor, OSU-HDAC42 also shows promising activity and sensitises platinum-resistant xenografts to cisplatin (Yang et al. 2009).

Further support for the use of this combination comes from a phase II randomised, double-blinded, placebo-controlled study which evaluated the efficacy of vorinostat in combination with carboplatin and paclitaxel in patients with advanced-stage NSCLC (Ramalingam et al. 2010). The confirmed response rate was 34 % with vorinostat versus 12.5 % with placebo ($p=0.02$). There was a trend toward improvement in median progression-free survival (6.0 months vs. 4.1 months; $p=0.48$) and overall survival (13.0 months vs. 9.7 months; $p=0.17$) in the vorinostat arm. Grade 4 platelet toxicity was more common with vorinostat (18 % vs. 3 %; $p<0.05$). Nausea, emesis, fatigue, dehydration and hyponatraemia also were more frequent with vorinostat.

The combination of a demethylating agent such as decitabine together with an HDAC inhibitor has been shown in tumour models to be more effective at reversing epigenetic silencing in vitro and in vivo than either agent alone (Steele et al. 2009; Cameron et al. 1999). A phase I study of the combination of decitabine with vorinostat in patients with advanced solid tumours or non-Hodgkin's lymphomas showed a maximum tolerated dose (MTD) of decitabine 10 mg/m^2/day on days 1–5 and vorinostat 200 mg three times a day on days 6–12 in a sequential schedule and decitabine 10 mg/m^2/day on days 1–5 with vorinostat 200 mg twice a day on days 3–9 on a concurrent schedule. However, the sequential schedule of decitabine 10 mg/m^2/day on days 1–5 and vorinostat 200 mg twice a day on days 6–12 was more deliverable than both MTDs with fewer delays on repeated dosing and was the recommended phase II dose of this combination. Disease stabilisation for ≥ 4 cycles was observed in 11/38 (29 %) evaluable patients.

There are various issues with HDAC inhibitors which will need to be addressed if they are to be used successfully in a solid tumour setting. Firstly, their often short pharmacokinetic half-life may be a problem, especially if being delivered to a solid tumour rather than a haematological malignancy. Although HDAC inhibitors do appear to have a reasonably long pharmacodynamic half-life, as measured, for instance, by histone acetylation of PBCs, it is not clear whether their half-life exceeds the time taken to infiltrate a solid tumour to execute function. Secondly, as discussed earlier there is also uncertainty whether histone acetylation really is the chemotherapeutic target since HDACs have multiple targets, amongst them crucial regulators of cell cycle and apoptosis. Establishing the underlying mechanism for the success of these agents in cutaneous T cell lymphoma (CTCL), and whether this is relevant to other tumours, may help identify the types of tumours likely to respond to HDAC chemotherapy (Khan et al. 2010).

13.4 Future Epigenetic Targets in Solid Tumours

Increasingly, it will be important to focus on epigenetic therapies that have the potential to act in a more targeted way than the currently available compounds. Although our knowledge of epigenetic mechanisms and their control in solid tumours is ever-increasing and will certainly continue to uncover potential targets for anticancer drug development, it is still not clear which exact events trigger and maintain the deregulation of the epigenetic code. This will make cancer-specific rational approaches to the discovery of novel epigenetic therapies challenging.

An alternative approach to demethylating agents that targets methylation-dependent silencing at CpG islands could be to inhibit the mediators of DNA methylation's effects on gene expression, rather than the mark itself (Chapman-Rothe and Brown 2009). Methyl binding domain (MBD) proteins have a crucial role in linking DNA methylation with transcriptional silencing and may be potential targets for epigenetic therapies which would reactivate gene expression by inhibiting the repressive effects of MBD-dependent epigenetic silencing (Sansom et al. 2007). MBD2 knockdown in tumour cell lines causes upregulation of specific epigenetically silenced genes, e.g. $p14^{ARF}$ (Martin et al. 2008). Furthermore, deficiency of MBD2 reduces adenoma burden on an $APC^{(Min/+)}$ background through Wnt signalling, and in contrast to DNMT1 hypomorphs, there is no predisposition to lymphomagenesis in these mice (Martin et al. 2008). Unlike nucleoside DNMT inhibitors, the reversal of methylation-dependent silencing by an MBD inhibitor would not be predicted to be dependent on DNA replication and may have a greater level of specificity to transcription of sets of key genes, without affecting the protective effect of DNA methylation, at non-transcribed regions, on genomic integrity.

Recent studies also demonstrated that the deregulation of histone lysine methyltransferases (HMKT) and histone lysine demethylases may be important targets for therapy in solid tumours (Mund and Lyko 2010). Polycomb group (PcG) proteins have been shown to be required for the maintenance of embryonic stem cells and could therefore also have a role in maintaining tumour stem/sustaining cells (Sauvageau and Sauvageau 2008; Lee et al. 2006; Boyer et al. 2005). Indeed, the key component of Polycomb repressive complex (PCR2) EZH2, a specific histone 3 lysine 27 (H3K27) methyltransferase, is essential for stem cell maintenance in glioblastoma and ovarian tumours (Rizzo et al. 2011; Suva et al. 2009). EZH2 plays a critical role in tumorigenesis and cancer progression through epigenetic gene silencing and chromatin remodelling (Simon and Lange 2008; Cao and Zhang 2004). There is increasing evidence that overexpression of the *EZH2* gene occurs in a variety of human malignancies, including oral, oesophageal, gastric, colon, hepatocellular, bladder, breast, prostate and endometrial cancers (Matsukawa et al. 2006; Bryant et al. 2007; Collett et al. 2006). Putative oncogenic and tumour suppressive roles for EZH2 have been suggested (Karanikolas et al. 2009; Nikoloski et al. 2010). Elevated expression of EZH2 has been shown to be associated with advanced stages of ovarian cancer and independently associated with short overall survival of ovarian cancer patients (Rao et al. 2010). Furthermore, EZH2 knockdown in ovarian cell lines leads to reduced cell growth/proliferation and inhibited cell migration and/or invasion in vitro (Rao et al. 2010), as well as resensitisation of drug-resistant ovarian cancer cells to cisplatin (Hu et al. 2010). Development of specific inhibitors of EZH2 and other HKMTs will have potential as drugs that target this key subpopulation of drug-resistant, tumour-sustaining cells. An overview of published trials with epigenetically active substances for solid tumors is provided in (Table 13.1).

Table 13.1 Published trials with epigenetically active substances for different solid tumour entities

Tumour entity	Substance	Phase	Patients number	Response	Median survival	Literature
Non-small cell lung cancer	Decitabine	I/II	15		OS 6.7 months OS >15 months in three patients	Momparler et al. (1997)
	Decitabine	Case report			81-month survival	Momparler and Ayoub (2001)
	Decitabine	I	35	Target gene induction in 36 %		Schrump et al. 2006)
	Decitabine + cisplatin	I II	8 14	No objective response	OS 3.7 months	Schwartsmann et al. (2000)
	DHAC	II	17	5 SD for ≥ 2 months		Holoye et al. (1987)
	Azacytidine + entinostat	I/II	19	1 CR, 1 PR 24 months	OS 6.4 months	Juergens et al. (2011)
	Romidepsin	II	16	3 SD	PFS 1.8 months OS 6 months	Otterson et al. (2010)
	Vorinostat	II	16	8 SD	OS 7.1 months	Traynor et al. (2009)
	Vorinostat or placebo + carboplatin + paclitaxel	II	62 vorinostat 32 placebo		PFS 6.0 versus 4.1 months OS 13.0 versus 9.7 months	Ramalingam et al. (2010)
	Vorinostat + sorafenib	I	15	1 PR, 8 SD	PFS 2.2 months	Dasari et al. (2012)
	Entinostat or placebo + erlotinib	II	67 entinostat 65 placebo	High E-cadherin expression levels at time of diagnosis indicate increased sensitivity to HDACi/EGFRTKI inhibition		Witta et al. (2012)
Mesothelioma	DHAC	II	41	1 CR, 2 PR		Yogelzang et al. (1997)

(continued)

Table 13.1 (continued)

Tumour entity	Substance	Phase	Patients number	Response	Median survival	Literature
Head and neck cancer	Decitabine	II	27	1 PR		Abele et al. (1987)
	Vorinostat	II	12	1 PR (not confirmed) 3 SD (9–27 weeks)		Blumenschein et al. (2008)
	Romidepsin	II	14	2 SD		Haigentz et al. (2012)
Gastric cancer	Vorinostat	I	10	4 SD >8 weeks	PFS 2.3 months	Doi et al. (2012)
Colorectal cancer	Decitabine	II	42	1 PR		Abele et al. (1987)
	Decitabine + vorinostat	I	11	2 SD		Stathis et al. (2011)
	VPA	I	10	MTD i.v. 60 mg/kg		Atmaca et al. (2007)
	Vorinostat + 5FU + leucovorin	II	58	1PR	2-month PFS 53 %, OS 6.5 months	Fakih et al. (2012)
	Belinostat	I	12	No objective responses		Steele et al. (2008)
Hepatocellular carcinoma	Resminostat	II	Ongoing study			Bitzer 2012 (2012)
Breast cancer	Vorinostat	I/II	26	UGT2B17*2 genotype increases vorinostat efficacy + toxicity		Wong 2011 (2011)
	Vorinostat	II	14	4 SD	PFS 2.6 months OS 24 months	Luu et al. (2008)
	Vorinostat + tamoxifen	II	43	19 % CR/PR, 21 % SD >24 weeks	OS 29 months	Munster et al. (2011)
	Vorinostat + doxorubicin	I	5	Max. dose 800 mg/day 2 PR, 2 SD >8 weeks		Munster et al. (2009a)
	VPA + epirubicin/FEC	I II	10 15	64 % CR/PR		Munster et al. (2009b)

Ovarian cancer	Azacytidine	Ib–IIa	29	1 CR, 3 PR, 10 SD	PFS 3.7 months, OS 14 months	Fu et al. (2011)
	Azacytidine + entinostat	I		2 PR, 11 SD (lung, ovarian)	PFS 2 months	Bauman et al. (2012)
	Decitabine + carboplatin	I	10	1 CR, 4 SD ≥6 months		Fang et al. (2010)
	Decitabine + carboplatin	II	17	1 CR, 5 PR, 6 SD ≥3 months	PFS 10.2 months	Matei et al. (2012)
	Vorinostat	II	22	1 PR	2 PFS ≥6 months	Modesitt et al. (2008)
	Belinostat	II	32	1 PR, 10 SD	PFS 13.4 months	Mackay et al. (2010)
	Belinostat + carboplatin	II	27	1 CR, 1 PR, 12 SD	PFS 3.3 months OS 13.7 months	Dizon et al. (2012a)
	Belinostat + carboplatin + paclitaxel	II	35	3 CR, 12 PR	6-month PFS 46 % OS n.r.	Dizon et al. (2012b)
	VPA + hydralazine	II	7	3 PR, 4 SD	PFS 3.3 months OS 6.1 months	Candelaria et al. (2007)
Prostate cancer	DAC	II	12	2 SD >10 weeks		Thibault et al. (1998)
	Panobinostat alone and + docetaxel	I	16	63 % > or = 50 % decline in PSA		Rathkopf et al. (2010)
	Vorinostat	II	27	2 SD	PFS 2.8 months OS 11.7 months	Bradley et al. (2009)
Renal cell carcinoma	Decitabine/IL-2	I	5	No objective response		Gollob et al. (2006)
	Vorinostat + sorafenib	I	8	6 SD	PFS 6.8 months	Dasari et al. (2012)
	Panobinostat	II	20	No objective response		Hainsworth et al. (2011)
Bladder cancer	Vorinostat	I	7	1 SD		Kelly et al. (2005)
	Vorinostat	II	Ongoing study			Quinn (2012)

(continued)

Table 13.1 (continued)

Tumour entity	Substance	Phase	Patients number	Response	Median survival	Literature
Malignant melanoma	Decitabine	II	18	1 PR		Abele et al. (2012)
	Decitabine	I	19	No objective response		Aparicio et al. (2003)
	Decitabine + IL-2	I	13	1 CR, 2 PR DAC enhances IL-2 activity		Gollob et al. (2006)
	DHAC	II	40	1 CR >11 months, 1 CR >4.7 months	1-month PFS 6.7-month OS	Creagan et al. (1993)
	Vorinostat + doxorubicin	I	6	2 SD ≥8 months		Munster et al. (2009a)
	Vorinostat + marizomib	I	17	SD 61, 39 % decreases in tumour size		Millward et al. (2012)
	Entinostat	II	28	7 SD	OS 8.84 months	Hauschild et al. (2008)
	VPA + karenitecin	I/II	39	47 % SD	OS 8.2 months	Daud et al. (2009)
Soft tissue sarcoma	Vorinostat	II	40	Ongoing		Egerer G (2012)
	Vorinostat	Case report	1	SD (18 months)		Lee and McGuire (2012)
Brain tumours	Vorinostat	II	66		OS 5.7 months	Galanis et al. (2009)
	Vorinostat + bortezomib	II	37	1 PR	OS 3.2 months	Friday et al. (2012)
	Vorinostat + bevacizumab + CPT-11	I	19		High-dose versus low-dose: OS 10.1 versus 5.7, PFS 4.25 versus 1.9	Chinnaiyan et al. (2012)
	Romidepsin	II	35		PFS 8 weeks, 1 PFS >6 months	Iwamoto et al. (2011)
	Panobinostat + bevacizumab	I	12	3 PR, 7 SD	3 (25 %) PFS >6 months PFS 4.3 months OS 8.2 months	Drappatz et al. (2012)
	VPA	Case report	1	CR after 10-month VPA (RCTX-refractory)	16-month PFS	Witt et al. (2004)

Conclusions

It is now clear that normal differentiation control breaks down during tumour development and that all tumour types show aberrant regulation of the epigenetic code, including changes in DNA methylation, histone modification and microRNAs. This has lead to much interest in the development of epigenetic cancer therapies to target this aberrant epigenetic regulation. Histone deacetylase (HDAC) and DNA methyltransferase (DNMT) inhibitors are now used in the treatment of certain haematological malignancies. However, their more general applicability to solid tumours remains unproven and may be limited by lack of specificity and delivery challenges. Novel approaches to overcome these limitations and to develop more specific drugs are required. Ultimately, improved specificity of epigenetic therapies will require increased mapping of the aberrant epigenetic landscape in cancer and cancer-specific target validation using chemical epigenetic approaches.

In addition to improved chemical epigenetic approaches, tumour biomarkers and an understanding of the biology will be key to improved epigenetic therapy approaches. As cancer results from a combination of epigenetic and genetic aberrations, it is anticipated that having combinations of therapeutic approaches available will be important. This raises additional challenges of optimising the dose and schedule of these agents when given in combination and of personalising therapies depending on the molecular characteristics of the patients' tumours. Defining the epigenetic and genetic landscape for individual patients may allow epigenetic therapies to be targeted to groups of patients who will particularly benefit from these therapies.

References

Abele R, Clavel M, Dodion P et al (1987) The EORTC Early Clinical Trials Cooperative Group experience with 5-aza-2′-deoxycytidine (NSC 127716) in patients with colo-rectal, head and neck, renal carcinomas and malignant melanomas. Eur J Cancer Clin Oncol 23:1921–1924

Aparicio A, Eads CA, Leong LA et al (2003) Phase I trial of continuous infusion 5-aza-2′- deoxycytidine. Cancer Chemother Pharmacol 51:231–239

Appleton K, Mackay HJ, Judson I, Plumb JA, McCormick C, Strathdee G, Lee C, Barrett S, Reade S, Jadayel D, Tang A, Bellenger K, Mackay L, Setanoians A, Schatzlein A, Twelves C, Kaye SB, Brown R (2007) Phase I and pharmacodynamic trial of the DNA methyltransferase inhibitor decitabine and carboplatin in solid tumors. J Clin Oncol 25:4603–4609

Atmaca A, Al-Batran SE, Maurer A et al (2007) Valproic acid (VPA) in patients with refractory advanced cancer: a dose escalating phase I clinical trial. Br J Cancer 97:177–182

Bandyopadhyay D, Mishra A, Medrano EE (2004) Overexpression of histone deacetylase 1 confers resistance to sodium butyrate-mediated apoptosis in melanoma cells through a p53-mediated pathway. Cancer Res 64:7706–7710

Bauman J, Verschraegen C, Belinsky S et al (2012) A phase I study of 5-azacytidine and erlotinib in advanced solid tumor malignancies. Cancer Chemother Pharmacol 69:547–554

Bi G, Jiang G (2006) The molecular mechanism of HDAC inhibitors in anticancer effects. Cell Mol Immunol 3:285–290

Bitzer M (2012) 4SC-201 (resminostat) and sorafenib in advanced hepatocellular carcinoma (Shelter). ClinicalTrials.gov: http://clinicaltrials.gov/ct2/show/NCT00943449?term=resminostat+hcc&rank=1

Blumenschein GR Jr, Kies MS, Papadimitrakopoulou VA, Lu C, Kumar AJ, Ricker JL, Chiao JH, Chen C, Frankel SR (2008) Phase II trial of the histone deacetylase inhibitor vorinostat (Zolinza, suberoylanilide hydroxamic acid, SAHA) in patients with recurrent and/or metastatic head and neck cancer. Invest New Drugs 26:81–87

Bolden JE, Peart MJ, Johnstone RW (2006) Anticancer activities of histone deacetylase inhibitors. Nat Rev Drug Discov 5:769–784

Boyer LA, Lee TI, Cole MF, Johnstone SE, Levine SS, Zucker JP, Guenther MG, Kumar RM, Murray HL, Jenner RG, Gifford DK, Melton DA, Jaenisch R, Young RA (2005) Core transcriptional regulatory circuitry in human embryonic stem cells. Cell 122:947–956

Bradley D, Rathkopf D, Dunn R, Stadler WM, Liu G, Smith DC, Pili R, Zwiebel J, Scher H, Hussain M (2009) Vorinostat in advanced prostate cancer patients progressing on prior chemotherapy (National Cancer Institute Trial 6862): trial results and interleukin-6 analysis: a study by the Department of Defense Prostate Cancer Clinical Trial Consortium and University of Chicago Phase 2 Consortium. Cancer 115:5541–5549

Brueckner B, Kuck D, Lyko F (2007) DNA methyltransferase inhibitors for cancer therapy. Cancer J 13:17–22

Bryant RJ, Cross NA, Eaton CL, Hamdy FC, Cunliffe VT (2007) EZH2 promotes proliferation and invasiveness of prostate cancer cells. Prostate 67:547–556

Cameron EE, Bachman KE, Myohanen S, Herman JG, Baylin SB (1999) Synergy of demethylation and histone deacetylase inhibition in the re-expression of genes silenced in cancer. Nat Genet 21:103–107

Candelaria M, Gallardo-Rincón D, Arce C et al (2007) A phase II study of epigenetic therapy with hydralazine and magnesium valproate to overcome chemotherapy resistance in refractory solid tumors. Ann Oncol 18:1529–1538

Cao R, Zhang Y (2004) The functions of E(Z)/EZH2-mediated methylation of lysine 27 in histone H3. Curr Opin Genet Dev 14:155–164

Chapman-Rothe N, Brown R (2009) Approaches to target the genome and its epigenome in cancer. Future Med Chem 1:1481–1495

Cheng JC, Matsen CB, Gonzales FA, Ye W, Greer S, Marquez VE, Jones PA, Selker EU (2003) Inhibition of DNA methylation and reactivation of silenced genes by zebularine. J Natl Cancer Inst 95:399–409

Chinnaiyan P, Chowdhary S, Potthast L et al (2012) Phase I trial of vorinostat combined with bevacizumab and CPT-11 in recurrent glioblastoma. Neuro Oncol 14:93–100

Collett K, Eide GE, Arnes J, Stefansson IM, Eide J, Braaten A, Aas T, Otte AP, Akslen LA (2006) Expression of enhancer of zeste homologue 2 is significantly associated with increased tumor cell proliferation and is a marker of aggressive breast cancer. Clin Cancer Res 12:1168–1174

Creagan ET, Schaid DJ, Hartmann LC et al (1993) A phase II study of 5,6-dihydro-5-azacytidine hydrochloride in disseminated malignant melanoma. Am J Clin Oncol 16:243–244

Dasari A, Gore L, Messersmith WA et al (2012) A phase I study of sorafenib and vorinostat in patients with advanced solid tumors with expanded cohorts in renal cell carcinoma and non-small cell lung cancer. Invest New Drugs. doi:10.1007/s10637-012-9812-z

Daud AI, Dawson J, DeConti RC et al (2009) Potentiation of a topoisomerase I inhibitor, karenitecin, by the histone deacetylase inhibitor valproic acid in melanoma: translational and phase I/II clinical trial. Clin Cancer Res 15:2479–2487

Dizon DS, Blessing JA, Penson RT et al (2012a) A phase II evaluation of belinostat and carboplatin in the treatment of recurrent or persistent platinum-resistant ovarian, fallopian tube, or primary peritoneal carcinoma: a Gynecologic Oncology Group study. Gynecol Oncol 125:367–371

Dizon DS, Damstrup L, Finkler NJ et al (2012b) Phase II activity of belinostat (PXD-101), carboplatin, and paclitaxel in women with previously treated ovarian cancer. Int J Gynecol Cancer 22:979–986

Doi T, Hamaguchi T, Shirao K et al (2012) Evaluation of safety, pharmacokinetics, and efficacy of vorinostat, a histone deacetylase inhibitor, in the treatment of gastrointestinal (GI) cancer in a phase I clinical trial. Int J Clin Oncol. doi:10.1007/s10147-011-0348-6

Drappatz J, Lee EQ, Hammond S et al (2012) Phase I study of panobinostat in combination with bevacizumab for recurrent high-grade glioma. J Neurooncol 107:133–138

Duvic M, Talpur R, Ni X, Zhang C, Hazarika P, Kelly C, Chiao JH, Reilly JF, Ricker JL, Richon VM, Frankel SR (2007) Phase 2 trial of oral vorinostat (suberoylanilide hydroxamic acid, SAHA) for refractory cutaneous T-cell lymphoma (CTCL). Blood 109:31–39

Duvic M, Olsen EA, Breneman D, Pacheco TR, Parker S, Vonderheid EC, Abuav R, Ricker JL, Rizvi S, Chen C, Boileau K, Gunchenko A, Sanz-Rodriguez C, Geskin LJ (2009) Evaluation of the long-term tolerability and clinical benefit of vorinostat in patients with advanced cutaneous T-cell lymphoma. Clin Lymphoma Myeloma 9:412–416

Egerer G (2012) Study on efficacy and tolerability of vorinostat in patients with advanced, metastatic soft tissue sarcoma (STS) (SAHA-I). ClinicalTrials.gov: http://www.clinicaltrials.gov/ct2/show/NCT00918489?term=sarcoma+vorinostat&rank=1

Fakih MG, Groman A, McMahon J et al (2012) A randomized phase II study of two doses of vorinostat in combination with 5-FU/LV in patients with refractory colorectal cancer. Cancer Chemother Pharmacol 69:743–751

Fang F, Balch C, Schilder J, Breen T, Zhang S, Shen C, Li L, Kulesavage C, Snyder AJ, Nephew KP, Matei DE (2010) A phase 1 and pharmacodynamic study of decitabine in combination with carboplatin in patients with recurrent, platinum-resistant, epithelial ovarian cancer. Cancer 116:4043–4053

Friday BB, Anderson SK, Buckner J et al (2012) Phase II trial of vorinostat in combination with bortezomib in recurrent glioblastoma: a north central cancer treatment group study. Neuro Oncol 14:215–221

Fu S, Hu W, Iyer R, Kavanagh JJ, Coleman RL, Levenback CF, Sood AK, Wolf JK, Gershenson DM, Markman M, Hennessy BT, Kurzrock R, Bast RC Jr (2011) Phase 1b-2a study to reverse platinum resistance through use of a hypomethylating agent, azacitidine, in patients with platinum-resistant or platinum-refractory epithelial ovarian cancer. Cancer 117:1661–1669

Galanis E, Jaeckle KA, Maurer MJ, Reid JM, Ames MM, Hardwick JS, Reilly JF, Loboda A, Nebozhyn M, Fantin VR, Richon VM, Scheithauer B, Giannini C, Flynn PJ, Moore DF Jr, Zwiebel J, Buckner JC (2009) Phase II trial of vorinostat in recurrent glioblastoma multiforme: a north central cancer treatment group study. J Clin Oncol 27:2052–2058

George RE, Lahti JM, Adamson PC, Zhu K, Finkelstein D, Ingle AM, Reid JM, Krailo M, Neuberg D, Blaney SM, Diller L (2010) Phase I study of decitabine with doxorubicin and cyclophosphamide in children with neuroblastoma and other solid tumors: a Children's Oncology Group study. Pediatr Blood Cancer 55:629–638

Gifford G, Paul J, Vasey PA, Kaye SB, Brown R (2004) The acquisition of hMLH1 methylation in plasma DNA after chemotherapy predicts poor survival for ovarian cancer patients. Clin Cancer Res 10:4420–4426

Glasspool RM, Teodoridis JM, Brown R (2006) Epigenetics as a mechanism driving polygenic clinical drug resistance. Br J Cancer 94:1087–1092

Glasspool RM, Gore M, Rustin G, Mcneish I, Wilson R, Pledge S (2009) Randomized phase Ii study of decitabine in combination with carboplatin compared with carboplatin alone in patients with recurrent advanced ovarian cancer. J Clin Oncol 27:15S

Gollob JA, Sciambi CJ, Peterson BL et al (2006) Phase I trial of sequential low-dose 5-aza-2′-deoxycytidine plus high-dose intravenous bolus interleukin-2 in patients with melanoma or renal cell carcinoma. Clin Cancer Res 12:4619–4627

Graham JS, Kaye SB, Brown R (2009) The promises and pitfalls of epigenetic therapies in solid tumours. Eur J Cancer 45:1129–1136

Haigentz M Jr, Kim M, Sarta C et al (2012) Phase II trial of the histone deacetylase inhibitor romidepsin in patients with recurrent/metastatic head and neck cancer. Oral Oncol 48:1281–1288

Hainsworth JD, Infante JR, Spigel DR et al (2011) A phase II trial of panobinostat, a histone deacetylase inhibitor, in the treatment of patients with refractory metastatic renal cell carcinoma. Cancer Invest 29:451–455

Hauschild A, Trefzer U, Garbe C et al (2008) Multicenter phase II trial of the histone deacetylase inhibitor pyridylmethyl-N-{4-[(2-aminophenyl)-carbamoyl]-benzyl}-carbamate in pretreated metastatic melanoma. Melanoma Res 18:274–278

Holleran JL, Parise RA, Joseph E, Eiseman JL, Covey JM, Glaze ER, Lyubimov AV, Chen YF, D'Argenio DZ, Egorin MJ (2005) Plasma pharmacokinetics, oral bioavailability, and interspecies scaling of the DNA methyltransferase inhibitor, zebularine. Clin Cancer Res 11:3862–3868

Holoye PY, Dhingra HM, Umsawasdi T et al (1987) Phase II study of 5,6-dihydro-5-azacytidine in extensive, untreated non-small cell lung cancer. Cancer Treat Rep 71:859–860

Hu S, Yu L, Li Z, Shen Y, Wang J, Cai J, Xiao L, Wang Z (2010) Overexpression of EZH2 contributes to acquired cisplatin resistance in ovarian cancer cells in vitro and in vivo. Cancer Biol Ther(10)

Issa JP, Kantarjian HM (2009) Targeting DNA methylation. Clin Cancer Res 15:3938–3946

Issa JP, Garcia-Manero G, Giles FJ, Mannari R, Thomas D, Faderl S, Bayar E, Lyons J, Rosenfeld CS, Cortes J, Kantarjian HM (2004) Phase 1 study of low-dose prolonged exposure schedules of the hypomethylating agent 5-aza-2′-deoxycytidine (decitabine) in hematopoietic malignancies. Blood 103:1635–1640

Iwamoto FM, Lamborn KR, Kuhn JG et al (2011) A phase I/II trial of the histone deacetylase inhibitor romidepsin for adults with recurrent malignant glioma: North American Brain Tumor Consortium Study 03-03. Neuro Oncol 13:509–516

Jones PA (1985) Altering gene expression with 5-azacytidine. Cell 40:485–486

Juergens RA, Wrangle J, Vendetti FP et al (2011) Combination epigenetic therapy has efficacy in patients with refractory advanced non-small cell lung cancer. Cancer Discov 1:598–607

Kantarjian HM, Issa JP (2005) Decitabine dosing schedules. Semin Hematol 42:S17–S22

Karanikolas BD, Figueiredo ML, Wu L (2009) Polycomb group protein enhancer of zeste 2 is an oncogene that promotes the neoplastic transformation of a benign prostatic epithelial cell line. Mol Cancer Res 7:1456–1465

Kelly WK, O'Connor OA, Krug LM et al (2005) Phase I study of an oral histone deacetylase inhibitor, suberoylanilide hydroxamic acid, in patients with advanced cancer. J Clin Oncol 23:3923–3931

Khan O, Fotheringham S, Wood V, Stimson L, Zhang C, Pezzella F, Duvic M, Kerr DJ, La Thangue NB (2010) HR23B is a biomarker for tumor sensitivity to HDAC inhibitor-based therapy. Proc Natl Acad Sci USA 107:6532–6537

Kim MS, Blake M, Baek JH, Kohlhagen G, Pommier Y, Carrier F (2003) Inhibition of histone deacetylase increases cytotoxicity to anticancer drugs targeting DNA. Cancer Res 63:7291–7300

Klisovic RB, Stock W, Cataland S, Klisovic MI, Liu S, Blum W, Green M, Odenike O, Godley L, Burgt JV, Van Laar E, Cullen M, Macleod AR, Besterman JM, Reid GK, Byrd JC, Marcucci G (2008) A phase I biological study of MG98, an oligodeoxynucleotide antisense to DNA methyltransferase 1, in patients with high-risk myelodysplasia and acute myeloid leukemia. Clin Cancer Res 14:2444–2449

Kristensen LS, Nielsen HM, Hansen LL (2009) Epigenetics and cancer treatment. Eur J Pharmacol 625:131–142

Lee J, McGuire C (2012) Clinical efficacy of vorinostat in a patient with leiomyosarcoma. Clin Med Insights Oncol 6:101–105

Lee TI, Jenner RG, Boyer LA, Guenther MG, Levine SS, Kumar RM, Chevalier B, Johnstone SE, Cole MF, Isono K, Koseki H, Fuchikami T, Abe K, Murray HL, Zucker JP, Yuan B, Bell GW, Herbolsheimer E, Hannett NM, Sun K, Odom DT, Otte AP, Volkert TL, Bartel DP, Melton DA, Gifford DK, Jaenisch R, Young RA (2006) Control of developmental regulators by polycomb in human embryonic stem cells. Cell 125:301–313

Luu TH, Morgan RJ, Leong L, Lim D, McNamara M, Portnow J, Frankel P, Smith DD, Doroshow JH, Wong C, Aparicio A, Gandara DR, Somlo G (2008) A phase II trial of vorinostat (suberoylanilide hydroxamic acid) in metastatic breast cancer: a California Cancer Consortium study. Clin Cancer Res 14:7138–7142

Lyko F, Brown R (2005) DNA methyltransferase inhibitors and the development of epigenetic cancer therapies. J Natl Cancer Inst 97:1498–1506

Mackay HJ, Hirte H, Colgan T et al (2010) Phase II trial of the histone deacetylase inhibitor belinostat in women with platinum resistant epithelial ovarian cancer and micropapillary (LMP) ovarian tumours. Eur J Cancer 46:1573–1579

Martin V, Jorgensen HF, Chaubert AS, Berger J, Barr H, Shaw P, Bird A, Chaubert P (2008) MBD2-mediated transcriptional repression of the p14ARF tumor suppressor gene in human colon cancer cells. Pathobiology 75:281–287

Matei D, Fang F, Shen C et al (2012) Epigenetic resensitization to platinum in ovarian cancer. Cancer Res 72:2197–2205

Matsukawa Y, Semba S, Kato H, Ito A, Yanagihara K, Yokozaki H (2006) Expression of the enhancer of zeste homolog 2 is correlated with poor prognosis in human gastric cancer. Cancer Sci 97:484–491

Millward M, Price T, Townsend A et al (2012) Phase 1 clinical trial of the novel proteasome inhibitor marizomib with the histone deacetylase inhibitor vorinostat in patients with melanoma, pancreatic and lung cancer based on in vitro assessments of the combination. Invest New Drugs 30:2303–2317

Modesitt SC, Sill M, Hoffman JS, Bender DP (2008) A phase II study of vorinostat in the treatment of persistent or recurrent epithelial ovarian or primary peritoneal carcinoma: a Gynecologic Oncology Group study. Gynecol Oncol 109:182–186

Momparler RL, Ayoub J (2001) Potential of 5-aza-2′-deoxycytidine (decitabine) a potent inhibitor of DNA methylation for therapy of advanced non-small cell lung cancer. Lung Cancer 34(Suppl 4):S111–S115

Momparler RL, Bouchard J, Onetto N, Rivard GE (1984) 5-aza-2′-deoxycytidine therapy in patients with acute leukemia inhibits DNA methylation. Leuk Res 8:181–185

Momparler RL, Bouffard DY, Momparler LF et al (1997) Pilot phase I-II study on 5-aza-2′-deoxycytidine (decitabine) in patients with metastatic lung cancer. Anticancer Drugs 8:358–368

Mund C, Lyko F (2010) Epigenetic cancer therapy: proof of concept and remaining challenges. Bioessays 32:949–957

Munster PN, Marchion D, Thomas S et al (2009a) Phase I trial of vorinostat and doxorubicin in solid tumours: histone deacetylase 2 expression as a predictive marker. Br J Cancer 101:1044–1050

Munster P, Marchion D, Bicaku E et al (2009b) Clinical and biological effects of valproic acid as a histone deacetylase inhibitor on tumor and surrogate tissues: phase I/II trial of valproic acid and epirubicin/FEC. Clin Cancer Res 15:2488–2496

Munster PN, Thurn KT, Thomas S et al (2011) A phase II study of the histone deacetylase inhibitor vorinostat combined with tamoxifen for the treatment of patients with hormone therapy-resistant breast cancer. Br J Cancer 104:1828–1835

Nikoloski G, Langemeijer SM, Kuiper RP, Knops R, Massop M, Tonnissen ER, van der Heijden A, Scheele TN, Vandenberghe P, de Witte T, van der Reijden BA, Jansen JH (2010) Somatic mutations of the histone methyltransferase gene EZH2 in myelodysplastic syndromes. Nat Genet 42:665–667

Oki Y, Aoki E, Issa JP (2007) Decitabine – bedside to bench. Crit Rev Oncol Hematol 61:140–152

Otterson GA, Hodgson L, Pang H et al (2010) Phase II study of the histone deacetylase inhibitor Romidepsin in relapsed small cell lung cancer (Cancer and Leukemia Group B 30304). J Thorac Oncol 5:1644–1648

Pediconi N, Ianari A, Costanzo A, Belloni L, Gallo R, Cimino L, Porcellini A, Screpanti I, Balsano C, Alesse E, Gulino A, Levrero M (2003) Differential regulation of E2F1 apoptotic target genes in response to DNA damage. Nat Cell Biol 5:552–558

Plumb JA, Strathdee G, Sludden J, Kaye SB, Brown R (2000) Reversal of drug resistance in human tumor xenografts by 2′-deoxy-5-azacytidine-induced demethylation of the hMLH1 gene promoter. Cancer Res 60:6039–6044

Plummer R, Vidal L, Griffin M, Lesley M, de Bono J, Coulthard S, Sludden J, Siu LL, Chen EX, Oza AM, Reid GK, McLeod AR, Besterman JM, Lee C, Judson I, Calvert H, Boddy AV (2009)

Phase I study of MG98, an oligonucleotide antisense inhibitor of human DNA methyltransferase 1, given as a 7-day infusion in patients with advanced solid tumors. Clin Cancer Res 15:3177–3183

Qian X, LaRochelle WJ, Ara G, Wu F, Petersen KD, Thougaard A, Sehested M, Lichenstein HS, Jeffers M (2006) Activity of PXD101, a histone deacetylase inhibitor, in preclinical ovarian cancer studies. Mol Cancer Ther 5:2086–2095

Quinn D (2012) Vorinostat in treating patients with locally recurrent or metastatic cancer of the urothelium. ClinicalTrials.gov: http://clinicaltrials.gov/ct2/show/NCT00363883?term=Bladder+cancer+vorinostat&rank=1

Ramalingam SS, Maitland ML, Frankel P, Argiris AE, Koczywas M, Gitlitz B, Thomas S, Espinoza-Delgado I, Vokes EE, Gandara DR, Belani CP (2010) Carboplatin and paclitaxel in combination with either vorinostat or placebo for first-line therapy of advanced non-small-cell lung cancer. J Clin Oncol 28:56–62

Rao ZY, Cai MY, Yang GF, He LR, Mai SJ, Hua WF, Liao YJ, Deng HX, Chen YC, Guan XY, Zeng YX, Kung HF, Xie D (2010) EZH2 supports ovarian carcinoma cell invasion and/or metastasis via regulation of TGF-{beta}1 and is a predictor of outcome in ovarian carcinoma patients. Carcinogenesis 31:1576–1583

Rathkopf D, Wong BY, Ross RW et al (2010) A phase I study of oral panobinostat alone and in combination with docetaxel in patients with castration-resistant prostate cancer. Cancer Chemother Pharmacol 66:181–189

Reid GK, Besterman JM, MacLeod AR (2002) Selective inhibition of DNA methyltransferase enzymes as a novel strategy for cancer treatment. Curr Opin Mol Ther 4:130–137

Rizzo S, Hersey J, Graham J, Zeller C, Huang TH, Yan P, Vass JK, Brown R, Paul J (2011) Ovarian cancer stem cell like side populations are enriched following chemotherapy and overexpress EZH2. Mol Cancer Ther 10:325–335

Sansom OJ, Maddison K, Clarke AR (2007) Mechanisms of disease: methyl-binding domain proteins as potential therapeutic targets in cancer. Nat Clin Pract Oncol 4:305–315

Sauvageau M, Sauvageau G (2008) Polycomb group genes: keeping stem cell activity in balance. PLoS Biol 6:e113

Schrump DS, Fischette MR, Nguyen DM et al (2006) Phase I study of decitabine-mediated gene expression in patients with cancers involving the lungs, esophagus, or pleura. Clin Cancer Res 12:5777–5785

Schwartsmann G, Schunemann H, Gorini CN, Filho AF, Garbino C, Sabini G, Muse I, DiLeone L, Mans DR (2000) A phase I trial of cisplatin plus decitabine, a new DNA-hypomethylating agent, in patients with advanced solid tumors and a follow-up early phase II evaluation in patients with inoperable non-small cell lung cancer. Invest New Drugs 18:83–91

Siegel D, Hussein M, Belani C, Robert F, Galanis E, Richon VM, Garcia-Vargas J, Sanz-Rodriguez C, Rizvi S (2009) Vorinostat in solid and hematologic malignancies. J Hematol Oncol 2:31

Simon JA, Lange CA (2008) Roles of the EZH2 histone methyltransferase in cancer epigenetics. Mutat Res 647:21–29

Stathis A, Hotte SJ, Chen EX et al (2011) Phase I study of decitabine in combination with vorinostat in patients with advanced solid tumors and non-Hodgkin's lymphomas. Clin Cancer Res 17:1582–1590

Steele NL, Plumb JA, Vidal L, Tjornelund J, Knoblauch P, Rasmussen A, Ooi CE, Buhl-Jensen P, Brown R, Evans TR, DeBono JS (2008) A phase 1 pharmacokinetic and pharmacodynamic study of the histone deacetylase inhibitor belinostat in patients with advanced solid tumors. Clin Cancer Res 14:804–810

Steele N, Finn P, Brown R, Plumb JA (2009) Combined inhibition of DNA methylation and histone acetylation enhances gene re-expression and drug sensitivity in vivo. Br J Cancer 100:758–763

Suva ML, Riggi N, Janiszewska M, Radovanovic I, Provero P, Stehle JC, Baumer K, Le Bitoux MA, Marino D, Cironi L, Marquez VE, Clement V, Stamenkovic I (2009) EZH2 is essential for glioblastoma cancer stem cell maintenance. Cancer Res 69:9211–9218

Takai N, Narahara H (2010) Histone deacetylase inhibitor therapy in epithelial ovarian cancer. J Oncol 2010:458431

Teodoridis JM, Strathdee G, Plumb JA, Brown R (2004) CpG-island methylation and epigenetic control of resistance to chemotherapy. Biochem Soc Trans 32:916–917

Teodoridis JM, Hall J, Marsh S, Kannall HD, Smyth C, Curto J, Siddiqui N, Gabra H, McLeod HL, Strathdee G, Brown R (2005) CpG island methylation of DNA damage response genes in advanced ovarian cancer. Cancer Res 65:8961–8967

Thibault A, Figg WD, Bergan RC et al (1998) A phase II study of 5-aza-2′-deoxycytidine (decitabine) in hormone independent metastatic (D2) prostate cancer. Tumori 84:87–89

Traynor AM, Dubey S, Eickhoff JC et al (2009) Vorinostat (NSC# 701852) in patients with relapsed non-small cell lung cancer: a Wisconsin Oncology Network phase II study. J Thorac Oncol 4:522–526

Winquist E, Knox J, Ayoub JP, Wood L, Wainman N, Reid GK, Pearce L, Shah A, Eisenhauer E (2006) Phase II trial of DNA methyltransferase 1 inhibition with the antisense oligonucleotide MG98 in patients with metastatic renal carcinoma: a National Cancer Institute of Canada Clinical Trials Group investigational new drug study. Invest New Drugs 24:159–167

Witt O, Schweigerer L, Driever PH et al (2004) Valproic acid treatment of glioblastoma multiforme in a child. Pediatr Blood Cancer 43:181

Witta SE, Jotte RM, Konduri K et al (2012) Randomized phase II trial of erlotinib with and without entinostat in patients with advanced non-small-cell lung cancer who progressed on prior chemotherapy. J Clin Oncol 30:2248–2255

Wong NS, Seah EZ, Wang LZ et al (2011) Impact of UDP-gluconoryltransferase 2B17 genotype on vorinostat metabolism and clinical outcomes in Asian women with breast cancer. Pharmacogenet Genomics 21:760–768

Xu WS, Parmigiani RB, Marks PA (2007) Histone deacetylase inhibitors: molecular mechanisms of action. Oncogene 26:5541–5552

Yang YT, Balch C, Kulp SK, Mand MR, Nephew KP, Chen CS (2009) A rationally designed histone deacetylase inhibitor with distinct antitumor activity against ovarian cancer. Neoplasia 11:552–563, 553 p following 563

Yogelzang NJ, Herndon JE 2nd, Cirrincione C et al (1997) Dihydro-5-azacytidine in malignant mesothelioma. A phase II trial demonstrating activity accompanied by cardiac toxicity. Cancer and Leukemia Group B. Cancer 79:2237–2242

Yoo CB, Jeong S, Egger G, Liang G, Phiasivongsa P, Tang C, Redkar S, Jones PA (2007) Delivery of 5-aza-2′-deoxycytidine to cells using oligodeoxynucleotides. Cancer Res 67:6400–6408

Zhou L, Cheng X, Connolly BA, Dickman MJ, Hurd PJ, Hornby DP (2002) Zebularine: a novel DNA methylation inhibitor that forms a covalent complex with DNA methyltransferases. J Mol Biol 321:591–599

Index

DOI 10.1007/978-3-642-38404-2, © Springer-Verlag Berlin Heidelberg 2014

MIX
Papier aus verantwortungsvollen Quellen
Paper from responsible sources
FSC® C105338

If you have any concerns about our products,
you can contact us on
ProductSafety@springernature.com

In case Publisher is established outside the EU,
the EU authorized representative is:
Springer Nature Customer Service Center GmbH
Europaplatz 3, 69115 Heidelberg, Germany

Printed by Libri Plureos GmbH
in Hamburg, Germany